英汉对照

English-Chinese Nursing Conversation

# 护理英语会话

（第2版）

主　编　王文秀　王　颖

人民卫生出版社

图书在版编目(CIP)数据

英汉对照护理英语会话/王文秀,王颖主编. —2 版.
—北京:人民卫生出版社,2017
ISBN 978-7-117-23732-1

Ⅰ.①英… Ⅱ.①王… ②王… Ⅲ.①护理学-英语-口语 Ⅳ.①R47

中国版本图书馆 CIP 数据核字(2016)第 283741 号



英汉对照护理英语会话
第 2 版

主　　编:王文秀　王　颖
出版发行:人民卫生出版社(中继线 010-59780011)
地　　址:北京市朝阳区潘家园南里 19 号
邮　　编:100021
E - mail:pmph @ pmph.com
购书热线:010-59787592　010-59787584　010-65264830
印　　刷:三河市宏达印刷有限公司
经　　销:新华书店
开　　本:787 × 1092　1/16　印张:42
字　　数:1048 千字
版　　次:2011 年 5 月第 1 版　2017 年 3 月第 2 版
2024 年 8 月第 2 版第10 次印刷(总第 16 次印刷)
标准书号:ISBN 978-7-117-23732-1/R · 23733
定　　价:98.00 元

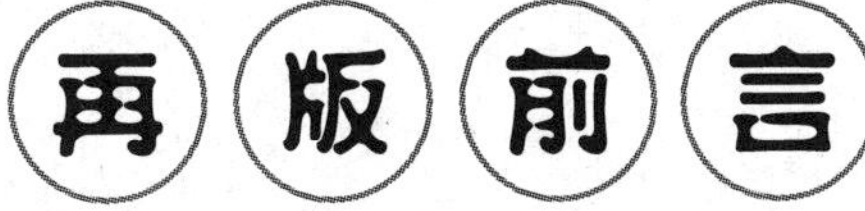

# 再版前言

《护理英语会话》一书自2011年出版以来颇受业界人士重视和广大读者的厚爱，多次重印，发行数万册。临床真实情境的再现及贴切英语的支持使本书成为国内外护理界同道顺畅交流沟通的专门书籍，更为诸多高等护理院校护理英语案例教学和青年护士“护理英语会话”培训和自修提供了丰富的素材。外国友人和境外同胞亦对本书给予了很高的赞誉。

考虑到本书受众人群不断扩大，为使本书更臻完善，在人民卫生出版社有关人员的指导下，进行了此次修订。

本次修订在保持原书“内容翔实，使用便捷，章节安排合理”的前提下，对原有的内容进行了筛选和补充。力求为广大读者提供一条更加科学的“读了即懂，懂了即用，用了即对”的学习护理英语会话的方便之路。在语言素材的筛选过程中我们的指导原则是：①脱口而出：尽量收录流行实用的语句；②触类旁通：一语多说，多种表达，举一反三；③对答如流：选用经典贴切的对话，使对话完全符合读者所处的语言环境。

为了使那些赴海外工作的护理人员尽快地能与以英语为母语的病人进行良好的沟通和交流，本书增加了“海外护理集锦”等篇章。这些篇章主要显现了在英、美等西方国家的护理工作中，当事人、病人及其家属所讲英语与赴海外工作的护理人员所用的英语之间的巨大差异。笔者期待，通过这些篇章的设立，帮助上述人员迅速熟悉所在英语国家的临床护理英语口语的特点，更好地为当地患者服务。

感谢承德医学院的各级领导和各位老师对本书编写工作的支持。

人民卫生出版社的贾旭编辑和各位同仁对本书进行了精心的策划和细致的指导；王珩教授和Dick Smith先生对本书进行了认真的审阅；李志红、张旭、张艳玲、冯永平、王涤清等人士亦为本书的编写提供了帮助，在此一并表示真挚的感谢。

期待修订后的《护理英语会话》能够为广大读者提供更优质的服务。

王文秀
2016年11月12日
于承德

# 前言

编写本书的目的是提高护理人员的英语口语能力，使涉外护理岗位的从业护士能使用娴熟的英语进行护患之间的沟通与交流，对发生于患者身上的问题感同身受，快速地进入有效沟通的情境，帮助患者解除病痛。本书以美国的《国际护士资格考试认证》的内容和要求为参照目标，强调了现代护理理念，体现了人文关怀和个性化护理。

本书的第一部分为《基础护理篇》，由 14 个单元组成，每一个单元有一个主题，包括了踏入医院，从导医台到挂号处，从急诊室到门诊处，住院和出院，各项检测和全面检查，巡诊和会诊等环节。每个单元都配有与该单元所涉及的典型情境有关的护理人员所需的“常用语”，可作为护理人员“急用先学”部分。“常用语”后面配备了与该节内容相关的情景会话，使读者通过反复排练牢记常用句型，在不同的语境中准确地脱口而出。

第二部分《护理个案篇》收集编写了 88 例典型护理个案。这些个案从不同角度展示了护理工作的学科特性和内涵，充分体现了“关爱生命，以人为本，以德施护”的人本护理观和运用护理程序对患者进行心身整体护理的科学方法论。

本书所选语句都是在医疗环境中护士的常用语，内容丰富新颖，语言简洁，并且巧妙地融入了西方当前的护理理念。使用本书，读者亦能学到很多新的、与护理工作相关的知识，从而更深地理解现代护理工作。

除了作为涉外护理岗位的从业护士的自修文本之外，本书还可用作指导新护士上岗以及护校在校高年级学生的学习参考书。

本书立项于 2005 年，历时六载，终于成书，不胜欣慰。本书的付梓为我课题组《医务英语系列》书籍的编写工作画上了一个圆满的句号。本课题组设立于 2000 年，所编书籍均于人民卫生出版社出版。十多年来，人民卫生出版社的各级领导对我们的编写工作给予了极大的支持，第一编辑室的各位同仁亦多次提供了睿智的指导，在此一并致以真诚的谢意。

尽管我们竭尽绵力，但书中一定还存在着不少缺点，甚至错误。我们诚挚地期待着读者的批评指正，以便再版修订时加以改进。

承德医学院

**王文秀**

二零一一年元月

# 目录

## Part One　Basic Nursing Care
## 基础护理篇



## Part Two　Nursing Cases
## 护理个案篇

## Part Three　Overseas Nursing Cases
## 海外护理集锦篇

## Part Four Model Sentences for Overseas Nursing
## 海外护理典型语句篇

# Part One

## Basic Nursing Care

## 基础护理篇

# 1. Meeting Patients in Hospital

# 医院会面

## A. Sentences Commonly used(常用语)

1. How are you?
   你好吗？
2. Glad to meet you.
   认识你我很高兴(见面时用，分手时说 Glad meeting you.)。
3. Good morning, Miss Paine. I am nurse Johnson.
   早上好，帕恩小姐。我是约翰逊护士。
4. Mr. And Mrs. Gates, my name is Miss White. I am a nurse.
   盖茨先生和盖茨太太好，我是怀特小姐，是名护士。
5. Hello, I am nurse Hunt. Are you Mrs. Bill?
   你好，我是亨特护士。你是比尔夫人吗？
6. Hi, Peter, I am your nurse. Who is here with you today?
   你好，彼得，我是负责你的护士。今天谁陪你来的？
7. Hello, Mr. George. Nice to see you again. How have you been?
   你好，乔治先生，很高兴再次见到你。最近还好吗？
8. You're looking better today.
   你今天看上去好多了。
9. Hello, I haven't seen you for a long time. How's everything going?
   你好，我很久没有见到您了，一切都好吗？
10. How are you feeling today?
    你今天感觉如何？
11. May I help you?
    我能帮助你吗？
12. What can I do for you?
    我能为你效劳吗？
13. What's the trouble?
    有什么不舒服吗？
14. Please come in and have a seat.
    请进，随便坐。

15. Please take a seat! / Please sit down!
请坐下!
16. Wait a moment, please.
请等一会儿。
17. Sorry to have kept you waiting.
对不起,让你久等了。
18. It's nice weather today. How did you come here?
今天天气真好,你怎么来这儿的?
19. Did you have any trouble finding us today?
今天来找我们还顺利吗?
20. How was the traffic?
路上交通状况怎么样?
21. How do you do! This way, please!
您好!请这边走!
22. Welcome to our hospital(ward)!
欢迎你到我们医院(病房)来。
23. What can I do for you?
你有什么事?
24. May I help you?
我能帮你什么忙吗?
25. Is there anything else you would like me to explain to you?
你还有什么不清楚的事情需要我为你解释吗?
26. Which department do you want to visit?
你要去哪个科室?
27. Put your medical card in the box at the reception desk.
请把就诊卡放在服务台的箱内。
28. Today the department of ophthalmology is closed.
今天眼科不开诊。
29. Surgery is open till noon every day.
外科每天只有上午半天门诊。
30. Please observe the clinical hours.
请按门诊时间来就诊。
31. Please come with me, I will show you the way to the Radiology.
请跟我来,我带你去放射科。
32. I will take you there.
我带你去那儿。
33. What's your problem?
你哪里不好?
34. What's wrong with you?
你怎么了?

35. When did your problem start?
你什么时候犯病的？
36. How long have you been sick?
你病了多长时间啦？
37. What do you find the most uncomfortable ?/What bothers you the most?
你哪最难受？
38. Is your pain bearable?
疼痛可以忍受吗？
39. Can you tolerate this pain?
疼痛能忍住吗？
40. You will be the third to be seen.
你是第三号。
41. Please wait for a moment.
请等一会儿。
42. Please be seated until your name is called.
没叫你前请在此静候。
43. When did you come to China?
你什么时候来中国的？
44. What was your profession in your country?
在贵国你做什么工作？
45. What are you doing in China?
你现在在中国做什么工作？
46. Thank you. Please wait a while.
谢谢，请等一会儿。
47. Please come to room No. 5 when your name is called.
听到叫你名字时，请到 5 号诊室就诊。

## B. Situational conversation（情景会话）

### (1)

Nurse： Hello，my name is Nurse Li Dehong. My English name is Linda. Please call me Nurse Linda. Can I help you? What's your problem?

护士： 你好，我是李德红护士。我的英文名叫琳达。请称呼我为琳达护士。请问有什么我能帮你的？你哪里不舒服？

Patient： I want to see a doctor，please. I don't feel very well，but I don't know what to do.

病人： 我想看医生。我有点不舒服，但是不知道该怎么办。

Nurse： What are your symptoms?

护士： 你有什么症状？

Patient： I have a temperature，I feel tired and aching and I just feel unwell.

病人：我发烧，感觉酸痛乏力，很不舒服。

Nurse: You need to see an Internal Medicine doctor. Do you understand Chinese?

护士：你应该挂内科。你会讲中文吗？

Patient: No.

病人：不会。

Nurse: I will help you to register first and take you to the Outpatient's Department.

护士：我会先帮你挂号，然后带你去门诊部。

Patient: Thank you very much.

病人：非常感谢。

**(2)**

Nurse: Hello, my name is Nurse Li Dehong. My English name is Linda. Please call me Nurse Linda. Can I help you? What is your problem?

护士：你好，我是李德红护士。我的英文名叫琳达。请称呼我为琳达护士。请问有什么我能帮你的？你哪里不舒服？

Patient: I have had severe diarrhea and vomiting since yesterday, I'd like to see a doctor.

病人：从昨天开始我一直腹泻呕吐，需要看医生。

Nurse: You need to go to the Emergency Room; I will show you where to go. You will have to register first and then you can see a doctor, I will help you.

护士：你需要去看急诊，我会告诉你怎么走。你需要先挂号才能看医生，我会帮助你完成这一切。

Patient: Thank you very much, you are very kind.

病人：非常感谢，你人真好。

※ ※ ※

Nurse: Hello, may I help you? My name is Nurse Lee.

护士：你好，我是李护士，请问有什么我能帮你的？

Patient: Yes, please. I have a severe headache, I need to see someone, where do I have to go?

病人：有，我头好痛，我要看医生，该怎么走？

Nurse: You need to see a neurologist, the Neurology Department is on the fourth floor, the elevators and stairs are over there in the corner, but you will need to register first.

护士：你需要看神经科医生，神经科在四楼，电梯和楼梯在那边拐角处，不过你需要先挂号。

Patient: Thank you, can you tell me how I do that?

病人：谢谢！你能告诉我怎么挂号吗？

**(3)**

Nurse: Hello, my name is Nurse Li Dehong. My English name is Linda. Please call me Nurse Linda. Can I help you?

护士：你好，我是李德红护士。我的英文名叫琳达。请称呼我为琳达护士。有什么我能帮你的？

Patient： Yes，please. I'm looking for an ATM machine，is there one in the hospital?

病人： 好的，谢谢。我在找自动取款机，请问医院里面有吗？

Nurse： Yes，there is. You'll find it down this corridor，(pointing) you'll find it on your right.

护士： 医院有！沿着走廊一直走，就在你的右手边。

Patient： Thanks.

病人： 谢谢。

## (4)

Nurse： Hello，my name is Nurse Li Dehong. My English name is Linda. Please call me Nurse Linda. Can I help you?

护士： 你好，我是李德红护士。我的英文名叫琳达。请称呼我为琳达护士。有什么我能帮你的？

Patient： I'm looking for the toilet/WC/cloakroom/bathroom/washroom.

病人： 请问卫生间在哪里？

Nurse： Yes，they are on the second floor. The stairs are over there (pointing) or you can take the elevator. You will find the toilets straight ahead of you，when you get out of the elevator.

护士： 卫生间在二楼。楼梯在那边，或者你可以坐电梯上去。从电梯出来后，正对着你的就是。

Patient： Thanks a lot.

病人： 非常感谢。

## (5)

Nurse： Hello，my name is Nurse Li Dehong. My English name is Linda. Please call me Nurse Linda. Can I help you?

护士： 你好，我是李德红护士。我的英文名叫琳达。请称呼我为琳达护士。有什么我能帮你的？

Patient： Yes，thank you. I'm looking for the X-ray Department.

病人： 好的，谢谢。我在找放射科。

Nurse： The X-ray Department is down that corridor，and you find it on your right hand. Please follow the orange line，that will take you to the X-ray Department.

护士： 沿着走廊走下去，在你的右手边就是。请沿着那条橙线一直走，你就能找到放射科。

Patient： Great，thanks.

病人： 太好了，谢谢。

## (6)

Nurse： Hello，my name is Nurse Li Dehong. My English name is Linda. Please call me Nurse Linda. Can I help you?

护士： 你好，我是李德红护士。我的英文名叫琳达。请称呼我为琳达护士。有什么我能帮你的？

Patient: Please can you tell me where the subway is from here?

病人：请问你能告诉我到地铁站怎么走？

Nurse: You will need to take a taxi or bus to get to the subway.

护士：你需要打的或者坐公交车到地铁口。

Patient: Oh, is it quite far from here?

病人：哦，离这儿很远吗？

Nurse: Yes, it is. To get a bus you need to go out of the hospital to the main road, cross over the road, the Bus Stop is on your left, you will need to get the No. 104 bus.

护士：是的，如果坐公交车，你需要出了医院到主路上去，穿过主路之后左手边就是公共汽车站，你需要坐104路。

Patient: How long will it take me to get to the subway?

病人：坐到地铁口需要多长时间？

Nurse: It will take about 15 minutes.

护士：大概15分钟。

Patient: OK. Where can I get a taxi?

病人：好的，在哪里乘出租车？

Nurse: If you go out of this door to the main road, there are taxis waiting.

护士：穿过这个门到主路上就有。

Patient: That's great, thanks.

病人：太好了，谢谢！

# 2. Registration and Appointment

# 挂号和预约

## A. Sentences Commonly Used(常用语)

1. Do you understand Chinese?
   请问你懂中文吗？
2. Is this your first visit to our hospital?
   你是第一次来我们医院吗？
3. Have you been here before?
   你以前来过吗？
4. Do you have medical health insurance?
   请问你有医疗保险吗？
5. If you do not have medical health insurance, you may have to pay for the medical bill.
   如果你没有医疗保险，你将自己支付医疗费用。
6. Even though you have medical health insurance, you may have to pay the bill and claim afterwards.
   即使你有医疗保险，你也可能需要自己支付费用再事后索赔。
7. Please tell me what your problem is?
   请告诉我你哪里不舒服？
8. You need to register first; the counter is over there.(pointing to the counter)
   你需要先挂号，挂号台在那边。(指向收费处)
9. You need to pay the cashier and then register, and the cashier counter is over there.
   你需要先交款然后再挂号，收费处在那边。
10. The registration form is in Chinese. I will help you.
    挂号表是中文的，我来帮你。
11. I will help you.
    我来帮你。
12. I will help you, please sit down. I will get you the form.
    我来帮你，请坐好。我去给你拿表。
13. Name
    名字
14. DOB —date of birth

出生日期

15. Address（Chinese address and home address for doctor's letter）
 地址（中国住址和方便医生寄信的家庭住址）
16. Nationality
 国籍
17. Telephone No.
 电话号码
18. Medical Insurance No.
 医疗保险单号
19. Have you a registration card?
 你有挂号卡吗？
20. Are you a medical or surgical case?
 你看内科还是外科？
21. Do you have your history sheet?
 你有病历吗？
22. Which department do you want to register with?
 你要挂哪科的号？
23. I think you should see a dermatologist first.
 我认为你应当先看皮肤科。
24. Please don't lose your registration card.
 请不要遗失你的挂号卡。
25. This is your registration card.
 这是你的挂号卡。
26. Bring it whenever you come.
 每次来时都带着它。

## B. Situational Conversation( 情景会话 )

### (1)

Nurse: Hello! Can I help you?
护士：你好！有什么可以帮你的吗？
Patient: Hi! I'm new here. I want to see a doctor. Can you show me the way to the registry?
病人：你好！我第一次来这里。我要看医生。请问挂号处往哪边走？
Nurse: Yes. It's just on the first floor of that tallest building over there.
护士：喔，挂号处在那座最高的楼里面，在第一层。
Patient: I'm sorry. Did you mean the ground floor or the second floor?
病人：抱歉，你是说第一层还是第二层？
Nurse: The ground floor.
护士：第一层。

Patient: Thank you very much.

病人： 非常感谢。

Nurse: You are welcome.

护士： 不客气。

**（2）**

Nurse: Good morning. What can I do for you?

护士： 早上好，我能为你做些什么？

Patient: Good morning. I have a bad cough, and I want to see an internist.

病人： 早上好。我咳嗽很严重，想挂个内科医生的号。

Nurse: OK! Have you ever been here before? Do you have a registration card?

护士： 好的。请问你以前来过吗？有没有挂号卡？

Patient: It's my first visit here. I'm a tourist.

病人： 我第一次来这里。我是观光客。

Nurse: Then you need to register a new card. Can I have a look at your ID card or passport? I need your name, age, occupation and address.

护士： 那么你得办张新卡。我可以看看你的身份证或者护照吗，我需要输入你的姓名、年龄、职业和地址。

Patient: Here you are.

病人： 给你。

Nurse: Thank you.

护士： 谢谢。

……

Nurse: Er, can I have your telephone number? If you have no, please tell me the phone number of your hotel room.

护士： 唔，你的电话是多少？如果没有，请告诉我你旅馆房间的电话。

Patient: The phone number of my hotel room is eight, one, double eight, seven, two, double three, extension three, eight, four, zero, three.

病人： 我旅馆房间的电话号码是 81887233-38403。

Nurse: Eight, one, double eight, seven, two, double three, extension three, eight, four, zero, three. Right?

护士： 81887233-38403，对吗？

Patient: Yes, you got it.

病人： 对。

Nurse: Good! Which kind of medicine do you prefer? Western medicine or traditional Chinese medicine?

护士： 好的。请问你想看中医还是西医？

Patient: Er, I have been longing to try the supernatural traditional Chinese medicine. It's very popular in China-town.

病人： 唔，我一直想试试神奇的中医。它在唐人街很吃香。

Nurse： That's a good idea. You'll find that Chinese herb can make magic. 7 yuan please.

护士： 好注意！你会发现中草药的神奇效果。请给我7元人民币挂号费。

Patient： OK!

病人： 给你。

Nurse： Here is your passport. Please make sure it's in safe keeping. Here is your registration card and receipt. I recommended a famous old herbalist doctor. His office is on the fifth floor of the building 2 at the east district. You can get there easily by yourself or you can ask a guide-nurse to help you.

护士： 请拿回你的护照，千万别弄丢了。这是你的挂号卡和收据。我向你推荐了一位著名的老中医，他的办公室在东区5楼，你很容易就能找到那儿，你也可以请一位导诊护士带你去那儿。

Patient： Thanks a million.

病人： 万分感谢。

Nurse： How long do you intend to stay in China?

护士： 你准备在中国待多久？

Patient： Two weeks or longer.

病人： 两周或更久。

Nurse： Wish you a great time and a safe travel.

护士： 祝你旅途愉快、一路顺风。

Patient： Thank you! Goodbye.

病人： 谢谢。再见。

**（3）**

Patient： Excuse me，which line should I stand in to register，please?

病人： 请问，我挂号该排哪一队？

Nurse： This is the line for new patients. The registration fee will be 7 yuan. Pay over there，and they will give you a registration card. Fill it in and bring it back to me.

护士： 初诊的病人站那条队。挂号费7元。排到那边后付了款，他们会给你一张挂号卡。填写后交到这儿。

Nurse： What's the problem?

护士： 你哪里不舒服？

Patient： Since this morning I've had high temperature，and I feel generally wretched.

病人： 今天早上开始，我发高烧，浑身疲乏无力。

Nurse： In that case，you'd better go to the Medical Department.

护士： 像你这样的情况，还是去看内科吧。

Patient： Which way do I go?

病人： 内科怎么走？

Nurse： Go up to the second floor，and you'll see the sign. Give the doctor your registration card.

护士： 上了二楼，你可以看到内科的牌子。把挂号卡给医生就行了。

Patient： Is it very busy?

病人： 内科病人多不多？
Nurse: Normally yes, but today you are lucky.
护士： 往日很多，可今天却不多。
Patient: Oh, good. Thank you.
病人： 谢谢。

**(4)**

Nurse: Do you want to see a doctor?
护士： 你要看病吗？
Patient: Yes.
病人： 是的。
Nurse: Have you ever been here before?
护士： 你以前来过这里吗？
Patient: No, this is my first visit.
病人： 没有，这是第一次来。
Nurse: Have you a registration card?
护士： 你有挂号卡吗？
Patient: Yes, I have.
病人： 有的。
Nurse: Do you remember your card number?
护士： 你记得你的挂号卡号码吗？
Patient: No, I can't remember it.
病人： 不记得了。
Nurse: I'll make a file (record) for you.
护士： 我要给你做一份病历。
Patient: Thank you.
病人： 谢谢你。
Nurse: Which department do you want to register with?
护士： 你要挂哪科的号？
Patient: I want to see a surgeon.
病人： 我要看外科。
Nurse: This is your file. Please don't lose it and bring it whenever you come.
护士： 这是你的病历。请不要遗失。每次来时带着它。
Patient: Yes, I will. But can you tell me how to get to the Consulting Room?
病人： 好的，我会带的。请问到诊疗室如何走？
Nurse: Go down this road until you come to the drugstore. Make a left turn and it's just there.
护士： 沿着这条路走到药房再向左拐就到了。

**(5)**

Nurse: Hello, I am Nurse Li Dehong. My English name is Linda. Please call me Nurse Linda.

Can I help you?

护士：你好，我是李德红护士。我的英文名叫琳达。请称呼我为琳达护士。有什么我能帮你的？

Patient: I want to see a doctor. I don't feel very well, but I don't know what to do.

病人：我想看医生。我有点不舒服，但是不知该怎么做。

Nurse: What are your symptoms?

护士：你有什么症状？

Patient: I have a temperature, feel very tired and my joints are aching and I just feel unwell.

病人：我发烧，感觉很累，关节疼痛，感觉很不舒服。

Nurse: You need to see an Internal Medicine doctor. Do you understand Chinese?

护士：你需要看内科。你会讲中文吗？

Patient: No.

病人：不会。

Nurse: You need to register first and then I will take you to Outpatients. The registration fee is 7 yuan. Please take a seat, I will get a form for you.

护士：你需要先挂号，然后我带你去门诊部。挂号费是 7 元，请坐一会儿，我去给你拿表。

Patient: Thank you.

病人：谢谢。

Nurse: Here is the registration form, and you need to write the answers to a few questions.

护士：这是挂号表，你需要填写一些信息。

Nurse: What is your name?

护士：你叫什么名字？

Patient: Linda Smith.

病人：琳达·史密斯。

Nurse: What is your date of birth?

护士：你的出生日期？

Patient: 3. 4. 1980.

病人：3. 4. 1980。

Nurse: Is that 3rd April 1980 or 4th March 1980?

护士：您指的是 1980 年 4 月 3 日还是 1980 年 3 月 4 日？

Patient: 3rd April 1980.

病人：1980 年 4 月 3 日。

Nurse: What is your address here in Beijing?

护士：你在北京的住址是哪里？

Patient: Hotel Lido, Chaoyang District.

病人：朝阳区丽都饭店。

Nurse: Are you a tourist?

护士：你是游客吗？

Patient: Yes, I am.

病人：是的。

Nurse: Please can I have your address in your own country?

护士：请问能告诉我你在你自己国家的住址吗？

Patient: 16，Trafalgar Square，Greenwich，London，E13 9DL.

病人：伦敦，格林威治区特拉法广场 16 号，邮编 E13 9DL。

Nurse: Please can you write that down on this form?

护士：请问你能在挂号表里填写吗？

Nurse: What is your nationality?

护士：你是哪国人？

Patient: British.

病人：英国人。

Nurse: What is your telephone number?

护士：你的电话号码是什么？

Patient: My mobile number is 1498765321.

病人：我的手机号码是 1498765321.

Nurse: Who is your next of Kin?

护士：你的近亲是哪位？

Patient: Mr. Alan Week.

病人：阿伦•维克先生。

Nurse: Please can you write his name and address and telephone number?

护士：请问你能填写一下他的姓名、地址和电话号码吗？

……

Nurse: Do you have health insurance?

护士：请问你有医疗保险吗？

Patient: Yes，I do.

病人：我有。

Nurse: Even though you have health insurance，you will have to pay the medical bill first and then claim. The hospital will give you a letter to give to your insurance company.

护士：即使你有医疗保险，你也需要先支付医疗费用，再进行索赔。医院会给你的保险公司开一份证明。

Patient: No，I don't.

病人：没有。

Nurse: You will have to pay your medical bill before you leave the hospital.

护士：你需要在出院之前付清医疗费用。

Nurse: I will take this form back to the counter and get your paperwork. Please can I have 7 yuan for the registration fee? Please stay here，I will come back.

护士：我会将挂号表送到收费处换你的电脑记录表。请给我 7 元挂号费。在原地等一会儿，我马上回来。

Patient: Thank you.

病人：谢谢。

Nurse: I will take you to Outpatients now, would you like a wheelchair?
护士：我会带你去门诊部，你需要轮椅吗？
Patient: No, thank you. I will be OK.
病人：不用，谢谢！我自己能行。
Nurse: We need to go to the third floor, the elevators are over there, please follow me.
护士：我们要到三楼，那边有电梯，请跟我来。
Nurse: Here is the Outpatient Department. I will tell the nurse you are here.
护士：门诊部到了。我会告诉护士你在这里。
Nurse: The nurse will come and take you to the doctor when he is ready for you. Is there anything else I can do for you? Is there anything else you would like to ask me?
护士：护士一会儿过来。轮到你的时候，她会带你到医生那里。还有什么需要我帮忙的吗？还有什么需要咨询的吗？
Patient: No, thank you. You've been very kind.
病人：不用了，谢谢。你已经帮了很大忙。
Nurse: You are welcome. I hope you get better soon. Goodbye.
护士：不用客气，希望你尽快康复，再见！

## （6）

Nurse: Hello, I am Nurse Li Dehong. My English name is Linda. Please call me Nurse Linda. Can I help you?
护士：你好，我是李德红护士。我的英文名叫琳达。请称呼我为琳达护士。有什么我能帮你的？
Patient: I want to see a doctor. I'm ill.
病人：我要看医生，我病了。
Nurse: What are your symptoms?
护士：你有什么症状？
Patient: I have had diarrhea and vomiting for the last couple of days.
病人：我两天来一直呕吐腹泻。
Nurse: You need to see a doctor in the Emergency Room. Do you understand Chinese?
护士：你需要看急诊。你懂中文吗？
Patient: No.
病人：不懂。
Nurse: You will need to register first and then see the emergency doctor. I will take you to the Emergency Department, would you like a wheelchair? The registration fee is 7 yuan. Please wait a moment, I will get a form for you.
护士：你需要先挂号再看急诊医生。我会带你去急诊科，你需要轮椅吗？挂号费是 7 元。请等一会儿，我去给你拿挂号表。
Patient: Thank you.
病人：谢谢。
Nurse: Here is the registration form, and you will need to write the answers to a few

questions.
护士：这是挂号表，你需要填写一些信息。
Nurse: What is your name?
护士：你叫什么名字？
Patient: Paula Jones.
病人：保拉•琼斯。
Nurse: What is your date of birth?
护士：你的出生日期是？
Patient: 8. 9. 1963.
病人：8. 9. 1963。
Nurse: Is that 8th September 1963 or 9th August 1963?
护士：1963 年 9 月 8 日还是 1963 年 8 月 9 日。
Patient: 8th September 1963.
病人：1963 年 9 月 8 日。
Nurse: What is your address here in Beijing?
护士：你在北京的住址是哪里？
Patient: Hotel Beijing, Wangfujing.
病人：王府井北京饭店。
Nurse: Are you a tourist?
护士：你是游客吗？
Patient: Yes, I am.
病人：是的。
Nurse: Please can I have your address in your own country?
护士：请问能告诉我你本国住址吗？
Patient: 16a, Crowthorne Crescent, Handscross, West Sussex, BN12 7RN.
病人：地址是：西苏塞克斯市（英）汉迪克罗斯区克劳索恩新月街 16 号 a 门邮编是：BN12 7RN。

※ ※ ※

Nurse: What is your nationality?
护士：你是哪国人？
Patient: British.
病人：英国人。
Nurse: What is your telephone number?
护士：你的手机号码是多少？
Patient: My mobile number is 7079857432.
病人：我的手机号码是 7079857432。
Nurse: Who is your next of Kin?
护士：你的近亲是哪位？
Patient: Mr. David Jones.
病人：大卫•琼斯先生。

Nurse： Please can you write his name and address and telephone number?

护士： 你能填一下他的姓名、地址和电话吗？

Patient： Yes，certainly.

病人： 当然可以。

Nurse： Do you have health insurance?

护士： 你有医疗保险吗？

Patient： Yes，I do.

病人： 有。

Nurse： Even though you have health insurance，you will have to pay the medical bill first and then claim. The hospital will give you a letter to give to your insurance company.

护士： 即使你有医疗保险，你也需要先支付医疗费用，再进行索赔。医院会开一份证明给你的保险公司。

Patient： No，I don't.

病人： 没有。

Nurse： You will have to pay your medical bill before you leave the hospital.

护士： 你需要在出院之前付清医疗费用。

Patient： OK.

病人： 好的。

Nurse： I will take this form back to the counter and get your paperwork. Please can I have 7 yuan for the registration fee? Please stay here，I will come back.

护士： 我会将挂号表送到收费处换你的电脑记录表。请给我七元挂号费。请原地等一会儿，我马上回来。

Patient： Thank you.

病人： 谢谢。

Nurse： I will take you to the emergency doctor now.

护士： 我现在带你去急诊医生那里。

Patient： Thank you.

病人： 谢谢。

Nurse： Is there anything else I can do for you? Is there anything else you would like to ask me?

护士： 还有什么需要我帮忙的吗？还有什么需要咨询的吗？

Patient： No，thank you. You've been very kind.

病人： 不用了，谢谢。你已经帮了很大忙。

Nurse： You are welcome. I hope you get better soon. Goodbye.

护士： 不用客气，希望你尽快康复。再见！

**（7）**

Nurse： Good morning.This is doctor Johnson's office. What can I do for you ?

护士： 早上好，这里是约翰逊医生的办公室。有什么需要帮忙的吗？

Mrs. Reed： Yes，this is Mrs.Reed. I'd like to make a appointment to see doctor this week.

雷德太太： 是的，我是雷德太太。我想本周预约看病。

Nurse： Well，let's see. I'm afraid he is fully booked on Monday and Tuesday.

护士： 好的，让我查看一下。约翰逊医生本周星期一和星期二都已经预约满了。

Mrs. Reed： How about Thursday？

雷德太太： 星期四怎么样？

Nurse： Sorry，but he is also booked on Thursday. Will Wednesday be OK for you，Mrs. Reed?

护士： 抱歉，周四也已经预约满了。雷德太太，星期三您方便吗？

Mrs. Reed： I have to work on Wednesday. By the way，is Dr. Johnson available on Saturday?

雷德太太： 星期三我得上班。顺便问一下，约翰逊医生周六有空吗？

Nurse： I'm afraid the office is closed on weekends.

护士： 我们周末不上班。

Mrs. Reed： Well，what about Friday?

雷德太太： 那么，星期五如何？

Nurse： Friday，let me check. Oh，great. Dr. Johnson will be available on Friday afternoon.

护士： 星期五，让我查一下。太好了，约翰逊医生星期五下午有空。

Mrs. Reed： That fine; I'll go on Friday afternoon then. Thank you.

雷德太太： 好，那我周五下午过去。谢谢你。

## （8）

Mrs. Lee： Can I speak to Dr. Johnson，please?

李太太： 请问约翰逊医生在吗？

Nurse： I am Dr. Johnson's nurse. What can I do for you?

护士： 我是他的护士，有什么需要帮忙的吗？

Mrs. Lee： This is Mrs. Lee. Please help me.

李太太： 我是李太太，请帮帮我。

Nurse： What the problem，Mrs. Lee?

护士： 您怎么啦，李太太？

Mrs. Lee： Oh，no，it's not me，My son Bill is sick.

李太太： 哦，不，不是我，我的儿子比尔病了。

Nurse： What happened?

护士： 比尔怎么了？

Mrs. Lee： he has red spots on his arms，his shoulders...

李太太： 他的手臂上、肩膀上长有红斑。

Nurse： Does he have red spots elsewhere on his body?

护士： 他是不是其他部位也长了？

Mrs. Lee： Yes，he dose.

李太太： 是。

Nurse： Dose he have a fever?

护士： 他有没有发热呢？

Mrs. Lee: Yes, he dose. This morning his temperature was 39 degrees Celsius.

李太太： 发热了。今天早上他烧到了39℃。

Nurse: Oh.

护士： 哦。

Mrs. Lee: What's the wrong with bill? He cried all day long. I just can't stop him.

李太太： 医生，比尔究竟怎么了？他哭一整天了，劝都劝不住。

Nurse: He may have an infection.

护士： 他可能是感染了。

Mrs. Lee: Infection? Oh, dear. Can Dr. Johnson come and see him now?

李太太： 感染了？天啊！约翰逊医生现在可以来看他吗？

Nurse: Dr. Johnson is going to have an operation this morning. But you should bring Bill to the ER (emergency room) as soon as you can.

护士： 今天上午约翰逊先生得给病人手术，你应该尽快带比尔去看急诊。

Mrs. Lee: Thank you very much.

李太太： 非常感谢。

Nurse: Goodbye.

护士： 再见。

## (9)

Patient: I would like to see a dentist.

病人： 我想看牙医。

Nurse: For a filling, a denture, or a cleaning?

护士： 补牙、镶牙、还是洗牙？

Patient: I want to have a denture fitted and my teeth cleansed; please make an appointment for me.

病人： 我要镶牙并洗牙，请给我约个时间。

Nurse: OK! Next Wednesday, do you prefer eight o'clock, or ten o'clock?

护士： 好吧！下周星期三，您愿意上午8点钟来还是10点钟来？

Patient: Ten o'clock is better.

病人： 10点钟对我更合适。

Nurse: All right, ten o'clock, next Wednesday. See you then.

护士： 好，下周星期三10点见。

(Next Wednesday, 9: 55 a.m.)

(下周三，上午9: 55)

Nurse: Please come with me.

护士： 请随我来。

Patient: How long do I have to wait?

病人： 我还需要等多久？

Nurse: You are next. The patient before you is a rather complicated case. I am afraid you will probably have to wait for at least half an hour.

护士： 下一个就轮到您了。您前面那个病人情况比较复杂。恐怕您至少还得等半个小时。

Patient: OK, I'll wait.

病人： 好的，我等着。

# 3. Admission into Hospital

# 住院

## A. Sentences Commonly Used(常用语)

1. Let's fill in an admission card.
   我们要填一张住院卡。
2. It says here, "Name and address of next of Kin". Who is your nearest relation?
   现在该填"近亲的姓名和地址"了，请问与你关系最密切的人是谁？
3. Do you know which doctor is in charge of your case?
   你知道你的责任医生是哪一位吗？
4. The call button is here.
   这是呼叫按钮。
5. You may push it if you need a nurse.
   如果你需要护士就按它。
6. This is your bedside table for such things as toilet articles.
   这是床头柜，你可以放洗漱用具等。
7. If you have any valuables, we'll keep them for you.
   如果你有贵重物品，我们可以代你保管。
8. My name is Helen. I'm your primary nurse.
   我的名字叫海伦。我是负责你的护士。
9. She is the head nurse of the ward.
   她是这个病房的护士长。
10. This is Ward 3 and here is your room.
    这是3号病房，是你的房间。
11. Patients usually get up at 7 a.m. and breakfast is at 8.
    病人一般早晨7:00起床，8:00吃饭。
12. We're serving breakfast right now.
    我们现在正在供应早餐。
13. Lunch is at 12:30. Patients can have a rest after that.
    午餐时间是12:30，饭后病人可以休息。
14. Bedtime is from 9:30 to 10 p.m.
    病人应在晚上9:30～10:00上床睡觉。

15. The ward rounds and treatment start at 9 a.m.
9：00 开始查房，做治疗。
16. You can watch TV，but please don't bother the others.
你可以看电视，但请不要妨碍其他人。
17. Your family may stay here with you from 9 a.m. to 9 p.m.
你的家人可以从早 9：00 到晚 9：00 在这里陪护你。
18. You can have your meals，watch television，and enjoy various recreations in the common room.
你可以在休息室里吃饭、看电视以及进行各种各样的娱乐活动。
19. The ward is your home during your stay in hospital.
在你住院期间，病房就是你的家。
20. Our clinical dietitian is available to advise on special diets.
我们有临床营养师指导特殊饮食。
21. I'm the nurse in charge of this ward.
我是这间病房的护士长。
22. Will you show me where the common room，bathroom and telephone are?
请告诉我休息室、浴室和电话在哪儿好吗？
23. By the way，which kind of food do you prefer，Chinese or Western?
顺便问一下，你喜欢吃中餐还是喜欢吃西餐？
24. How is your appetite?
你的胃口怎么样？
25. What are your eating habits?
你的饮食习惯怎么样？
26. Hello，I'm on duty tonight.
你好，今天晚上我值班。
27. I'm your nurse. My name is Li Yanhua.
我是你的责任护士，我叫李燕华。
28. This is your wardmate，called ××. You can exchange your experience with him/her.
这是某某病友，你们多交流下。
29. The doctor makes their morning rounds at nine.
医生上午 9 点查房。
30. I'll tell you something about our hospital and its regulation.
我来告诉你一些我们医院的情况以及制度。
31. I'll show you the washroom a little while.
一会儿我带你去盥洗室。
32. Go straight and then turn right，the first room is the man's room.
往前走右拐第一间就是男卫生间。
33. Do you have any valuables to deposit?
你有什么贵重物品需要寄存吗？
34. Please do not smoke. It will affect your health.

请您不要吸烟，以免影响您的健康。

35. No spitting.
请勿随地吐痰。
36. Mind you don't drop your groceries about.
请注意环境卫生，不要乱丢杂物。
37. Please put your things into the garbage, thank you.
请你将杂物放进卫生箱里，谢谢合作。
38. Please keep the ward quiet!
请保持病房安静。
39. If you have any question, please tell me.
有任何问题，都请告诉我。

## B. Situational Conversation（情景会话）

### (1)

Nurse: The doctor says you need to be hospitalized for further tests. Here is your admission form, please come with me and I will show you what to do and show you where your bed is.

护士：医生说你需要住院接受进一步检查。这是住院表，请跟我来，我会告诉你床位在哪里和该怎么做。

Patient: Can I go home to collect some wash things, there are things I need to do.

病人：我能回家拿些换洗衣服吗？我回家有点事情。

Nurse: Certainly (Of course), but please follow me now so you will know where your bed is and you can come back in a couple of hours.

护士：当然可以。不过请先跟着我来，这样你会知道你的床在什么地方，然后你出去两个小时内回来就可以。

Patient: Will I see that doctor on the ward?

病人：我在病房里会再见到那位医生吗？

Nurse: No, the ward doctor will see you when you come in and ask you questions and examine you, he will explain what is going to happen.

护士：不会，你去病房的时候，病房的医生会过去看你，并问你一些问题和进行检查，他会告诉你该怎么做。

Patient: Will I be in hospital long?

病人：我需要住院很久吗？

Nurse: I'm sorry I can't say, it will depend on our investigations and diagnosis.

护士：很抱歉，现在还不好说，主要是取决于我们的检查和诊断结果。

### (2)

Head Nurse: Welcome, Miss Brown. I'm the nurse in charge of this department. Please make yourself at home. Someone is now tidying up the patient-bed for you. You can check in at the reception desk and then have a rest in the waiting room.

护士长： 你好布朗太太，欢迎你。我是这个病区的护士长。请把这里当做您自己的家。现在工作人员正为你整理病床，你可以先办理登记然后在等候室稍事歇息。

Patient： Thank you. I'm sorry to trouble you so much.

病人： 谢谢。非常不好意思给你们带来麻烦。

Head Nurse： Don't mention it. It's just our job.

护士长： 不客气，这些都是我们的工作。

※ ※ ※

Patient： Oh, it's a little honey room.

病人： 噢，是个像家一样温馨的小房间。

Nurse： I'm glad you like it.

护士： 很高兴你喜欢它。

Patient： Can I have your name?

病人： 能告诉我你的名字吗？

Nurse： My name is Wang Lin. If you need anything, you can press this button. Each of the nurses is at your service.

护士： 我叫王琳。如果有什么需要，就按这个呼叫铃。每位护士都随时为你服务。

Patient： That's very kind of you.

病人： 你们真好。

Nurse： Are you Moslem?

护士： 你是穆斯林吗？

Patient： No, I'm not.

病人： 不是的。

Nurse： Then which kind of food do you prefer? Chinese or Western?

护士： 那么你喜欢什么样的食物呢？中餐还是西餐？

Patient： It depends. Both are my favorite. What about the mealtime?

病人： 都喜欢，看情况。用餐时间如何？

I prefer western food.

我更喜欢西餐。

Nurse： Patients usually get up at 7: 00 a.m. Breakfast is at 7: 30, lunch at noon, and supper at 6: 30 p.m. The ward rounds and treatment start at 8: 30. 3: 00-5: 00 p.m. is the visiting time.

护士： 病人一般在 7: 00 起床。早餐时间是 7: 30，午餐是 12: 00，晚餐是下午 6: 30。早上 8: 30 开始查房和治疗。下午 3: 00 到 5: 00 是探视时间。

Patient： I got it.

病人： 我知道了。

Nurse： How is your appetite?

护士： 胃口怎么样？

Patient： Just so so.

病人：过得去。

Not so good.

一般，不太好。

Not so bad.

还可以。

Just as good as ever.

跟生病前没什么不同。

I have no appetite at all.

一点胃口都没有！

Patient：How about the food here?

病人：这里的吃食味道如何？

Nurse：There's no accounting for tastes. Actually，many foreign patients liked it.

护士：萝卜青菜各有所爱。不过说起来，很多外国病人挺爱吃的。

Patient：Ok，I'd like to try.

病人：那我也不妨试试。

Nurse：Are you allergic to certain foods such as seafood?

护士：你对什么食物过敏吗，比如海鲜？

Patient：No，never.

病人：还没发现有什么让我过敏的食物。

Nurse：Do you have any special demands?

护士：你对食物有什么特殊要求吗？

Patient：Yes，please give me some fruit with each meal.

病人：是的。我想每餐都来点水果。

I don't like greasy food.

我不喜欢肥甘厚腻的食品。

I prefer more vegetables than meat.

少来点肉，多来点青菜。

I eat little，but I'd like to have a snack in the afternoon and before going to bed.

我吃得不多，不过我喜欢在下午和睡前来点小吃食。

Nurse：Please eat more during the treatment. It will help you recover more quickly.

护士：治疗期间还是多吃点东西好，能帮助你尽快恢复健康。

Patient：I don't like sweet/ salty things.

病人：我不爱吃得太甜/咸。

Nurse：Do you prefer a normal soup or a cream soup?

护士：你要例汤还是要奶油汤？

Do you prefer milk or sour milk?

你喜欢喝牛奶还是酸奶？

Do you prefer black tea，green tea，jasmine tea，or coffee?

你喜欢红茶、绿茶、茉莉花茶还是咖啡？

Patient：I like rice gruel（porridge/ noodles/ toast）.

病人： 我喜欢大米粥(麦片、面条、烤面包)。

I want some fruit juice(iced water/ mineral water/ strawberry juice/ apple juice).

我想要点果汁(冰水/矿泉水/草莓汁/苹果汁)。

I don't like soda-crackers. I just want to eat cakes.

我不吃苏打饼干。我只吃蛋糕。

Since my teeth are not good, I can only take soft food and eat soup.

我的牙不好,只能吃柔软的食物和汤。

Nurse: You can make a concrete choice for each meal when the worker of the refectory comes here.

护士： 食堂工人来的时候你可以具体选择每一餐的食物。

Patient: OK!

病人： 那行。

Nurse: Mr. Li is your doctor. He will come to see you 10 minutes later. There are some very common exams that an inpatient must take, and there are some special examinations based on your disease. Dr. Li must be talking about it.

护士： 李医生是你的主管医生,他10分钟后来看你。有一些住院病人必须做的基本检查和一些根据你的病情安排的特殊检查。一会儿李医生会同你谈这些。

Patient: I'll be here waiting for him.

病人： 我在这里等他来。

Nurse: Dr. Li is very good at the diagnosis and treatment on this kind of disease. I'm sure you'll get a speedy recovery. If you need anything, don't hesitate to let me know.

护士： 李医生非常擅长这种疾病的诊断和治疗。我相信你很快就会恢复健康。如果你需要什么,尽管告诉我。

Patient: Must I be confined to this area?

病人： 我只能在病房范围活动吗?

Nurse: Not exactly. You can go to the garden downstairs for a walk, but you must let us know before that.

护士： 不一定。你可以去楼下的花园走走,不过去之前要告知我们。

Patient: OK.

病人： 好。

Nurse: You can have a rest now. See you later.

护士： 那你休息吧。一会儿见。

Patient: See you later.

病人： 回头见。

**(3)**

Patient: Excuse me. I'd like to know where I should go for the admission procedures.

病人： 请问在哪儿办理住院手续?

Nurse: In the inpatient department. It's not in this building. It's in the opposite building.

护士： 在住院部办理。住院部不在本楼,在对面楼里。

※ ※ ※

Patient: May I go through the admission procedures?
病人: 可以办住院手续吗?
Nurse: Yes, please show me your inpatient appointment card.
护士: 可以,请出示你的住院证。
Patient: What shall I do next?
病人: 下一步我该怎么做?
Nurse: You have to fill in this form carefully and I'll make you a record of hospitalization.
护士: 你仔细填写这张表格,我给你建个住院病历。
Patient: Can I be admitted now or later?
病人: 现在住院还是过一会儿?
Nurse: Not now, I'm afraid. There is no bed available now.
护士: 恐怕现在不行。现在没有空床位。
Patient: When can I get a bed?
病人: 什么时候有床位?
Nurse: A patient will be discharged at noon, so you may be admitted this afternoon.
护士: 中午有位病人出院,所以你只能下午来住院。
Patient: That's great. To be honest, I'm not prepared.
病人: 太好了,说老实话,我还没准备好。
Nurse: Please come this afternoon and not later than 4: 00 p.m. You are in ward 8.
护士: 请下午来,不要超过 4 点。你在 8 号病房。
Patient: I've never been in a hospital, so I'm a little scared.
病人: 这是我第一次住院,所以我有点害怕。
Nurse: Don't worry about it. I hope you'll feel at home here.
护士: 别担心。希望你在这儿不要感到拘束。
Patient: What daily articles should I bring along?
病人: 我需要带些什么日常用品?
Nurse: You'd better bring toothbrush, toothpaste, comb, slippers, and towels.
护士: 你最好带牙刷、牙膏、梳子、拖鞋和毛巾。
Patient: What else should I bring?
病人: 还有其他的吗?
Nurse: No more. There are quilt, bed sheet and hospital pajama in the ward.
护士: 不用了。病房里备有被子、床单和病服。
Patient: Could you tell me the visiting hours?
病人: 您能告诉我探视时间吗?
Nurse: The visiting hours are from 3: 00 to 8: 00 p.m.
护士: 探视时间是下午 3 点至 8 点。

※ ※ ※

Patient: Are there any beds available now? I've got registered this morning.
病人: 有空床位了吗?我今天早上已经办好手续。

Nurse： Yes，please follow me. Let's go to your ward.

护士： 有的，请跟我来。我们去你住的病房吧。

Patient： Is this my bed?

病人： 这是我的床位吗？

Nurse： Yes. Look，the panel on the head of the bed is equipped with a nurse-call system.

护士： 是。瞧，床头墙上的控制板上装有呼叫护士装置。

Patient： What's the use of it?

病人： 这个装置有什么用？

Nurse： If you have something emergent，please press the button by the bedside. A nurse will come as soon as possible.

护士： 如有什么紧急事情，请按床头边的按钮，护士会立即赶来。

Patient： When will the morning ward round begin?

病人： 早上查房什么时候开始？

Nurse： The ward round and treatment start at 8：00 a.m. every morning.

护士： 每天早上8点开始查房和治疗。

Patient： Will the nurse watch the patients at night?

病人： 护士晚上也观察病人吗？

Nurse： Yes，the nurse on duty makes two rounds of the wards during the night.

护士： 值班护士每夜查两次房。

## （4）

Nurse： Excuse me. Is this Miss Xie?

护士： 请问，你是谢小姐吗？

Patient： Yes.

病人： 是的。

Nurse： How do you do!

护士： 你好！

Patient： How do you do!

病人： 你好！

Nurse： I'm your nurse. My name is Huang Sisi. Welcome to our ward!

护士： 我是你的责任护士。我叫黄思思，欢迎你到我们病房来。

Patient： Excuse me. Where is my bed?

病人： 请问哪张床是我的？

Nurse： This way，please. Your bed is No. 309.

护士： 你的床号是309，就在这儿。

Patient： Oh，Thanks.

病人： 谢谢！

Nurse： Dr. Zhang is responsible for your treatment. Dr. Qian is the chief of this ward. They are very kind and considerate. So you are in good hands. And they make their morning rounds at 8 every day.

护士：张医生是你的主治医生，钱医生是病房主任。他们人都很好，很负责。你会得到很好的照顾。他们每天早晨 8 点来查房。

Patient: Oh. I forgot to bring my washbowl.

病人：呀，我忘了带脸盆来。

Nurse: Don't worry. Everything is ready for you in the ward. Here is your washbowl，beside cupboard and chair. And this is calling lamp. Press this button any time you need me.

护士：没关系，我们病房为你准备了所有的生活用品，这是你的床头柜、椅子和脸盆。如果你有任何需要，请按墙上的呼叫器。

Patient: Where is the washroom?

病人：请问卫生间在哪？

Nurse: Go straight and take the second turning on the left. The third room is washroom.

护士：一直往前走，在第二个转弯处向左拐，第三间就是卫生间。

Patient: Thank you!

病人：谢谢 .

Nurse: And this is your wardmate，called Huang Lu. You can change your experience with her. By the way，mind you don't drop your groceries about.

护士：这是你的病友，她叫黄路，你们可以互相交流。顺便说一下，请注意环境卫生，不要乱丢杂物。

Patient: Oh，I got it.

病人：哦，知道了。

Nurse: Please stay here for a while. The doctor will check you soon.

护士：请你稍等片刻，医生马上过来为你检查。

Patient: OK.

病人：知道了。

## (5)

Patient: Excuse me，nurse. Is this the Central surgical Ward?

病人：打扰了，护士，请问这是普外科病房吗？

Nurse: Yes，it is.

护士：是的。

Patient: I'm Wang Yi. I was notified to be here at half past 2.

病人：我叫王义，你们通知我今天两点半到这儿住院。

Nurse: Mr. Wang，please come in and take a rest. Let's fill in an admission card.

护士：噢，王先生，请进来坐。我们要填一张入院卡。

Nurse: Your surname is Wang. Would you mind spelling it，please?

护士：你姓王，是吗？

Patient: W-A-N-G.

病人：是的，三横王。

Nurse: Thank you. And your first name?

护士：谢谢，你的名是？

Patient: Yi.
病人：义。
Nurse: Your address?
护士：你的地址？
Patient: 256 Fuxing Road，Shanghai.
病人：上海复兴路 256 号。
Nurse: And your telephone number?
护士：你的电话号码？
Patient: 65709664，Extension 408.
病人：65709664，分机号码 408。
Nurse: The date of your birth?
护士：你的出生日期？
Patient: 22nd November 1965.
病人：1965 年 11 月 22 日。
Nurse: And what's your occupation?
护士：你的职业？
Patient: I'm an engineer.
病人：工程师。
Nurse: It says here，"Name and address of your Kin." Who is your nearest relation?
护士：现在该填"近亲的姓名和地址"了，请问与你关系最密切的人是……？
Patient: My parents.（My wife，Li Li.）
病人：我父母。（我妻子李莉）
Nurse: And you live at the same address?
护士：你们住在一起吗？
Patient: Yes.
病人：是的。
Nurse: Now，who is your family doctor?
护士：你的家庭医生是哪一位？
Patient: Dr. Zhang.
病人：是张医生。
Nurse: And his address?
护士：他的地址？
Patient: 75 Huaihai Road.
病人：淮海路 75 号。
Nurse: Do you know which doctor is in charge of your case?
护士：你知道你的责任医师是哪一位吗？
Patient: I don't know.
病人：不知道。
Nurse: It's Dr. Liu.
护士：是刘医生。

Patient： I see. Thank you.

病人： 我知道了，谢谢。

Nurse： If you would just wait here for a few minutes，I'll get a nurse to take care of you.

护士： 请你在这儿稍等一下，我请一位护士来照顾你。

## （6）

Nurse： Is this Mr. Li? Welcome to our ward. Please take this bed. Everything is ready. Let me help you get into bed.

护士： 你是李先生吗？欢迎你来我们病房。请睡这个床。一切都准备好了。

Patient： Thank you very much. I'd like to sit a while before lying down. Where have you put my clothes?

病人： 十分感谢。我想先坐一会儿再躺下。你把我的衣服放在哪里了？

Nurse： They have been given to your relatives at the Admission Office. They have been told to bring them back for you to wear when you leave the hospital.

护士： 住院处已交给你的家属了。已告知他们在你出院时带回来给你。

Patient： I've forgotten to bring my cup.

病人： 我忘记带杯子了。

Nurse： Don't worry. Here is a little teapot for you. The ward attendant will bring you hot water twice a day. I hope that will be enough for you.

护士： 别着急。这里有小茶壶备你用。病房工人每天给你送两次热水。我想够了吧。

Nurse： Now take a rest. I'll come back later to tell you something about our hospital and its regulations.

护士： 现在该休息了。等一会儿我再来，告诉你一些我们医院的情况和制度。

Patient： Good. Thanks a lot.

病人： 好。多谢你。

（The nurse returning）

（护士返回）

Nurse： This is No. 3 ward of the Internal Medicine Department. Your bed is No. 302. Dr Zhang is the chief of this ward but Dr Li is responsible for your treatment. He is kind and considerate. So you are in good hands.

护士： 这是内科三病房，你是 302 床。病房主任姓张，但李医生负责你的治疗。他人很好，并且很负责。你会得到很好的照顾。

Patient： When are my relatives allowed to visit me?

病人： 我的家属几时可以来探视？

Nurse： From three to four in the afternoon.

护士： 每天下午 3～4 点钟。

Patient： An hour is too short. Why do you limit the visits only to one hour?

病人： 为什么探视时间仅限制为一小时？我感到太短了。

Nurse： It is necessary to give patients a quiet environment for their treatment and rest. Besides，longer visits will be too tiring for them. Your meals are：breakfast at seven， lunch at twelve, and super at six in the evening. The doctors make their morning rounds at nine. Another round is made in the evening.

护士： 这是因为必须让病人有安静的治疗和休养环境。时间太长会使病人感到疲劳。这里吃饭的时间是早饭 7 点，午饭 12 点，晚饭在傍晚 6 点。医生在上午 9 点查房。另外一次查房在晚上。

Patient: Where is the washroom?

病人： 盥洗室在哪里？

Nurse: We will show you after a little while. By the way, we will also show you our nurse's station and treatment room.

护士： 等一会儿我们带你去看。顺便还要让你认认护士办公室和治疗室。

Patient: Thank you. Oh, I have also forgotten to bring my bowls and chopsticks. What can I do?

病人： 谢谢。啊，我忘记带碗筷了。怎么办？

Nurse: Never mind. The hospital furnishes everything for your meals. These have to be sterilized every time they are used. The doctor has ordered a soft diet for you. We will put you on the regular diet when your condition has improved.

护士： 不要紧。医院为你们准备好了餐具。每次用后都消毒。医嘱给你软食。在你的病情改善后给你正常饮食。

Patient: That's fine. I hope I will not get any injections. I've never had them before.

病人： 好。我不希望打什么针。我还没有打过针。

Nurse: Don't be afraid. It feels just like a mosquito bite. Anyway, you may not even need injections. The doctor may prescribe other treatment for you.

护士： 别怕。打针就像蚊子叮一下。而且，你也可能不打针。医生也许给你用其他方法治疗。

Nurse: My name is Wang Ying. I am the head nurse of this ward. Press this button any time you need me. But someone will always come if I am not there.

护士： 我叫王英。我是本病房的护士长。如果要找我，可按一下电钮。如果我不在，其他人也会来的。

Patient: Thank you for all the information. You have made me feel much easier.

病人： 谢谢你的介绍。你使我感到很安心。

Nurse: When I have time I will come back to find out more about your condition and what we can do to make you comfortable. See you later.

护士： 等我有时间时再来进一步了解你的情况，我们会让你感到更舒服些。再见。

Patient: Good-bye. Thank you.

病人： 谢谢。再见。

# 4. Discharging a Patient

# 出院

## A. Sentences Commonly Used(常用语)

1. The doctor has prescribed some medication for you; you will need to take...
   医生给你开了些处方药，你需要吃……。
2. The doctor is going to discharge you today/ this morning/this afternoon.
   医生今天/今天上午/今天下午给你办理出院。
3. You will need to take some medication home with you.
   你需要带一些药回家。
4. You will need to come back for a check up on...
   你需要在……时回医院复查。
5. You will need to come back to have your sutures removed on...
   你需要在……时回医院拆线。
6. Please remember you will need to re-register again when you come back.
   请记住，当你回医院的时候需要再次挂号。
7. You need to keep the dressing on for...days.
   你需要留着包扎……天。
8. Please do not get the dressing wet.
   不要把包扎弄湿。
9. Please rest when you get home.
   回家之后好好休息。
10. Please do not lift anything heavy for a few weeks.
    这几个星期内不要提重的东西。
11. If you are concerned about your health, please phone us, a nurse will give you the telephone number.
    如果你担心健康情况，请给我们来电，护士会给你我们的电话号码。
12. If you feel that there are any complications/ problems, please contact the hospital immediately.
    如果你感到有什么并发症出现，请立刻与医院联系。
13. Please come to the Emergency room straight away if you are...
    如果你……，请直接到急诊室。

Wound breaks open.
伤口破裂。
Wound is oozing.
伤口渗出。
Pain comes back.
又开始疼。
Having chest pain.
胸痛。
Breathless.
喘不过气。
Medication doesn’t seem to be working.
吃药没有效果。
Health deteriorates.
健康恶化。
Feeling unwell.
感觉难受。

14. Have you any questions you would like to ask?
    你有什么问题需要询问？
15. The doctor will write a letter for you to give to your doctor，explaining the treatment you have had.
    医生会给你的私人医生写信，告知你所接受的治疗。
16. Do you need a letter for your health insurance company?
    你需要医院给你的医疗保险公司写信吗？
17. Before you leave，I’d like to give you some good suggestions.
    在你出院前，我想给你一些好的建议。
18. Please remember to settle your account before you leave hospital.
    在你出院之前请记着结账。
19. I think I’m quite all right now.
    我似乎已经完全好了。
20. You are going to be discharged the day after tomorrow.
    你后天就要出院了。
21. You have been in hospital for two weeks.
    你住院两个星期了。
22. But the doctor told me that I still had to rest for one more week.
    但医生告诉我仍需要再休息一周。
23. First，avoid any mental stress and have a good rest.
    第一，避免精神紧张，好好休息。
24. Secondly，examinations of fasting blood sugar and an ECG should be done regularly.
    第二，定期查空腹血糖和做心电图检查。
25. Wait a minute I’ll go to the Admission Office to get your bill at once.

请稍候，我马上去住院处给你拿账单。

26. Have you made sure you haven't left anything behind?
你确信没有忘记什么东西吗？
27. How time flies. You have been in the hospital for two weeks and you have gotten a complete recovery.
时间过得真快。你在我们医院已经住了一周了，病也已经痊愈了。
28. You are going to be discharged tomorrow.
明天你就出院了。
29. You can leave hospital now，but you must rest at home for at least one week.
你现在可以出院了，不过至少还得在家休养一周。
30. Please come with me to the discharge office to pay your bill/ settle accounts.
请随我到出院处去结账。
31. Our president has given you an 8% discount because you are our honored guest，then you will pay ￥7,200 all together for your hospitalization.
由于您是我们的贵宾，因此院长给了您 8% 的折扣，折后住院费是 7200 元。
32. You can pay by credit card or in cash.
你可以用信用卡或现金付账。
33. Here is the change，please check it before leaving.
这是找给你的钱，请在离开柜台前清点一次。
34. Are you sure that you haven't left anything behind?
确定没有落下什么东西吗？
35. Welcome to China again.
欢迎再到中国来。

## B. Situational Conversation(情景会话)

### (1)

Nurse： The doctor is going to discharge you later this morning.
护士： 医生早上过些时候安排你出院。
Patient： That's marvelous，thanks.
病人： 太感谢了！
Nurse： You will need to come back to have your sutures removed in 3 days.
护士： 你需要 3 天后过来拆线。
Patient： Do I come back here to the ward?
病人： 我需要回来这个病房吗？
Nurse： No，you need to go back to Outpatients，please remember you will need to re-register again when you come back.
护士： 不用，你需要去门诊部，请记住当你回来的时候你需要重新挂号。
Patient： Oh，OK，who do I ask for?

病人：哦，好的，我该找谁？

Nurse：I will write the doctor's name down for you，so you can give it to the registration nurse.

护士：我会把医生的名字写给你，你把它交给挂号处的护士就可以。

Patient：That will be great，thanks.

病人：非常感谢！

Nurse：You need to keep the dressing on until you have your sutures removed，please do not get the dressing wet.

护士：你要一直绑着绷带直到拆线，请不要弄湿了。

Patient：Will you give me some clean ones to take home with me?

病人：你会给我一些干净的绷带吗？

Nurse：Yes，I will. You will need to rest when you go home and please do not lift anything heavy for a few weeks and only gentle exercise for a while.

护士：是的，我会给你一些。回到家之后多休息，请在这几周内不要提重的东西，可以做一些轻微的运动。

Patient：Great，no housework then.

病人：太好了，可以不做家务了。

Nurse：The doctor will prescribe some medication for you to take home.

护士：医生会给你开些药回到家里吃。

Patient：What medicine do I need?

病人：我需要什么药？

Nurse：He will prescribe some painkillers and antibiotics for you to take.

护士：他会给你开些止痛药和抗生素。

Patient：OK，will you get these for me or do I need to go the pharmacy?

病人：好的，是你准备好给我还是我去药房取？

Nurse：The doctor will give you the prescription，and you will need to go to the Pharmacy Department，I will show you where to go.

护士：医生会给你处方，你需要自己去药房，我会带你过去。

Patient：OK，I'll do that on my way out of the hospital.

病人：我出院时自己能办好。

Nurse：You must come to the Emergency Room straight way if your wound breaks open，is oozing or the pain comes back.

护士：当遇到如下情况，请直接到急诊室：伤口破裂、往外渗水、疼痛发作。

Patient：OK，where do I go to pay the hospital bill，will the hospital give me a letter for my insurance company?

病人：好的，我到哪里去交住院费？医院给我的医疗保险公司写信了吗？

Nurse：The doctor will write a letter for you to give to your doctor，explaining the treatment you have had. And also a letter for your health insurance company，the cashier will give you a list of your expenses and a receipt.

护士：医生会给你的私人医生写信，告知给你所做的治疗，还会给你的医疗保险公司写信，收费处会给你一张费用清单和收据。

Patient: OK, that's fine. I don't need anything else, thanks very much, nurse.

病人：好的，那很好。我没别的要求了，非常感谢你，护士小姐。

Nurse: You are welcome.

护士：不客气。

**(2)**

Patient: The doctor says that the tests were OK, does that mean I can go home?

病人：医生说检测结果显示没有问题，是不是意味着我现在可以回家了。

Nurse: The doctor is going to discharge you this afternoon.

护士：医生今天下午安排你出院。

Patient: Oh, that's great.

病人：噢，太好了！

Nurse: You will need to take some medication home with you, he has prescribed some tablets for your blood pressure and you need to take one twice a day morning and evening, he has also prescribed a sub-lingual tablet which you should take when the pain comes in your chest, put one tablet under your tongue and let it dissolve, you must only take a maximum of two tablets a day.

护士：你需要带一些药回家，他给你开了些治疗高血压的药片，每天早晚各吃一片。另外，他还开了舌下锭，当你胸部痛时，请放一片在你的舌头下面让其慢慢融化，每天最多吃两片。

Patient: OK, do I need to come back for a check up?

病人：噢，我还需要回来复查吗？

Nurse: You will need to come back for a check up in two weeks.

护士：你需要两周后回来复查。

Patient: Where will I have to go for the check up, in Outpatients?

病人：我将到哪儿去复查，门诊部？

Nurse: Yes, you will need to register first, like the last time and then go and see the doctor in Outpatients. I'll write the doctor's name down for you, so you can give it to the registration nurse.

护士：是的，你需要先挂号，像上次一样到门诊部看医生。我将把医生的姓名给你写下来以便你给挂号处的护士。

Patient: That will be really helpful, thanks a lot.

病人：真的太有帮助了，谢谢！

Nurse: You will have to rest when you go home, just gentle exercise at first and do not lift anything heavy for a few weeks.

护士：你回家后需要好好休息，在几个星期内可以做一些轻微的运动，但不要提重的东西。

Patient: Can I go out shopping? It's just walking.

病人：我可以去逛街吗？就像散步一样。

Nurse: Yes, but do not lift anything heavy for a few weeks.

护士：可以，但在几周之内不要提重的东西。

Patient: OK.

病人：好的。

Nurse: If you are concerned about your health, you must please phone us, someone will give you the telephone number before you leave.

护士：如果你担心健康情况，请务必给我们打电话。你离开之前，会有人将电话号码告诉你。

Patient: No, I'm sure I'll be fine.

病人：不会，我肯定没问题。

Nurse: You must go to the Emergency Room straight away if you are having severe chest pain, and the medication isn't working, or if you are feeling breathless.

护士：如果有剧烈的胸痛，或者药不起作用，或者呼吸不畅，请务必到急诊室就医。

Patient: OK, I will.

病人：好的，我会的。

Nurse: Have you any questions you would like to ask?

护士：有什么问题需要问的吗？

Patient: No, I don't think so, I'll wait till I see the doctor, and ask him some questions, thanks a lot.

病人：我觉得没有了。我会等医生来了之后问他一些问题，非常感谢你。

Nurse: The doctor will write a letter for you to give to your doctor, explaining the treatment you have had and give you a letter for your health insurance company if you need one.

护士：医生会给你的私人医生写信，介绍你曾经接受过的治疗情况。如果你需要给保险公司开证明，医生会给你开一个。

Patient: Just a copy of the letter to my doctor will be fine and the bill for my stay here, when I have to pay.

病人：把给我的私人医生的信复印一下就可以了，另外就是住院费账单包括须付款的时间。

Nurse: Someone will show you where to go, and the cashier will give you a bill with a list of your expenses and she will give you a receipt when you pay.

护士：待会会有人将你带过去。出纳会给你住院的花费清单，并在你付钱的时候给你收据。

Patient: OK, great. I can give all that to my insurance company when I go home, thanks a lot.

病人：好的。我可以在回家后把所有的东西给我的保险公司。非常感谢！

Nurse: You're welcome. I'll see you later.

护士：不要客气，一会儿见！

### (3)

Nurse: You have been in the hospital for two weeks, haven't you?

护士：你住院两个星期了，是吧？

Patient： Exactly，but the doctor told me I still have to rest for one more week.

病人： 对的，可是医生说我还得休息一个星期。

Nurse： The doctor has written a certificate for you. There are two suggestions. First，avoid any mental stress and have a good rest. Second，examinations of fasting sugar and an ECG should be done regularly.

护士： 医生已经给你开好了证明书。里面有两条建议。第一，避免精神紧张，好好休息。第二，定期查空腹血糖和做心电图检查。

Patient： My family doctor needs my medical history. May I have it tomorrow?

病人： 我的家庭医生需要我的病史，明天能给我吗？

Nurse： Certainly.

护士： 当然可以。

Patient： Please give me my account.

病人： 请给我结一下账。

Nurse： I'll go to the admissions' office to get your bill at once.

护士： 我立即到住院处去给你结账。

※　※　※

Patient： How much do I owe you? May I pay it by check?

病人： 我欠多少钱？能用支票付款吗？

Nurse： Altogether three thousand and five hundred yuan，seventy-five fen. You may pay either in cash or by check.

护士： 总共3500元7角5分，你付现金或开支票都行。

Patient： I must go now. Will you call a taxi for me?

病人： 我该走了。请给我叫辆出租汽车，好吗？

Nurse： Have you made sure you haven't left anything behind?

护士： 你没有遗留下什么东西吗？

Patient： I don't think so. I'm really very grateful to you all. You were so kind to me.

病人： 我想没有。我十分感谢你们大家。你们对我都这么好。

Nurse： Don't mention it. That is our job.

护士： 不必客气，那是我们的职责。

Nurse： The taxi has come.

护士： 出租车来了。

# 5. Inquiring Symptoms

# 询问病情

## A. Sentences Commonly Used（常用语）

1. How are you feeling today?
   今天你感觉怎么样？
2. How do you feel today? Is there anything wrong?
   你今天感觉怎么样？有什么不舒服吗？
3. What's matter with you?
   你怎么不舒服？
4. What's bothering you?
   你哪儿不舒服？
5. Can you tell me about your problem?
   你能告诉我你的问题吗？
6. What kind of difficulties are you having?
   你最近有什么问题？
7. What sort of problem have you been having?
   你现在有什么问题？
8. What symptoms do you have?
   你有些什么样的症状？
9. Tell me about your trouble, please.
   请告诉我你哪儿不舒服？
10. Tell me what's wrong?
    告诉我哪儿不好？
11. Tell me why you came today?
    告诉我你今天为什么来这儿？
12. What do you think is wrong with you?
    你认为自己有什么问题？
13. You don't look well. Is there anything wrong?
    你看起来气色不好，哪儿不舒服吗？
14. You look very pale. What trouble do you have?
    你看上去很苍白，哪儿不舒服吗？

15. How did it happen?
这是怎么发生的？
16. How long have you felt sick?
你病了多久了？
17. What do you think causes the symptom?
你觉得引起这个症状的原因是什么？
18. What do you think provokes it?
你认为是什么诱发出这种症状的？
19. When did it begin (start)?
什么时候开始的？
20. When did you begin feeling sick?
你是什么时候开始觉得身体不舒服的？
21. When did you begin to notice these symptoms?
你是什么时候开始发现这些症状的？
22. When did you first complain?
第一次是什么时候发生的？
23. Have you noticed any of these symptoms recently?
最近你注意到有这些症状吗？
24. When did you first notice it?
你第一次注意到这种情况是什么时候？
25. Has this happened before?
这种情况以前发生过吗？
26. Have you had similar trouble before?
你以前有过类似的毛病吗？
27. Have you ever felt anything like this before?
以前你有过类似的感觉吗？
28. Have you noticed any change recently?
最近你注意到有什么变化没有？
29. Was it better or worse during the summer?
夏天时这个症状是好些还是更糟？
30. How often are the attacks?
多久发作一次？
31. How long does each episode last?
每次发作持续多久？
32. How long has this been a problem?
这个问题有多长时间了？
33. How long have you been like this?
你这种症状持续多长时间了？
34. How often does it happen, once a day, a week, or a month?
这种情况多久发生一次，一天一次，一周一次还是一月一次？

35. Is the condition serious?
病情严重吗？
36. Has it gotten worse?
病情加重了吗？
37. Do you feel you have a serious illness?
你觉得你得了重病吗？
38. Have you noticed anything that makes it worse?
你注意到有什么事情让这种症状加重吗？
39. Is the problem getting worse，better，or staying the same?
这个问题变得更糟了，好些了，还是保持原样？
40. How bad is it?
有多糟？
41. Would you explain how bad it is?
你能描述一下它有多糟吗？
42. Are you feeling better?
你感觉好些了吗？
43. When did you last feel well?
你最近一次感觉良好是什么时候？
44. We need just a little more information.
我们需要了解更多的情况。
45. Do you have a fever?
你发热吗？
46. Do you sweat a lot?
你出汗多吗？
47. Do you feel weak?
你感觉虚弱吗？
48. Are you feeling very tired lately?
你最近感觉很疲劳吗？
49. Do you become easily fatigued?
你是否变得很容易疲劳？
50. Please say it again.
请再说一遍。
51. Calm down! Say it slowly and clearly，please!
请不要着急，慢慢讲！
52. Please sit down!
请坐下！
53. May I ask you a question?
我可以问你一个问题吗？
54. What’s wrong with you?
请问你哪儿不舒服？

55. What's your name, please?
请问，你叫什么名字？
56. How old are you?
你有多大年纪？
57. You look younger than your age.
你看上去比实际年龄要年轻。
58. Where are you from?
你在什么地方出生的？
59. What's your address, please?
请告诉我你的地址，好吗？
60. What's your work?
你做什么工作？
61. Are you married or single?
你结婚了，还是独身？
62. Because of the nursing needs, I need know how many children you have.
因为护理需要，我想知道你有几个小孩？
63. Can you tell me exactly what symptoms you have?
你能明确告诉我你有哪些症状吗？
64. Have you had any illness before?
你以前曾经有过什么病吗？
65. Has anybody in your family got heart disease (kidney disease) in the past?
你的家庭成员有人得过心脏病（或肾脏病）吗？
66. Did you run a fever or have a sore throat?
你发烧吗？嗓子痛吗？
67. Did you bring up phlegm when coughing recently?
最近你咳嗽有痰吗？
68. Do you suffer from heartburn stomachaches (chest pains)?
你的胃有过烧灼感（胸痛）吗？
69. We need to know more information.
我们需要了解更多一些情况。
70. Are you feeling nausea?
你感到恶心吗？
71. Do you often belch (hiccup)?
你经常嗳气（或反酸）吗？
72. Have you vomited? What did you vomit? Food or blood?
你出现呕吐吗？吐的是什么？食物还是血？
73. Does anybody in your family suffer from urinary system disease?
你家里有人得泌尿系统疾病吗？
74. How do your eyes feel when looking far away?
你眼睛看远处如何？

75. How about your hearing?
你两耳听力如何？
76. How long have you had furuncles?
什么时候开始长疖子？
77. Is there anybody in your family having the same experience?
你的亲人中有没有患同样病的？
78. How about your appetite?
你的食欲如何？（胃口如何？）
79. Do you like fry or deep fry food?
你喜欢吃油煎、炸的食物吗？
80. Please weigh yourself.
请你称一下体重。
81. Does your weight lose or put on recently?
你最近体重减轻了还是增加了？
82. What's the color of the urine?
尿是什么颜色的？
83. Do you have trouble urinating?
排尿有问题吗？
84. Do you need to void (urinate) at night?
你夜间需要起来小便吗？
85. Are your bowels acting properly? /Are your bowels regular?
每天都解大便吗？
86. What kind of stool did you notice, watery or mucous?
你注意大便的样子了吗？是水样还是黏液样？
87. Do you feel abdominal pain when you go to the toilet?
你上厕所时感到腹痛吗？
88. When did your diarrhea start?
你什么时候开始腹泻？
89. Do you like smoking and drinking?
请问你平时喜欢喝酒、吸烟吗？
90. How much alcohol do you drink everyday?
你每天要喝多少酒？
91. How many cigarettes do you smoke everyday?
你每天抽多少支香烟？
92. I advise you to give up smoking and keep off any alcohol.
我建议你戒烟、戒酒。
93. When did your period start?
你第一次月经是什么时候？
94. Are your menstrual cycles regular?
来月经有规律吗？

95. Have you got any disease before you are pregnant?
怀孕前你得过什么病吗？
96. How about your sleep at night? Making dreams?
你夜间睡眠如何？做梦吗？
97. Have you ever taken sleeping pills?
服用过安眠药吗？
98. Did you take this kind of medicine before?
请问你以前用过这种药吗？
99. Are you allergic to penicillin?
你对青霉素过敏吗？
100. Has anyone in your family had been allergic to penicillin?
你家里人有没有对青霉素过敏的？
101. I wonder if anyone in your family has hypertension?
你的家里还有高血压患者吗？
102. Have you ever taken blood pressure?
你以前量过血压吗？
103. Have you ever taken any antihypertensive drugs?
你服用过降压药物吗？
104. Have you been coughing lately?
你最近咳嗽过吗？
105. Have you had a cold recently?
你最近感冒过吗？
106. Have you been short of breath?
你是否呼吸急促？
107. Do you often feel light-headed?
你经常会头晕吗？
108. In which ear can't you hear properly?
你哪一只耳朵听不见声音？

## B. Situational Conversation(情景会话)

### (1)

Nurse： Mrs. Smith, can you tell me what the problem is?
护士： 史密斯夫人，请问你哪里不舒服？
Mrs. Smith： I have had a severe stomachache now for a few days.
史密斯夫人： 我胃痛好几天了。

### (2)

Nurse： Mr. Jones, where does your knee hurt?

护士：琼斯先生，你的膝盖哪里痛？
Mr. Jones：It hurts just behind my kneecap.
琼斯先生：膝盖骨后面。

**（3）**

Nurse：Can you tell me what the problem is?
护士：请问你哪里不舒服？
Miss Davis：I have an aching feeling in my shoulder，and tingling in my fingers.
戴维斯小姐：我肩膀疼痛，而且手指发麻。
Nurse：Can you show me where?
护士：你能指给我看是哪里吗？
Miss Davis：Yes，it's just near my collarbone.
戴维斯小姐：可以，就在我的锁骨附近。

**（4）**

Ms. Rose：I have a red，blotchy rash on my body; I have had it for two days now.
罗斯女士：我身上起了红色疱疹，有两天时间了。
Nurse：Is it itching? Does it cause you any pain?
护士：你感觉痒吗？痛不痛？
Ms. Rose：No，it doesn't really hurt. It stings if I scratch it.
罗斯女士：不，不是很痛。但是挠的时候有刺痛感。
Nurse：Do you have any other problems? Abdominal pain?
护士：除此之外还有什么症状吗？例如腹痛？
Ms. Rose：No，there is nothing else wrong.
罗斯女士：没有了。

**（5）**

Nurse：Have you been feeling breathless，since you have had this chest pain?
护士：你胸痛以来有没有感到气短？
Ms. Smith：Yes，I have been feeling a little breathless.
史密斯女士：是的，一直感觉有点气短。
Nurse：How bad is your chest pain? What does it feel like?
护士：你胸痛程度如何？感觉像什么样的？
Ms. Smith：It feels like a sharp pain when I breathe in.
史密斯女士：当我吸气的时候感觉锐痛。

**（6）**

Nurse：How can I help you?
护士：有什么我能帮你？
Mr. Jones：I fell over and I have cut my arm quite badly，I think I may need a suture.

琼斯先生： 我摔了下来，手臂严重裂伤，我想可能需要缝合。

Nurse： OK, let me have a look.

护士： 好的，让我看一下伤势。

## (7)

Nurse： You're looking quite pale, Mrs. Smith. Do you have any abdominal pain?

护士： 史密斯夫人，你看起来脸色苍白。你感到肚子痛吗？

Mrs. Smith： Only a slight ache on the right side.

史密斯夫人： 仅仅是右边有点痛。

Nurse： Do you have bowels open regularly? What color are your stools?

护士： 你大便正常吗？粪便什么颜色？

Mrs. Smith： Yes, quite regularly. I'm not sure what color they are, but they are a bit pale.

史密斯夫人： 是的，大便正常。我没留意什么颜色，不过有点白。

Nurse： What do you mean by regularly? How many times a day?

护士： 你指的正常是什么意思？一天几次？

Mrs. Smith： I have my bowels open usually once a day, sometimes every other day.

史密斯夫人： 通常是一天一次，有时候是两天一次。

## (8)

Nurse： So tell me what is your problem.

护士： 那么你告诉我你哪里不舒服。

Ms. Rose： I have vomited a few times, and I feel nauseous though I don't know why.

罗斯女士： 我呕吐了几次，我感到恶心，但是不知道什么原因。

Nurse： Have you eaten anything that might have made you feel this way?

护士： 你是否吃了什么东西导致这样？

Ms. Rose： No, I don't think so.

罗斯女士： 我想没有。

Nurse： Do you have any other symptoms? Abdominal pain or headache?

护士： 你还有其他症状吗？例如腹痛或头痛？

Ms. Rose： No.

罗斯女士： 没有。

Nurse： Are you on any medication?

护士： 你现在吃什么药吗？

## (9)

Nurse： Thanks for calling SR hospital. This is nurse Wu speaking.

护士： 欢迎垂询SR医院，我是吴护士。

Patient： This is George Clooney. Is that the inquiry desk of SR hospital?

病人： 我是乔治•科洛里。是SR医院的咨询台吗？

Nurse： Yes. What can I do for you, Sir?

护士：是的，有什么可以帮助你的吗，先生？

Patient: Can I speak to Miss Li? I'm calling for some medical questions.

病人：我想跟李小姐通话，可以吗？ 我有一些医疗问题要咨询。

Nurse: She's just on another line. I'm the nurse for medical consultation too. Can I serve you, Mr. Clooney?

护士：她此刻正在接另一个电话。我也是负责医疗咨询的护士，有什么能为你效劳的吗，科洛里先生？

Patient: My wife has been pregnant for more than 39 weeks. When I consulted last time, Miss Li Said the ECD (expected date of confinement) was supposed to be around these days, but until now there is no evidence that my wife will deliver the baby. So I'd like to know what to do.

病人：我太太已经怀孕 39 周了。上次向李小姐咨询的时候，她说预产期是在这几天，但是现在我太太一点生产的迹象都没有。所以我想问一问该怎么处理。

Nurse: I suggest that your wife come and accept thorough exams. The OB could help your wife proceed the labor if necessary.

护士：我建议你太太过来做个全面检查。如果有必要的话，产科医生会人工破膜启动产程。

Patient: OK, I'll take your advice.

病人：好的，我接受你的建议。

Nurse: Are you driving by yourself?

护士：你会自己开车来吗？

Patient: Yes.

病人：是的。

Nurse: Drive slowly and be careful. Just in case of the rupture of membrane on the way.

护士：开慢一点，当心一点，以防在路上发生破裂。

Patient: Thanks. I think we will go to your hospital this Friday, just the day after tomorrow, is that OK?

病人：多谢提醒。我想这个周五，也就是后天到你们医院，你看可以吗？

Nurse: Yes, it's OK. The OB service is available everyday in our hospital.

护士：可以。我们这里每天都有产科医生在提供服务。

Patient: Thanks. And may I ask another quick question?

病人：谢谢。我能快速地问另外一个问题吗？

Nurse: Just go ahead.

护士：请便。

Patient: I have a slight back-leg pain, so I want to see an orthopedist. Is there any famous specialist on Friday?

病人：我有轻微的腰腿痛，想看看骨科医生。周五那天有名专家吗？

Nurse: Let me see. Yes, Doctor Wang is on service that morning. He is a very famous orthopedist. But you must register as soon as possible, because he is very popular.

护士：让我看看。有的。王医生在周五上午会出诊，他是一个非常著名的骨科医生。但你必须尽早挂号，因为他很抢手。

Patient: Must I go to the hospital for registration?

病人： 我必须到医院去挂号吗？

Nurse: No，you needn't. You can log on the web page of our hospital. The domain name is www.SRH.com.cn.

护士： 不用。你可以登录我们医院的网页进行挂号。网址是 www.SRH.com.cn。

Patient: Thanks again，Miss Wu. You are so kind.

病人： 再次多谢吴小姐。你真好。

# 6. Examination and Test

# 检查和检测

## A. Sentences Commonly Used(常用语)

1. I am going to take your temperature.
   我要量一下你的体温。
2. Please open your mouth and I will place this thermometer under your tongue for 3 minutes.
   请张开嘴，我把这个体温计在你的舌头下放 3 分钟。
3. Please let me feel your pulse.
   请让我摸摸你的脉搏。
4. I am going to feel your pulse on your wrist.
   我要在你的手腕上摸一下脉搏。
5. Let me take your blood pressure.
   让我给你量血压。
6. I am going to take your blood pressure now. It's one hundred and forty over ninety mmHg.
   现在我要给你量血压。你的高压是 140mmHg，低压是 90mmHg。
7. Get on the scales and I'll see how much you weigh.
   请站到磅秤上，我要看看你的体重。
8. Look right at me, please.
   请看着我。
9. Would you come toward me just a little?
   请稍微向我靠近一点好吗？
10. Let me examine you.
    让我给你检查一下。
11. Now open your mouth.
    现在张开你的嘴。
12. Open your mouth just as wide as you can.
    尽量把嘴张大。
13. Open your mouth and say"ah".
    张开嘴说"啊"。
14. I'll look into your mouth.

我看看你的嗓子。

15. Please stick out your tongue.
请伸出舌头。
16. Take a few deep breaths.
做几次深呼吸。
17. Breathe in /out.
吸气 / 呼气。
18. Now I want to look in your throat.
现在我要检查你的咽喉。
19. Please breathe deeply /normally.
请深呼吸 / 正常呼吸。
20. Let me take a look in your ears，first.
首先，让我看一下你的耳朵。
21. Now let me examine your nose.
现在让我检查你的鼻子。
22. Please unbutton your shirt and loosen your belt.
请解开上扣子，松开腰带。
23. Please take off your trousers /jacket.
请脱下裤子 / 夹克衫。
24. Please take off your shirt and socks，and lie down on your back.
请脱掉衬衣和袜子，然后仰面躺下。
25. Please take off your shoes and lie down.
请脱鞋，躺下。
26. Please take your clothes off and put this sheet over you.
请脱下你的衣服，盖上被单。
27. Now would you lie down?
现在请你躺下好吗？
28. Please lie on your left，facing the wall.
请朝左侧躺，面对墙壁。
29. Now the other side.
现在请换另一侧。
30. Please lie on your stomach.
请俯卧。
31. Please hold your breath.
请屏住呼吸。
32. You may breathe now.
现在你可以呼吸了。
33. Please cough.
请咳一下。
34. I just want to feel under your arm.

我只需要在你的腋下摸一摸。

35. Please bend your knees.
请屈膝。
36. Please lift your left leg /right leg.
请抬起你的左腿 / 右腿。
37. Please relax and don’t move.
请放松，不要动。
38. It will be finished in 3 minutes.
检查将在三分钟内完成。
39. It’s finished. You can get dressed.
做完了，你可以穿上衣服了。
40. We’re changing the bed linen immediately.
我们马上就换被褥。
41. You need a thorough examination.
你需要做一个全面检查。
42. Please hold your son. Don’t let him move.
请按住你儿子，别让他动。
43. Please do what I do.
请跟着我做。
44. Please walk to the door and back towards me.
请走到门那儿，然后走回来。
45. You need a blood test.
你需要验血。
46. I will prick your thumb.
我要刺一下你的拇指。
47. I’d like to take some blood from your arm.
我要从你手臂（静脉）取血。
48. I would like to draw your blood. /Let me draw your blood.
我将给你抽血 / 让我来给你抽血。
49. Give me your arm.
把手臂伸给我。
50. Please roll up your sleeve.
请把你的袖子卷起来。
51. Don’t worry. It doesn’t hurt you.
别担心，不会弄痛你的。
52. Tell me if I hurt you too much.
如果我弄得你很痛，请告诉我。
53. I’d like to shave off the air around the operation area.
我要刮掉你手术区皮肤上的毛。
54. You are doing perfectly.

你配合得很好。

55. It will finish in seconds.
马上就完了。

56. Okay, that's all.
好的，完了。

57. Okay, it's done. Did it hurt?
好了，完了，痛吗？

58. Please hold the gauze for a few minutes.
请按几分钟纱布。

59. I would like to test your urine.
我要检查你的尿液。

60. Please bring your urine in this cup.
请把你的尿液盛在这个杯子里拿来。

61. Please collect your urine in the middle part of urination.
请收集你的中段尿。

62. I'll come back in a minute.
我一会儿就回来。

63. The doctor is coming to see you soon.
医生很快就来看你。

64. Please take this paper to your doctor.
请把这张单子拿给你的医生。

65. Please wait until we get the result of the blood test.
请等到血检结果出来。

66. It is normal /essentially normal.
结果正常 / 基本正常。

67. Shall I explain it again?
要我再解释一遍吗？

68. Please turn around and show me your back.
请转过来让我看看你的背。

69. Please bend forward as far as you can.
请尽量向前倾。

70. Please bend back as far as you can.
请尽量向后仰。

71. Please lift your arms to the side.
把手臂水平侧向伸出。

72. Please put your arms forward.
手臂前伸。

73. Please raise your right /left arm as high as you can.
请将右臂（左臂）尽量抬高。

74. Can you touch your shoulder blade with your right/ left hand?

你能用右手(左手)摸着你的肩胛骨吗?

75. Can you raise your arms/ hands in front of you?
你能平举着你的手吗?

76. Can you bend your right/ left arm?
你能弯一下右(左)臂吗?

77. Can you move your fingers/ thumbs?
你能动一下你的手指(拇指)吗?

78. Can you squeeze my fingers?
你能用力握我的手指吗?

79. Can you turn your head to the right/ left?
你能头往右(左)转吗?

80. Please bend your neck forward/ backward/ right side/ left side.
请将你的脖子往前/后/右/左转。

81. Can you straighten your right/ left leg?
你能将右(左)腿伸直吗?

82. Can you bend your right/ left knee?
你能弯一下右(左)膝盖吗?

83. Can you move your ankle/ toes?
你能动一下你的脚踝(脚趾)吗?

84. I need a stool specimen.
我需要粪便样本。

85. Here is the specimen pot.
这是样本瓶。

86. When you have done the specimen please take it to the Bacteriology Department.
当你取样之后带到细菌室去。

87. Here is the form, I will tell you where to go.
这是化验单,我会告诉你怎么过去。

88. Please bring the results back to me.
请将化验结果带来给我。

89. You need to have an X-ray.
你需要拍一下X光。

90. You need an X-ray of your...
你需要拍一下……部位的X光。

91. You will have to go to the X-ray Department, please take this form.
你需要去放射科室,请带着这张化验单。

92. I will show you where to go, please bring the results back to me.
我会带你过去,化验结果出来后请拿给我。

93. You need to have an ultra-scan of your...
你需要做一下……部位的超声扫描。

94. Please take this form.

请带着化验单。

95. I will show you where to go, please bring the results back here.
我会带你过去，化验结果出来后请拿给我。

96. You will need to have a full bladder before the ultra-scan.
在做超声波扫描前，请憋尿，使膀胱充盈。

97. Please can you drink...glasses of water before you have the scan.
请在做超声波扫描前喝……杯水。

## B. Situational Conversation(情景会话)

### (1)

Nurse: How long have you had this problem?
护士：你有这个病多久了？
Patient: On and off for ages, I can't remember.
病人：断断续续多年了，我记不太清了。
Nurse: It is March now, have you had this problem just this year?
护士：现在是三月，你只是今年才有这个病的吗？
Patient: Longer, I think.
病人：还要长。
Nurse: Did you have it at Christmas time?
护士：是否在去年圣诞期间？
Patient: Yes, I did. I remember that it spoilt the day for me.
病人：对。我记得是在圣诞节发作的。
Nurse: Can you remember how long you had it before then, did you have the problem in the summer?
护士：你还能记得之前发作多长时间吗？你在夏天的时候有同样的毛病吗？
Patient: No, I didn't. It started after my holiday, and I had my holiday in September.
病人：没有，夏天时没有。它是我休假之后出现的，我休假在九月。
Nurse: So you think you may have had this problem for about 6 months then?
护士：所以现在你有这个毛病快6个月了？
Patient: Yes, I think so, about 6 months.
病人：对。我认为大约就6个月时间。
Nurse: You say you have the pain on and off, does that mean the pain is there everyday?
护士：你说时而发痛，这是否意味着在同样一个地方天天都断断续续地痛？
Patient: No, I wouldn't say it was everyday.
病人：不。不是天天都有。
Nurse: How many days between each attack of pain would you say?
护士：两次发作间隔多久？
Patient: Maybe every couple of days or so.

病人： 大约每两天一次。

Nurse: And when you get a day of pain, how many times do you get the pain throughout the day?

护士： 痛的那天，整天下来疼痛多少次？

Patient: It's usually after I've had breakfast and then a few more times during the day.

病人： 通常在早饭之后一次，白天再发作三四次左右。

Nurse: So would you say when you have the pain it can be four times a day?

护士： 你的意思是一天四次吗？

Patient: Yes, that's right.

病人： 对，是这样的。

Nurse: OK, thanks.

护士： 好的，谢谢。

**（2）**

Nurse: Good morning, Mrs. Jones, how are you this morning?

护士： 早上好，琼斯夫人，你早上觉得怎么样？

Patient: Not too bad, thank you.

病人： 不太坏，谢谢！

Nurse: Did you have your bowels open in the night?

护士： 你昨晚上厕所了吗？

Patient: Yes, I did several times.

病人： 是的，上了几次。

Nurse: How many times exactly?

护士： 具体是几次？

Patient: Oh about 4 or 5 times.

病人： 哦，大概四五次吧。

Nurse: OK, thank you, I'll tell the doctor.

护士： 好的，谢谢，我会告诉医生的。

**（3）**

Nurse: Mrs. Jones, I need to give you an injection of antibiotics.

护士： 琼斯夫人，我要给你打抗生素。

Patient: OK, nurse. Where are you going to give it to me?

病人： 好的，护士小姐。你要在什么地方打？

Nurse: In your right buttock, please will you turn over onto your front?

护士： 臀部右边，请转身趴着。

Patient: Sure, OK.

病人： 没问题。

Nurse: I'm just going to clean your skin, it will feel a bit cold, and you will feel a sharp prick. OK, finished now, you can turn back.

护士： 我将要给你清洁皮肤，会有一点冷和刺痛。好了，现在完成了，你可以转过来了。

Patient： Thanks，nurse.

病人： 谢谢你，护士小姐。

**(4)**

Nurse： Mrs. Jones，I need to do an ECG test.

护士： 琼斯夫人，我需要给你做心电图检测。

Patient： OK，when? Now?

病人： 好的，什么时候？是现在吗？

Nurse： Yes，will you follow me please to the treatment room?

护士： 是的，你可以跟着我到治疗室吗？

Patient： OK.

病人： 好的。

Nurse： Can you sit on the examination couch for me?

护士： 你可以坐到检查台上面吗？

Patient： Sure.

病人： 当然可以。

Nurse： Please unbutton your top.

护士： 请将上衣脱掉。

Patient： Do you want me to take off my bra?

病人： 我需要将乳罩也脱掉吗？

Nurse： No，just your top.

护士： 不用，上衣就可以。

Nurse： I am going to put these pads on your chest，and these jelly will feel cold.

护士： 我接下来将这些电极片放到你的胸部，会感觉有点冷。

Nurse： OK，I've finished now，you can get dressed.

护士： 好的，我现在完成了，你可以穿衣服了。

Patient： Thanks.

病人： 谢谢。

**(5)**

Nurse： Good morning，Miss Smith. How is your foot today?

护士： 早上好，史密斯小姐。你的脚今天感觉怎么样？

Patient： Hi，nurse. Better than I think.

病人： 你好，护士小姐。我觉得好多了。

Nurse： May I have a look?

护士： 我能看一下吗？

Patient： Sure.

病人： 当然。

Nurse： Can you lift your foot up onto the stool for me?

护士：你能将脚抬到凳子上吗？
Nurse：Can you bend your ankle and move your toes?
护士：你能扭动脚踝、移动脚趾吗？
Patient：Yes，sure. The ankle is a bit stiff but my toes can move great now.
病人：是的，当然。脚踝还是感觉有点僵硬，不过脚趾现在可以很好地移动了。
Nurse：Yes，that's good. Your foot is getting better，and you must try and keep your foot up when you are sitting down.
护士：那太好了。你的脚正在恢复，当你坐着的时候尽量将脚抬起来别着地。
Patient：OK，I'll try to remember.
病人：好的，我会记住的。

## （6）

**Normal Urine Sample（Specimen）（Inpatient） 常规尿样（住院病人）**

Nurse：Mrs. Jones，the doctor wants you to have a urine specimen.
护士：琼斯夫人，医生要你做尿液检测。
Patient：What，you want a urine specimen now?
病人：什么？你是现在要尿样吗？
Nurse：Yes，please. Here is the bottle. The toilets（washroom）are over there.
护士：是的，这是样本瓶，厕所在那边。
Patient：What shall I do with the specimen when I have done it?
病人：取了尿液样本之后我该怎么做？
Nurse：Please bring it back to me，and I will take it to the Bacteriology Department.
护士：请带回来给我，我会将它送到细菌室。
Patient：When will the results be back?
病人：结果什么时候能拿到？
Nurse：In a couple of hours，the doctor will come and tell you the results.
护士：两个小时内，医生会过来告诉你结果。
Patient：OK，thanks.
病人：好的，谢谢！

## （7）

Nurse：Mrs. Jones，the doctor wants you to have a urine specimen.
护士：琼斯夫人，医生要求你做尿样检测。
Patient：What，you want a urine specimen now?
病人：什么？你是现在要尿样吗？
Nurse：Yes，please. Here is the bottle. The toilets（washroom）are over there.
护士：是的，这是样本瓶，厕所在那边。
Patient：What shall I do with the specimen when I have done it?
病人：取了尿液样本之后我该怎么做？
Nurse：Here is the form，please take the specimen and form to the Bacteriology Department.

Wait for the results and bring them back to me.

护士：这是化验单，请将尿样和化验单带到细菌室。等结果出来后带回来给我。

Patient: Where is the Bacteriology Department?

病人：细菌室在哪里？

Nurse: It is on the third floor. Take the elevator or stairs, and the Bacteriology Department is on your left, and go to the first counter.

护士：细菌室在三楼，你可以坐电梯或走楼梯上去，你左手边的第一个窗口就是。

Patient: OK, and do I wait there for the results?

病人：好的，我需要在那儿等结果吗？

Nurse: No, you need to go to the second floor. When you come out of the elevator the counter straight ahead of you will have the results, you need to give them your receipt.

护士：不是，你需要到二楼，电梯出来正对着的那个窗口就是，你需要将领结果的条子交给他们。

Patient: How long will this all take?

病人：做完这些需要多长时间？

Nurse: The results take about 30 minutes.

护士：结果出来大概需要等30分钟。

Patient: Then what shall I do, come back here?

病人：那么我接着做什么？回来吗？

Nurse: Yes, come back here and I can tell the doctor you have your results.

护士：是的，回到这里，我会告诉医生你的化验结果出来了。

Patient: OK, thanks. See you later.

病人：好的，谢谢，一会儿见。

**(8)**

Nurse: Mrs. Smith, the doctor needs a stool specimen. Here is the specimen pot.

护士：史密斯夫人，医生需要你的粪便样本，这是样本瓶。

Patient: I don't know if I can give you a specimen right now.

病人：我不知道现在是不是能够给你。

Nurse: If you can't do a specimen now, please take the pot and collect a specimen when you get home, and bring it back later or tomorrow.

护士：如果你现在不能给的话，请将瓶子带回家取样，你可以晚点或明天带过来。

Patient: If I bring it back another time, what do I have to do, where shall I take it?

病人：如果我下回带过来，我该怎么做，我需要带到哪里？

Nurse: When you have done the specimen, please take it to the Bacteriology Department. Here is the form, I will tell you where to go, you will have to wait for the results and bring them back to me.

护士：你取样之后带到细菌室。这是化验单，我会带你过去，你需要等待结果出来之后拿来给我。

Patient: What if I bring the specimen back tomorrow, do I wait for the results and bring it back to you?

病人：如果我明天才带样本过来呢，我也要等结果出来后带给你吗？

Nurse: Yes, when you get the result, if it is positive or shows you have something wrong, you will have to register again as you will need to come back and see the doctor.

护士：是的，如果检测结果呈阳性或者表明你有疾病的话，你需要重新挂号回来看医生。

Patient: OK, and if it's negative, I can just leave?

病人：好的，如果是阴性，我就可以走了，是吗？

Nurse: Yes, if it's negative, you don't need to see the doctor.

护士：是的，如果是阴性你就不用看医生了。

Patient: OK, thanks.

病人：好的，谢谢！

## (9)

Nurse: Mrs. Jones, the doctor says you need to have an X-ray.

护士：琼斯夫人，医生说你需要做X线检查。

Patient: Yes, I do. Can you tell me where I have to go?

病人：是的，你能告诉我该去哪里吗？

Nurse: X-ray Department is on the first floor, if you go down the stairs turn left and follow the signs or follow the yellow line on the floor, it will take you to the X-ray Department. If you take the elevator, turn right.

护士：放射科在一楼，走楼梯的话，你下楼之后左转，沿着箭头或地上的黄色指示线就能找到。如果是坐电梯就出来后右转。

Patient: OK, thanks. Do I come back here when I've had the X-ray?

病人：好的，谢谢。拍了片之后我需要回到这里吗？

Nurse: No, you must wait for the results and then bring them back to me.

护士：不，你必须在那等结果，然后将结果带回来给我。

Patient: How long do I have to wait?

病人：我需要等多久？

Nurse: Not long, about 30 minutes, there are chairs where you can sit and wait.

护士：不是很久，大约30分钟。那里有椅子，你可以坐着等。

Patient: OK, thanks. See you later.

病人：好的，谢谢，一会儿见。

## (10)

Nurse: Miss. Smith, the doctor says you need an ultra sound of your abdomen.

护士：史密斯小姐，医生需要你做腹部的超声波扫描。

Patient: Yes, that's right. Can you tell me where I have to go, and what I have to do?

病人：好的，没问题。你能告诉我将要去哪里以及怎么做吗？

Nurse: I will show you where the department is; you will need to drink some water before the test.

护士：我会带你过去，你在检测之前需要喝些水。

Patient: Oh, sure, how much?

病人：哦，好的，要喝多少？

Nurse: The nurse in the department will give you 3 glasses of water to drink before they do the test. You will need to wait for the results and bring them back to me.

护士：检测之前，那里的护士会给你 3 杯水。你需要在那等结果出来后拿给我。

Patient: How long do I have to wait?

病人：我需要等多久？

Nurse: Not very long, about 30 minutes.

护士：不是很久，30 分钟左右吧。

Patient: OK, see you later.

病人：好的，再见。

## （11）

Patient: The doctor suggested I have a series of gastro-intestinal tests made. What shall I do?

病人：医生建议我做个胃肠造影。我该怎么做呢？

Nurse: I'll make an appointment for you at once. Come next Friday morning at 8 o'clock. Please don't eat or drink any thing after midnight.

护士：我现在就给您约定。下星期五早晨 8：00 来。到后半夜就不要再吃东西或者喝水了。

Patient: Not even water?

病人：水也不行吗？

Nurse: A sip of water is all right.

护士：小口水还是可以的。

Patient: When can I get the result?

病人：我什么时候能知道检查结果？

Nurse: Right away.

护士：马上就可以。

Patient: May I ask our interpreter to call for the result?

病人：可以请我们翻译打电话问结果吗？

Nurse: Yes, you may. You can have all the results next Monday when you come to see the doctor.

护士：是的，可以。您下周一看病的时候，所有结果都会出来的。

Patient: If my symptom get worse, I can come at any time, can't I? Or should I call first?

病人：如果我病情转重，我随时都可以来，是吗？要不要先打个电话？

Nurse: If you have time, it is better to notify us before you come. If you are too weak, we can do a home visit. Our doctor and nurse can go to your home by ambulance. In case you need to be hospital, we will bring you back.

护士：假如有时间，最好在来之前打个电话。假如您太虚弱，我们可以出诊。我们的医生和护士可以乘坐救护车到您家去。假如您需要到医院，我们就把您带回医院来。

# 7. Description of Pain

# 描述疼痛

## A. Sentences Commonly Used(常用语)

1. Do you get this pain all the time?
是一直疼痛吗？
2. Do you get this pain all the time or intermittently?
是一直的还是间歇性的疼痛？
3. Do you get this pain all the time or on and off?
是一直的还是间歇性的疼痛？
4. Do you get this pain often?
你经常这样痛吗？
5. How often do you get this pain?
你经常这样痛吗？
6. Have you had this pain before?
以前有过这种痛吗？
7. When did you last have an attack like this?
上次发作是什么时候？
8. When was the last time you had this pain?
上次发作是什么时候？
9. How long since the last attack?
距离上次发作有多长时间了？
10. When do you have this pain?
什么时候开始痛的？
11. How long does the pain last for?
疼痛持续多久了？
12. Do you have this pain at certain times of the day?
疼痛是每天在固定时间发作吗？
13. Do you have this pain after eating?
当你吃完饭之后疼痛发作吗？
14. Do you have this pain after exercise?
当你运动之后疼痛发作吗？

15. Do you have this pain when you are feeling upset, angry or anxious?
当你心烦、生气或焦虑的时候疼痛发作吗？
16. What do you mean by that?
你指的是什么？
17. Please explain what you mean by that.
请给我详细描述一下你具体指的是什么。
18. If I say to you that 1 means no pain, and 10 means severe pain, what number would you give your pain?
如果1代表不疼，10代表剧烈疼痛的话，你觉得你是属于哪个级别？
19. Do you take any pain relief? / Do you take any painkillers?
你吃过什么止痛药？
20. Did the tablets relieve the pain?
止痛药有效吗？
21. Do you have pain?
你有疼痛感吗？
22. Does it still hurt?
还疼吗？
23. Are you in much pain?
你疼得厉害吗？
24. How long have you had this pain?
你感到这种痛有多久了？
25. Have you ever had this pain before?
以前你有过这种疼痛吗？
26. Can you describe the pain?
你能描述一下怎么个疼法吗？
27. What does your pain feel like?
你的疼痛是什么样的感觉？
28. What kind of pain is it?
是什么样的疼痛？
29. What sort of pain have you been having?
你的疼痛是哪种类型的？
30. Does the pain come on after or before meals?
疼痛出现在饭前还是饭后？
31. Did the pain come on suddenly?
疼痛是突然出现的吗？
32. Does the pain wake you from sleep?
把你疼醒了吗？
33. Does the pain keep you from working?
疼痛是否让你无法工作？
34. Does the pain move?

疼痛有转移吗？

35. Is there any radiation of the pain to the shoulder?
疼痛放射到肩部吗？
36. Does this happen more at night or in the morning?
这种情况夜间发生的多还是白天发生的多？
37. Where is the pain?
哪儿痛？
38. Where does it hurt?
哪儿痛？
39. Where do you feel a pain?
你哪里痛？
40. Do you have headaches?
你头痛吗？
41. Where do you get the headaches?
你头的哪个地方感到痛？
42. Do you have migraines?
你是偏头痛吗？
43. Do you have any pain in your eyes?
你眼睛痛吗？
44. Do your ears ache?
你耳朵疼吗？
45. Do you have sore throats?
你咽喉/嗓子痛吗？
46. How long have you been having sore throats?
你嗓子疼有多长时间了？
47. Does it hurt when you open your mouth?
你张嘴的时候痛吗？
48. Do you have toothaches?
你牙痛吗？
49. Have you ever had chest pain or discomfort?
你曾经有过胸痛或胸部不适感吗？
50. Do you have abdominal pain?
你腹痛吗？
51. Is your tummy still sore?
你肚子还痛吗？
52. Are your breasts painful?
你乳房痛吗？
53. Does your back ache?
你背部疼痛吗？
54. Does the pain seem to move to your shoulder or back?

疼痛是不是转移到你的肩膀或者后背去了？

55. Do your legs hurt when you walk?
你走路时腿痛吗？
56. Do you ache all over?
你感到全身都痛吗？
57. Do you have pain when you urinate?
你排尿时痛吗？
58. Does it hurt when I press here?
我按这里时你感到痛吗？
59. Show me where it hurts.
给我看看哪儿痛？
60. Will you point to me where it hurts?
你能给我指一下哪儿痛吗？
61. Please point with your finger where it hurts the most.
请用手指出最痛点在什么部位。
62. Tell me exactly where it hurts.
告诉我疼痛的准确部位。
63. Does it hurt when you move?
活动时痛吗？
64. Do it help if you lie still?
如果你躺着不动，是不是感觉好一些？
65. Does any position help you to feel more comfortable?
有什么姿势会使你感到稍微舒服一些吗？
66. Is there anything you do that makes it better?
有没有什么减轻疼痛的方式？
67. What sort of things have you tried to make it better?
你试过用什么方法可以让这种症状好些吗？
68. Does it get better the more you move around?
是不是活动越多感觉越好？
69. Is the pain getting less?
疼痛减轻一些吗？

## B. Situational Conversation(情景会话)

### (1)

Nurse: Mrs. Smith, you look flushed, are you feeling OK?
护士：史密斯夫人，你看起来脸很红，没事吧？
Mrs. Smith: Yes, thank you, I'm just feeling hot.
史密斯夫人：是的，谢谢你。我就是有点热而已。

**(2)**

Nurse： Mr. Jones，does your knee hurt?
护士： 琼斯先生，你的膝盖痛吗？
Mr. Jones： No，nurse，it doesn't hurt，it feels numb.
琼斯先生： 不痛，就是有点麻。

**(3)**

Nurse： Can you tell me what the problem is?
护士： 请问你能告诉我哪里不舒服？
Miss Davis： I have an aching feeling in my shoulder and tingling in my fingers.
戴维斯小姐： 我的肩膀疼痛，手指发麻。

**(4)**

Ms. Rose： I have a red，blotchy rash on my body; I have had it for two days now.
罗斯女士： 我身上起了红色疱疹，有两天时间了。
Nurse： Is it itchy? Does it cause you any pain?
护士： 你感觉痒吗？痛不痛？
Ms. Rose： No，it doesn't really hurt. It stings when I scratch it.
罗斯女士： 不，不是很痛。但是挠的时候有刺痛感。
Nurse： Do you have any other problems?
护士： 除此之外还有什么症状吗？
Ms. Rose： No，there is nothing else wrong.
罗斯女士： 没有了。
Nurse： OK，I'll tell the doctor to come and see you.
护士： 好的，我叫医生过来看你。

**(5)**

Nurse： Have you been feeling breathless，since you have had this chest pain?
护士： 你胸痛以来有没有感到气短？
Ms. Smith： Yes，I have been feeling a little breathless.
史密斯女士： 是的，一直感觉有点气短。
Nurse： How bad is your chest pain? What does it feel like?
护士： 你胸痛程度如何？感觉像怎么样的？
Ms. Smith： It feel like a sharp pain when I breathe in.
史密斯女士： 当我吸气的时候感到锐痛。

**(6)**

Nurse： How can I help you?
护士： 有什么我能帮你？

Mr. Jones: I think I have damaged my elbow.

琼斯先生： 我想我的肘部受伤了。

Nurse: Why, what is the problem with it?

护士： 你的肘部怎么了

Mr. Jones: It is very painful when I straighten my arm.

琼斯先生： 当我伸直手臂的时候感到很痛。

Nurse: What does the pain feel like?

护士： 是怎么样的一种痛？

Mr. Jones: It feels like a sharp stabbing pain every time I stretch my arm out.

琼斯先生： 我的手臂每次伸直的时候都感到强烈的刺痛。

Nurse: How long have you had this?

护士： 你这样持续多久了？

Mr. Jones: A few days now.

琼斯先生： 有好几天了。

Nurse: Have you had an accident or done any exercise that could have damaged your elbow?

护士： 你有遇到什么意外伤害或者进行过可能伤到肘部的运动吗？

Mr. Jones: No, not that, I can remember.

琼斯先生： 没有，我记得没有。

Nurse: I'll get the doctor to examine your elbow.

护士： 我让医生过来检查一下你的肘部。

## (7)

Nurse: So tell me how you are feeling in yourself.

护士： 那么告诉我你现在是什么感觉。

Ms. Rose: I feel rather tired and a bit depressed, though I don't know why.

罗斯女士： 我感到很困，而且莫名其妙的抑郁。

Nurse: Has anything happened in your life to make you feel this way?

护士： 最近生活上有遇到什么变故吗？

Ms. Rose: No, I don't think so.

罗斯女士： 没有，我不这么认为。

## (8)

Nurse: You tell me you have a pain in your left shoulder and neck, what does the pain feel like?

护士： 你说你的左肩膀和脖子痛，是怎么样的一种痛？

Mr. Brown: It feels like a dull ache, and when I move my neck or arm it feels like a sharp pain.

布朗先生： 感觉像钝痛，当我扭脖子或者手臂的时候感到锐痛。

Nurse: Does the pain radiate down your arm?

护士： 疼痛放射到你的手臂吗？

Mr. Brown： Yes，it does sometimes; it makes my upper arm muscle feel bruised to touch and it aches some days.

布朗先生： 是的，有时候是这样。我的上臂摸起来像是挫伤了，痛好几天了。

Nurse： Is the pain in your arm there all the time?

护士： 你的手臂一直这么痛吗？

Mr. Brown： No，not all the time，on and off.

布朗先生： 不是，时痛时不痛。

Nurse： I'll tell the doctor to examine your neck，and you may need a neck X-ray.

护士： 我让医生过来检查一下你的脖子，你可能还需做X线检查。

Mr. Brown： OK，thanks.

布朗先生： 好的，谢谢！

## （9）

Nurse： You told me that you gave your pain a score of 8，have you taken painkillers I gave you?

护士： 你跟我说你的背很疼，并且形容你的疼痛程度是8，你吃止痛药吗？

Mrs. White： Yes，I have.

怀特夫人： 是的，我吃了。

Nurse： Did the tablets relieve the pain?

护士： 止痛药减轻疼痛了吗？

Mrs. White： No，not really.

怀特夫人： 没有，不是很有效。

Nurse： Did they reduce the pain at all?

护士： 一点效果都没有吗？

Mrs. White： Maybe some.

怀特夫人： 可能有点吧。

Nurse： If your score for pain was 8 before taking pain relief，what number is it after taking the painkillers?

护士： 如果在吃药之前疼痛程度是8，那么吃了药之后是多少呢？

Mrs. White： Oh，maybe about 6.

怀特夫人： 哦，大概是6.

# 8. Daily Nursing Care

# 日常护理

## A. Sentences Commonly Used(常用语)

**Greeting a Patient　问候病人**

1. Good Morning, how are you feeling today?
   早上好，你今天感觉怎么样？
2. Hello, how are you today?
   你好，你今天好吗？
3. Are you feeling comfortable?
   你感觉舒服吗？
4. Did you sleep well?
   你睡得好吗？
5. Are you in any pain or discomfort?
   你感到哪里疼或不舒服吗？
6. How are you today? / How was your sleep last night? / How is your appetite?
   你今天怎么样？ / 你昨晚睡得怎么样？ / 你的食欲怎么样？
7. What did you eat last evening? / last supper?
   你昨天晚饭吃了些什么？
8. You look (a little) tired. Didn't you sleep well last night?
   你看上去比较疲惫，昨晚是不是休息得不好？
9. Thank you for your cooperation.
   谢谢你的合作。
10. That is our job.
    这是我们应尽的义务。

**Cleanness and Sponge Bath　擦洗和擦浴**

11. You need to go to the bathroom for a wash / shower.
    你需要去浴室擦洗 / 冲洗一下。
12. Do you need to go to the bathroom for a wash / shower?
    你需要去浴室擦洗 / 冲洗一下吗？
13. Do you need to go to the bathroom / toilet?
    你需要上洗手间吗？

14. Do you need a bedpan / bottle?
你需要便盆吗？
15. You can't get up today.
你今天不能起床。
16. I'll rub your back with a warm towel and then massage it with alcohol and talcum powder.
我要用热毛巾给你擦背，然后用酒精和爽身粉按摩。
17. May I help you to clean up?
请问你需要我协助洗漱吗？
18. I'm sure that I'll be gentle and careful.
我保证动作很轻很仔细。
19. Do you need me to get you a bowl to wash yourself?
你需要我给你盆水擦洗吗？
20. Would you like a bowl, so you can wash yourself?
你需要盆水来擦洗吗？
21. Do you need a mouthwash?
你需要漱口水吗？
22. Would you like a mouthwash?
你需要漱口水吗？
23. Would you like a glass of water so you can clean your teeth?
你需要一杯水来漱口吗？
24. Would you like your wash bag?
你需要拿你的洗漱袋子吗？
25. Do you need clean clothes?
你需要干净衣服吗？
26. Do you have everything you need?
你还需要什么东西？
27. Here are some water, your tooth-brush and tooth paste.
这儿有水，你的牙刷和牙膏。
28. Now, please inhale, and split out the mouthwash into the tray.
现在你吸一口气，漱口水吐在弯盘里。
29. Right, you are a good cooperator.
对，你配合得很好。
30. Now, I'll massage you for protecting you from bedsore occurring.
现在，我给你做预防褥疮护理。
31. Please lie on your right / left side.
请把身子侧过去。

**Bed Making　整理床铺**

32. Now, we will clean your bed.
我们现在为你整理床铺。
33. Let me fluff up your pillow.

让我给你拍松枕头。

34. I need to make your bed.
我需要整理你的床。
35. I need to change your bed sheets.
我需要给你换床单。
36. Please can you get out of bed and sit in the chair?
请问你能离开床坐到椅子上吗？
37. Sit on the edge of the bed for a while and steady yourself.
请在床边坐一会，别摔了。
38. Get up slowly.
慢慢地起来。
39. Do you need any help?
你需要什么帮助吗？
40. Please roll / turn onto your right side.
请转到右侧躺着。
41. Please roll / turn onto your left side.
请转到左侧躺着。
42. Please roll/turn onto you back.
请转过来平躺着。
43. Please sit forward so I can do your pillows.
请往前坐，这样我可以整理你的枕头。
44. Are your pillows comfortable?
你的枕头枕着舒服吗？
45. Do you feel comfortable?
你感到舒服吗？
46. Are you comfortable?
你感觉舒服吗？
47. You need to get into bed now.
你现在需要躺在床上。
48. Please sit on the edge of the bed near the pillows.
请坐到靠近枕头的床边上。
49. Lean back on the pillows and raise your legs onto the bed.
靠在枕头上，把腿抬起放到床上。
50. Bend you knees and push yourself up the bed.
膝盖弯起来往后靠着床。
51. Do you need any help?
你需要什么帮助吗？
52. Please wait while I get another nurse to help me.
请稍后，我再找个护士过来帮忙。
53. Do you have everything you need?

你有什么需要拿的吗？

**Eating and Drinking　饮食**

54. Here is your breakfast.
    这是你的早餐。
55. Here is your lunch / dinner（supper）.
    这是你的午餐 / 晚餐。
56. Would you like your meal now?
    你想现在进食吗？
57. Would you like something to eat?
    你想吃点什么吗？
58. Is the food OK for you?
    食物可以吗？
59. Would you like something else?
    你还需要别的什么吗？
60. What would you like?
    你想要什么？
61. Would you like something to drink?
    你想喝些什么？
62. Would you like a cold drink or hot drink?
    你想喝点冷饮还是热饮？
63. Would you like a spoon or fork?
    你想要汤匙还是叉子？
64. Do you drink alcohol?
    你喝酒吗？
65. How much alcohol do you drink in a day?
    你一天喝多少酒？
66. Any vomiting?
    你吐了吗？
67. Do you vomit?
    你呕吐了吗？
68. What did you bring up?
    你吐的是什么？
69. When did the vomiting start?
    呕吐是什么时候开始的？
70. What foods don't you like to eat?
    你不爱吃什么食物？
71. Does any particular food upset you?
    有什么食物使你不舒服吗？
72. Did you eat any unusual food last night?
    你昨天晚上吃过什么不寻常的食物吗？

73. Do you think you eat a well-balanced diet?
你认为你的饮食均衡吗？
74. Are you allergic to any food?
你对食物过敏吗？
75. Do you have difficulty swallowing?
你吞咽有困难吗？

**Fluids 流质**

76. Would you like drink of...?
你想喝……吗？
77. How much have you had to drink?
你喝了多少？
78. What have you drunk today?
你今天喝了什么饮料？
79. What have you had to drink this morning /afternoon/evening?
你今天早上/下午/晚上喝了什么？
80. You need to drink more fluids.
你需要喝更多的流质。
81. Please could(can)you drink more?
请问你能再喝些吗？
82. I would like you to drink more fluids.
我想你再多喝些流质。
83. I need to check how much you have had to drink today.
我需要检查一下你今天喝了多少。

**Nausea and Vomiting 恶心、呕吐**

84. Please stay calm, I'll get you a vomit bowl.
请镇静，我去给你拿痰盂。
85. Take nice deep even breaths.
请深呼吸。
86. Inhale through the nose, and slowly out the mouth.
用鼻子吸气，慢慢地用嘴呼出来。
87. I'll get you a wet(damp)towel for your face.
我会给你一条湿毛巾敷脸。
88. I'll get the doctor to prescribe an anti-emetic tablet.
我会告诉医生给你开些止呕吐的药。
89. I'll get the doctor to prescribe an anti-emetic injection(shot)for you.
我会告诉医生给你开些止呕吐的注射液。
90. Would you like a mouthwash to rinse your mouth?
你需要漱口水漱口吗？

**Administrating Medication 药物治疗**

91. The doctor has prescribe for you...

医生给你开了……。

92. The doctor has prescribe for you a course of antibiotics.
医生给你开了一个疗程的抗生素。

93. You will need a course of injections，tablets.
你需要一个疗程的注射/药片。

94. The medication is called...
药物名称叫……。

95. The medication is used for...
药物用于……。

96. You need to take this medication...
你需要服……药。

97. Here is your medication.
这是你的药。

98. Please take these tablets.
请服下这些药片。

99. I need to give you an injection / a shot of...
我需要给你注射……。

100. I need to give you the injection in your arm / bottom / hand.
我需要在你的手臂/臀部/手部进行注射。

101. Here is your inhaler，please put the oxygen mask over your nose and mouth.
这是吸入器，请把氧气罩盖着鼻子和嘴。

102. Can you feel it?
你能感觉到吗？

103. Please remove the mask when it is finished.
完成之后，请将面罩移开。

104. This medication is for...
这些药用于治疗……。

105. Are you in any pain?
你感到痛吗？

106. Is the medication working?
药物有效吗？

107. Would you like some pain relief?
你需要止痛药吗？

108. Would you like some medication to help you with the pain?
你需要止痛的药吗？

**Checking Temperature，Pulse Rate，Respiration and Blood Pressure 量体温、脉搏、呼吸和血压**

109. It’s time to take your temperature.
到了给你测量体温的时间。

110. Did you drink any hot water within the half hour?

你在半小时内喝过热水吗？

111. OK, Let me take your temperature.
好，让我来给你测量体温。

112. Now, please put the thermometer under your arm.
请将体温计夹在你的腋下。

113. Put your arm out, I'll check your pulse rate.
请伸出手，我给你数数脉搏。

114. I have checked your respiration without telling you so that breathing would be more natural.
我测呼吸时没告诉你，这样你呼吸会更自然。

115. Now, give me the thermometer.
现在将体温计给我。

116. Would you roll up sleeves, and lie in the bed?
请你卷起衣袖，躺在床上，好吗？

117. I'm going to take your blood pressure now.
请伸出胳膊，我给你量血压。

118. Your blood pressure is a little high, and I'll examine you a step further.
你的血压是高了点，我来为你做进一步检查。

## B. Situational Conversational(情景会话)

### (1)

**Greeting a Patient　问候病人**

Nurse: Good morning, Mrs. Smith. How are you feeling today?
护士：早上好，史密斯夫人，你今天感觉怎么样？
Patient: I'm fine, thank you.
病人：我感觉很好，谢谢你。
Nurse: Did you sleep well?
护士：你睡得好吗？
Patient: Yes, thank you.
病人：是的，谢谢你。
Nurse: Are you feeling comfortable?
护士：你觉得舒服吗？
Patient: My pillows are a bit uncomfortable.
病人：我的枕头有点不舒服。
Nurse: OK, let me help you, can you bend forward, is that better for you?
护士：好的，让我帮你。你能向前弯一下吗？现在感觉好点了吗？
Patient: Yes, thanks very much.
病人：是的，非常谢谢。
Nurse: Are you in any pain or discomfort?

护士：　你感到痛或者不舒服吗？

Patient：　No pain at all，thank you.

病人：　一点疼痛也没有，谢谢你。

Nurse：　OK，that's great. I'll come and see you later.

护士：　好的，那太好了。我过一会儿过来看你。

※　　　※　　　※

Nurse：　Good morning，Mrs. Smith. How are you feeling today?

护士：　早上好，史密斯夫人，你今天感觉怎么样？

Patient：　Not so good.

病人：　不是很好。

Nurse：　Oh，I'm sorry to hear that，what's the problem?

护士：　哦，我很难过。有什么问题吗？

Patient：　I don't feel very well at all today.

病人：　我觉得今天一点都不舒服。

Nurse：　Are you in any pain or discomfort?

护士：　你感到疼痛或不舒服吗？

Patient：　I'm in a lot of pain.

病人：　我感到很痛。

Nurse：　Oh dear，have the painkillers not worked?

护士：　天哪，止痛药没有效果吗？

Patient：　No，and I haven't slept very well.

病人：　没有，而且我睡得一点都不好。

Nurse：　OK，I'll ask the doctor to prescribe some stronger painkillers for you，Is there anything else you would like?

护士：　好的，我会告诉医生给你开些强力的止痛药。你需要别的什么东西吗？

Patient：　Do you think I could have some cold water with ice in?

病人：　你觉得我能喝些加冰块的凉水吗？

Nurse：　Yes，of course，I'll go and get you some.

护士：　当然可以，我过去给你拿些过来。

## （2）

**Cleanness and Sponge Bath　擦洗和擦浴**

Nurse：　Mrs. Smith，do you need to go to bathroom?

护士：　史密斯夫人，你要去浴室吗？

Patient：　Yes please，I would like to have a shower，is that OK?

病人：　是的，我想冲个澡，可以吗？

Nurse：　Yes，it's OK. Would you like your wash bag?

护士：　当然可以。你需要洗漱包吗？

Patient：　No，thanks，just my facecloth，soap，toothpaste and toothbrush.

病人：　不用，有面巾、肥皂、牙刷和牙膏就可以。

Nurse: Where are they?
护士: 放在什么地方了?
Patient: In my cupboard.
病人: 在我的食橱里。
Nurse: Here you are, Mrs. Smith. Let me help you to the bathroom.
护士: 史密斯夫人,给你。让我扶你走到浴室。
Patient: Thanks, nurse.
病人: 谢谢你,护士小姐。

※ ※ ※

Nurse: You can't get up today, Mrs. Smith. Would you like a bowl so you can wash yourself?
护士: 史密斯夫人,你今天不能起床。你需要脸盆来洗漱吗?
Patient: Yes, please, nurse.
病人: 是的,护士小姐。
Nurse: Do you need a bedpan?
护士: 你需要便盆吗?
Patient: No, not right now, thanks, maybe later.
病人: 不用,现在不用,谢谢,可能待会才会用到。
Nurse: Would you like your wash bag?
护士: 你需要洗漱包吗?
Patient: Yes, you'll find it in the locker.
病人: 是的,洗漱包在锁柜里面。
Nurse: Would you like a glass of water, so you can clean your teeth?
护士: 你需要一杯水吗?你可以用来刷牙。
Patient: Yes, that would be great, do you have a mouthwash?
病人: 是的,那太好了。你有漱口水吗?
Nurse: Yes, I'll go and get you one.
护士: 有,我去给你拿。
Patient: Thanks, nurse.
病人: 谢谢你,护士小姐。

## (3)

**Morning Care 晨间护理**

Nurse: Good Morning. Did you sleep well last night?
护士: 早安,你昨晚睡得好吗?
Patient: Thanks you. I slept very well.
病人: 谢谢你。我睡得很好。
Nurse: May I help you to clean up?
护士: 让我帮你梳洗好吗?
Patient: All right.
病人: 好的。

Nurse: Here are some water, your toothbrush and toothpaste.

护士：这儿有水，你的牙刷和牙膏。

（Brushing teeth）

（刷牙）

Patient: I feel some soreness in my mouth.

病人：我感到嘴里有些痛。

Nurse: Don't worry. I'll take a look after you have finished brushing your teeth.

护士：不要紧。等你刷好牙，让我看看你的嘴。

（After examination）

（检查以后）

Nurse: I think there are small ulcerations on account of the fever.

护士：这是因为发烧而引起的几块小溃疡。

Patient: Can you do something about it?

病人：你怎么来治疗这些溃疡呢？

Nurse: I will give you some solution to rinse your mouth. That will help to clear them up.

护士：我将给你一些药水漱口。这些药水能促使溃疡愈合。

Nurse: Now, since you can't move easily. I will help you to clean up and make you comfortable.

护士：因为你行动不便，现在，让我帮忙给你整理整理。使你舒服一些。

Patient: Thank you.

病人：谢谢。

Nurse: Let me fluff up your pillow.

护士：让我给你拍松枕头。

Patient: That's wonderful.

病人：太好了。

Nurse: Please turn over to the other side. I will rub your back with a hot towel and then massage it with alcohol and talcum powder.

护士：请翻身到那边去。我要用热毛巾给你擦背，然后用酒精和爽身粉按摩。

Patient: What for?

病人：为什么？

Nurse: It is mainly to stimulate your blood circulation to prevent bedsore that generally results from persistent pressure on your back.

护士：主要是促进血液循环，预防通常会在受压部位发生的褥疮。

Patient: I see. My clothes are all wet from sweating during the night. Can I have them changed now?

病人：噢！明白了。我昨夜出汗衣服都湿透了。现在能换换吗？

Nurse: Of course. I have already brought some clean ones for you. I'll help you to change.

护士：当然可以。我已为你带来一些干净的衣服。让我帮你换上。

Patient: Fine.

病人：好。

Nurse: I am also going to change the sheets on your bed.

护士： 我还要给你换床单。

Patient： Do we have to make a complete change? Should I get out of bed?

病人： 是全部换吗？要不要我下床？

Nurse： No you needn't. You are very weak. I can do the change without you getting out of bed. You needn't exert yourself either. I can do everything for you.

护士： 不用。你很虚弱。你不用起床我就可以给你换好床单。你不需要费劲。我可以为你做任何事。

Patient： Good.

病人： 好的。

（After changing sheets）

（换床单后）

Nurse： Are you comfortable now?

护士： 现在你感到舒服些吗？

Patient： Yes. Thank you very much. I am quite comfortable.

病人： 是的。太感谢你了。我很舒服。

Nurse： You may rest now. Do you mind if I open the windows to air the room a little?

护士： 现在你该休息了。我开一会儿窗户换换气可以吗？

Patient： Sure.

病人： 当然可以。

Nurse： I will come back to close them for you later.

护士： 等一会儿我就来把窗户关上。

Patient： Thank you.

病人： 谢谢。

## （4）

### Eating and Drinking 饮食

Nurse： Good morning，Mrs. Smith，here is your breakfast.

护士： 早上好，史密斯夫人，这是你的早餐。

Patient： Thank you，nurse.

病人： 谢谢你，护士小姐。

Nurse： Is the food OK for you?

护士： 感觉饭菜还可以吗？

Patient： Yes，the food is fine，thank you.

病人： 是的，饭菜很不错，谢谢你。

※ ※ ※

Patient： Please may I have something to eat?

病人： 请问我能要些吃的吗？

Nurse： What would you like?

护士： 你想吃什么？

Patient： Do you have any bread?

病人：你有面包吗？

Nurse: No，I'm sorry we don't，would you like something else?

护士：没有，很抱歉我们没有。你想要别的什么吗？

Patient: I'd like something light，do you have any eggs?

病人：我想要些口味清淡的，你有鸡蛋吗？

Nurse: I don't know，I'll go and find out for you.

护士：我不清楚，我过去给你看一下。

Patient: Thanks very much，nurse. I appreciate it. I can't face any other food right now.

病人：非常感谢你，护士小姐。我很感激。我现在不愿意吃任何其他的食物。

Nurse: OK，I understand.

护士：好的，我明白。

※ ※ ※

Nurse: Hi，Mrs. Smith，here is your lunch.

护士：你好，史密斯夫人，这是你的午餐。

Patient: OK，thanks，nurse.

病人：好的，谢谢你，护士小姐。

Nurse: Would you like a spoon or fork?

护士：你需要汤匙或叉子吗？

Patient: No，chopsticks are fine，thanks.

病人：不用，筷子就可以，谢谢。

Nurse: Mrs. Smith，you haven't eaten your lunch，is the food OK for you?

护士：史密斯夫人，你还没有吃午饭，食物还好吗？

Patient: I'm sorry，but I don't like this meal.

病人：很抱歉，我不喜欢这些食物。

Nurse: Would you like something else?

护士：你想要些别的东西吗？

Patient: Please can I have something cold to drink?

病人：请问我能要些冷饮吗？

Nurse: OK，I'll go and get it for you，would you like something else to eat?

护士：好的，我过去给你拿些冷饮，你想吃些别的东西吗？

Patient: No，thank you，I'm not hungry now.

病人：不用，谢谢。我现在不饿。

Nurse: OK，Mrs. Smith，I'll go and get you your drink.

护士：好的，史密斯夫人，我过去给你取冷饮。

Patient: Thanks，nurse.

病人：谢谢你，护士小姐。

## (5)

**Fluids 流质**

Nurse: Hello，Mrs. Smith，I need to check how much you have had drunk today?

护士：你好，史密斯夫人，我需要检查一下你今天喝了多少流体。

Patient: I've drunk about 3 glasses of water and had a cup of coffee.

病人：我已经喝了三杯水和一杯咖啡。

Nurse: You need to drink more fluids, please can you drink more?

护士：你需要喝更多的流体，请问你能再多喝些吗？

Patient: OK, but can I have some ice in the water? This water is too warm.

病人：好的，但是我能在水里加冰吗？水不够凉。

Nurse: I'll ask someone to bring you some.

护士：我会叫人给你拿些。

Patient: Thanks, nurse.

病人：谢谢你，护士小姐。

※ ※ ※

Nurse: Mrs. Smith, you are having surgery later, you must not eat or drink anything from now.

护士：史密斯夫人，你今天要进行手术，从现在开始你不能进食也不能喝水。

Patient: Oh no, what happens if I get really thirsty, it's very hot in here.

病人：噢，不要啊。如果我口渴了怎么办，这里太热了。

Nurse: If you are very thirsty, please tell me, I can give you a mouthwash to gargle, but please do not swallow any of it.

护士：如果你非常口渴，请告诉我，我会给你些水漱口，但是请不要吞下去。

Patient: OK, nurse, thanks.

病人：好的，谢谢你，护士小姐。

※ ※ ※

Nurse: Mrs. Smith, because of your bowel operation, you can only drink small amounts of fluids today.

护士：史密斯夫人，由于你进行了肠手术，你今天只能喝少量的流体。

Patient: What do you mean by small amounts?

病人：你指的少量是多少？

Nurse: You can only drink 50 ml an hour.

护士：你每小时只能喝 50 毫升。

Patient: What! That's hardly anything, I already feel very dry.

病人：什么！那根本不算什么，我已经感到很渴了。

Nurse: I'm sorry, but you have to give your digestive tract a rest for a few days, you are on intravenous fluids, so your fluids will be fine.

护士：很抱歉，不过你需要让你的消化道休息几天，你在进行静脉输液，所以不要担心身体会缺水。

Patient: But my mouth feels very dry.

病人：但是我感到口渴啊。

Nurse: I can give you water to gargle, but please do not swallow it, and I will give you the amount you are allowed to drink every hour, is that OK?

护士： 我可以给你一些水含着，但是请不要吞下去。每小时我都按你能喝的量给你一些水，可以吗？

Patient: OK, I guess.

病人： 好的，我想。

**（6）**

**Nausea and Vomiting 恶心、呕吐**

Patient: Nurse, I'm going to be sick.

病人： 护士，我感到恶心、想吐。

Nurse: It's OK, Mrs. Smith, please stay calm, I'll get you a vomit bowl.

护士： 别紧张，请镇静，我去给你拿痰盂。

Patient: Thanks, nurse.

病人： 谢谢你，护士小姐。

Nurse: Take nice deep even breaths, inhale through the nose and slowly out the mouth.

护士： 请慢慢地深呼吸，用鼻孔大力吸气，用嘴慢慢地呼出来。

Nurse: OK, do you feel better?

护士： 好的，你现在感觉好点了吗？

Patient: Yes, thanks.

病人： 是的，谢谢。

Nurse: I'll get you a damp towel for your face, and I'll get the doctor to prescribe an anti-emetic shot for you.

护士： 我会给你一条湿毛巾敷脸，然后我会叫医生开些治疗呕吐的注射液给你。

Patient: Thanks, nurse. Can I have some water to sip?

病人： 谢谢你，护士小姐。我能喝口水吗？

Nurse: Yes, of course, I'll get you some.

护士： 当然可以，我去给你拿。

**（7）**

**Medication 药物治疗**

Nurse: Hello, Mrs. Smith, how are you feeling?

护士： 你好，史密斯夫人，你感觉怎么样？

Patient: Not too well, nurse, I'm still in some pain.

病人： 不太好，护士小姐。我仍然感到疼。

Nurse: Would you like some medication to help you with the pain?

护士： 你需要一些药物来治疗疼痛吗？

Patient: Yes, please, if you wouldn't mind.

病人： 是的，请给我一些，如果你不介意的话。

Nurse: I'll go and ask the doctor to prescribe a stronger painkiller for you.

护士： 我会过去叫医生开些强力止痛药给你。

Patient: Thanks, nurse. I appreciate it.

病人：谢谢你，护士小姐。我很感激。

Nurse：Mrs. Smith, the doctor has prescribed an injection for you to help with your pain, please can you turn over, I need to give you the injection in your bottom (buttock).

护士：史密斯夫人，医生给你开了注射液来治疗疼痛，请问你能转过身来吗，我要在你的臀部打针。

Patient：Thanks, nurse.

病人：谢谢你，护士小姐。

Nurse：You're welcome, I'll come back in 30 minutes to see if the injection has worked and you are feeling better.

护士：不客气。我30分钟后过来看注射液是否有效，看你是否会好转。

Patient：OK.

病人：好的。

## （8）

**Checking Temperature, Pulse Rate and Respiration　测量体温、脉搏和呼吸**

Nurse：Good afternoon, Mr. Li. Did you drink any hot water in the last half an hour?

护士：下午好，李先生。你半小时前喝过热水吗？

Patient：No, I don't.

病人：没有。

Nurse：Good. Then I will take your temperature. Now, put the thermometer under your arm, please. I'll also check your pulse rate and respiration.

护士：很好，我来给你测体温。请把体温表放在腋下，我还要测量你的脉搏和呼吸。

Patient：How is my pulse rate?

病人：我的脉搏怎样？

Nurse：A bit fast, because you had a fever this morning. But the rhythm is normal. That means your heart is pumping regularly without skipping.

护士：有点快。那是因为你今早发烧了。但呼吸是正常的，这说明你的心律正常，也就是说你的心脏跳动正常，并且没有间歇。

Patient：Well, have you checked my respiration?

病人：啊，你已经测量了我的呼吸？

Nurse：Yes, I did it without telling you so that your breathing would be more normal. The count is more accurate this way. Now give me the thermometer.

护士：是的，为了让你正常呼吸，我没有告诉你。这样测量就更准确。好了，请把体温表给我。

Patient：Here you are. Do I have any temperature?

病人：给你。我发烧了吗？

Nurse：Just a little. It usually follows a major operation. But it will certainly go down soon. Don't worry.

护士：有一点，通常术后会发烧。但很快就会退的，别担心。

Patient：Is there any other method to take temperature?

病人： 还有其他测量体温的方法吗？

Nurse： Yes，There are two other ways—under the tongue or by rectum. The temperature got under the arm would be half a degree lower than by mouth，and that by rectum half a degree higher. Of course，the oral measurement is easier and more accurate.

护士： 是的，还有两种其他的测量方法：口测和直肠测量法。腋下测量得到的体温比口测得到的体温低半度，而由直肠测得的体温比口测的高半度。当然，口测法既简单又准确。

Patient： Thanks you. I've learned a lot today.

病人： 谢谢你，我今天学到不少。

Nurse： Don't mention it. I'll take your temperature again this evening. See you then.

护士： 不用谢。今晚我会再来为你测一次体温。再见。

※ ※ ※

Doctor： Do you have a fever?

医生： 您发烧了吗？

Patient： Yes，I do. I feel ghastly. My cheeks are burning. It started with a chill and fever.

病人： 是的，我觉得很不好，我的两颊很烫，开始时又冷又热。

Doctor： You look ghastly，too. You must have a high temperature. I'd better take your temperature. Where's the thermometer?

医生： 您看起来是很不好，您肯定发高烧，我来量一下您的体温。体温表在何处？

Nurse： Let me take his temperature. Please，put this thermometer under your tongue. Let me feel your pulse. ...Give me the thermometer.

护士： 我来量吧。请把这体温计放在您的舌下，让我摸摸您的脉搏。……把体温表给我。

Doctor： What is it?

医生： 多少度？

Nurse： Thirty nine point eight degrees centigrade.

护士： 39.8℃。

Doctor： Pretty high. I expect it's flu. Many people have it.

医生： 高了，我看是流感，现在很多人患流感。

Nurse student： How many times a day should this patient have his temperature taken，nurse?

护士生： 老师，这个病人一天量几次体温？

Nurse： The patient should take his temperature twice a day at least. If it still pretty high it must be taken every four hours or even every two hours.

护士： 这个病人应该一天量两次体温。如果仍然很高，应该每四小时或两小时量一次。

Nurse student： When I take his temperature should I count his pulse too?

护士生： 我量体温时还要数他的脉搏吗？

Nurse： Yes，you take the pulse and count his respiration. It is necessary to be careful when using the thermometer! Because should the patient break it and swallow the glass or mercury it would be very dangerous.

护士： 应该数，不仅要数脉搏还要数他的呼吸。用体温计时必须小心。因为如果病人把体温表咬碎，吞下了玻璃或水银，那是很危险的。

Nurse student： Some patients are delirious. How shall I take his temperature?

护士生： 有些病人是谵妄，我如何测他们的体温呢？

Nurse： Take it by rectum. Be careful that the anus is clean. Hold the thermometer in for three to five minutes. If the patient's mouth is sore.Take his temperature by axilla.

护士： 可以通过直肠量体温，但应该小心，肛门要清洁。把体温计放置 3～5 分钟。如果病人口腔有疮，可以通过腋下测体温。

Nurse student： How long shall I leave the thermometer in the axilla?

护士生： 在腋下测体温需放置多久？

Nurse： Ten minutes.

护士： 10 分钟。

Nurse student： What are the different kinds of fever，doctor?

护士生： 医生，体温类型有几种？

Doctor： There are continuous fever like pneumonia，scarlet fever and typhus; remittent fever like typhoid and septic fever and intermittent fever like malaria.

医生： 有稽留热，如肺炎、猩红热和斑疹伤寒；弛张热如伤寒；脓毒性热和间歇热如疟疾。

Patient： What kind of fever is my temperature?

病人： 我的体温属于哪一种？

Doctor： It may be continuous fever. Flue is also continuous fever. We should give you an injection of penicillin and some medicine which will lower the fever. It should bring your fever down.

医生： 是稽留热，流感通常是持续性发热。我们要给您注射青霉素和口服一些退烧药，您的体温会降下来的。

Nurse student： Will his temperature come down by lysis?

护士生： 他的体温是渐退的吗？

Doctor： Yes，it will soon be normal after treating with medicine.

医生： 是的，用了药后会很快降到正常。

Nurse： Here is your medicine. Take one tablet three times daily after meal. Swallow them with a little boiled water.

护士： 这是您的药，1 天 3 次，1 次 1 片，饭后服。要用开水服药。

Patient： Thank you.

病人： 谢谢您。

Doctor： Don't mention it. You should have a good rest. Good-bye.

医生： 不客气，您要好好休息，再见。

# 9. Injection

# 注射

## A. Sentences Commonly Used(常用语)

1. Would you hand me your medical record, the sheet of the injection and drugs?
   请把病历、注射单和药品给我好吗?
2. Did you take this kind of medicine before?
   请问你以前用过这种药吗?
3. I'm going to do a tetanus hypersensitive test for you.
   我要给你做破伤风皮试。
4. I'll do a skin test to see if you have sensitivity streptomycin.
   现在我给你做链霉素过敏测试。
5. Well, it's not very painful, is it?
   嗯,不太痛,是吗?
6. You need to wait here for twenty minutes to get the result of the test.
   你需要在这等20分钟观察结果。
7. Don't leave here and please don't touch the injection spot.
   请不要离开,也别用手触摸注射部位。
8. Twenty minutes later, I'll have a look at your reaction.
   20分钟以后,我来看皮试结果。
9. If you have any discomfort, please tell me in time.
   如果有不舒服的感觉请及时告诉我。
10. You have been given an intravenous injection. Don't move this arm.
    你的静脉针已经打好了。请你别动这只胳膊。
11. Please lie on your right side and raise your left leg to relax gluteal muscle.
    请你向右侧卧,伸直左腿使臀部肌肉放松。
12. Can you put down your pants a little and I'll give you a shot?
    请你把裤子往下拉一点,我来给你打针。
13. Please don't be nervous, you may feel a bit sour and swollen, but it will be right soon.
    请不要紧张,可能有点酸胀感,一会儿就好。
14. Please press for 3～5 minutes with a cotton stick and don't scratch.
    请用棉签压3～5分钟,不要抓。

15. It's the first time you have used penicillin so please wait for 30 minutes to be observed.
你是第一次使用青霉素，请在这里等 30 分钟观察一下。
16. You could leave if you don't feel any discomfort.
如果没有反应和不适，你再离开。
17. According to the medical order, I have to get blood from the vein of your upper limb.
根据医嘱，我要从你的前臂静脉抽点血。
18. Please take off your overcoat, and roll up your sleeves.
请你脱掉外衣，卷起袖子。
19. Could you put your arm here and clench your fits, OK?
请你将手臂放在这儿，像这样我紧拳头好吗？
20. OK, release your fits.
好了，请松拳。
21. Please press here for a moment with a cotton stick.
这里请用棉签按压片刻。
22. In order to prevent dehydration, we must give you venous transfusion.
为了防止你脱水，我们必须给你静脉输液。
23. It'll take nearly 6 hours to give you transfusion. It's better for you to go to the washroom.
现在要给你输液，大约需要 6 小时。你最好先去一趟洗手间？
24. Please stretch out your hands and let me choose the part to inject.
请伸出你的手，我为你选择注射部位。
25. I'm sorry to your pain. Could you cooperate with me for your own good?
对不起，给你增加痛苦了，请你配合一下好吗？
26. Now rest your arm on mine.
现在把你的手臂放在我的手臂上。
27. If there is anything wrong with you (Whatever you need), please press the button, I'll come soon.
如果有什么不适（或有什么需要），请你按传呼器，我会立刻来看你。
28. As your heart isn't in a good condition, the speed of infusion will be slower.
你心脏不好，输液速度要慢一些。
29. We'll use more antibiotics for you.
我们还要给你用点抗生素。
30. Hi, kid. I'll give you a shot. I'm sure you are brave.
小朋友，阿姨给你打针，勇敢点好吗？
31. Did you feel better after the injection last time?
上次打针以后你感觉好些吗？
32. Better put hot towels on it. Twice a day for fifteen minutes.
最好用热毛巾敷。一天两次，每次 15 分钟。
33. Did you feel uncomfortable at the injection spot?
请问你打针的地方有什么不舒服吗？

## B. Situational Conversation（情景会话）

### (1)

Patient: How often should I have the injection?
病人：这针多久注射一次？
Nurse: Once a day (twice a day).
护士：每天一次(每天两次)。
Patient: Where do you give it?
病人：在哪个部位注射呢？
Nurse: In the buttocks (in the arms).
护士：在臀部(在手臂上)。
Patient: I discovered a lump on my buttock yesterday. What shall I do?
病人：我昨天发现我的臀部有个硬块。该怎么办呢？
Nurse: Let me have a look. Better put hot towels on it. Two times a day for fifteen minutes. If it doesn't get better, we'll try physiotherapy.
护士：让我看一下。最好用热毛巾敷。一天敷两次，每次 15 分钟。假若不见好，我们可以做做理疗。

### (2)

Nurse: Good morning. Mrs.Hu. It's time for me to give you IV fluids.
护士：早晨好，胡太太，我要给你静脉输液了。
Patient: Could you tell me about the use of the IV fluids?
病人：你能告诉我静脉输液的作用吗？
Nurse: Of course. The fluids can provide energy for heart functions and prevent you from electrolytic imbalances after operation.
护士：当然。这液体能为心肌提供能量。并预防术后电解质失衡。
Patient: Why don't you let the fluid drop more quickly?
病人：能不能让液体滴快些？
Nurse: Your IV fluids must be given slowly so as not to overload you.
护士：不行，你的静脉液必须要慢以免使你的心脏负担过重。
Patient: Nurse, don't give me the injection again.
病人：护士，别给我打针了。
Nurse: What's happen?
护士：为什么？
Patient: I think it is no use.
病人：我想打针也没用。
Nurse: Don't say that. You'll soon be well after the operation.
护士：别这么说，术后情况会迅速好转的。

Patient: Perhaps you're right, but I'm always feeling anxious. I think I'm a heavy burden on others. Don't bother any more.

病人：也许你说的对，可我总感到难过，我觉得自己对别人而言是沉重的负担，你别麻烦了。

Nurse: Mrs. Hu, you know we all care for you, especially your husband and children. Do what you're told, then, you can live a full, useful, and happy life.

护士：胡太太，你知道大家都关心你，特别是你丈夫和孩子们。按我们的话做，你会生活得充实又幸福的。

Patient: No, I feel that everything in the world is meaningless. So I don't want to live in the world to bother others.

病人：不，我觉得一切都没有意思，我不想活在世上给人添麻烦。

Nurse: Mrs. Hu, everyone has his own trouble, but he shouldn't see the world through dark-colored glasses. He can correctly deal with matters. Don't worry about too much. I'm sure your condition will soon be better if you cooperate with us.

护士：胡太太，每个人都有自己的烦恼。只要不用灰色眼镜看世界，就能正确处理这些事。别太担心，我保证你只要和我们合作，你的情况很快会好转的。

Patient: Thank you for your kindness.

病人：多谢你的好意。

Nurse: Look at the people around you. They are all full of confidence. Mr. Li's condition was worse than yours before operation, but you see he can do everything for him now.

护士：看看你周围的人，他们都那么自信，李先生术前情况还不如你，可你看他现在完全可以自理了。

Patient: I see, nurse. Please give me the shot.

病人：我懂了，请给我打针吧。

## （3）

Patient: Is this injection room?

病人：这是注射室吗？

Nurse: Yes. Could you show me your prescription, please?

护士：是的，请给我你的处方。

Patient: Here you are. Well, could you tell me how many injections I have got to take?

病人：在这，请问我要打几针？

Nurse: Let me see. One every other day for two weeks. From today on, you need to come to the hospital to get a shot every other day. The treatment will last for two weeks.

护士：让我看看处方，每两天一次，连续两周。从今天开始，你每隔一天来医院打一针，要持续两周。

Patient: In the morning or in the afternoon?

病人：上午来还是下午来？

Nurse: You can decide yourself whether mornings or afternoons. But you should be consistent in your visit, and it should be around the same time every time.

护士： 随便你，但你一定要坚持来，每次要在同一时间。

Patient： I will. What happens if I can't come?

病人： 我知道。假如我不来会怎样？

Nurse： It's very important that you don't skip a day. You should come here consistently. Otherwise the course may not be effective，all the former treatment may be in vain.

护士： 任何一天都不能忘记打针，这很重要。你一定要坚持来，否则以前做的治疗都无效。

Patient： I understand.

病人： 我懂了。

Nurse： Do you know if you're allergic to any antibiotics?

护士： 你对抗生素过敏吗？

Patient： No，definitely not.

病人： 不会，绝对不会。

Nurse： Fine. Is there anybody else in your family allergic to penicillin?

护士： 你家里有人对青霉素过敏吗？

Patient： I can't think of anyone who is allergic to it.

病人： 没有。

Nurse： Could you tell me when you used penicillin last time?

护士： 能告诉我上次使用青霉素是什么时候？

Patient： Well，let me see. It could be three or four years ago when I...Actually I don't quite remember the exact time.

病人： 让我想想，大概是三或四年前，……我记不清了。

Nurse： Are you allergic to any other particular drugs?

护士： 你对其他药物过敏吗？

Patient： No，as far as I can remember.

病人： 不会。

Nurse： OK. Now I'll give you a small injection first. Please roll up your sleeve and stretch out your left arm. Don't be nervous. It's just a small shot.

护士： 我先给你做个皮试，请挽起袖子伸出你的左臂。别紧张，只是个小小的皮试。

Patient： Shall I sit down?

病人： 我能坐下来吗？

Nurse： Yes，rest your arm on the table and relax. Hold still please. If you feel any discomfort，such as dizziness，sweating or chest distress，please tell me.

护士： 可以，把胳膊放在桌子上，放松。坚持一会。如果你感到任何不舒服，如头晕、出汗或是胸闷的话就告诉我。

Patient： Yes，I will. I don't understand why I still need to have a penicillin allergic test. You know，you give an allergic test of this kind every time before a penicillin injection. I have never been found allergic to it. I'm wondering if it's necessary.

病人： 知道。我真不明白为什么每次打青霉素都要做皮试，我对青霉素从不过敏。有必要吗？

Nurse：Some of the patients may become allergic to some types of penicillin even though they have used penicillin before. Though it's rather rare，we must be very careful of this，since the allergy to penicillin can cause serious consequences and sometimes it's life threatening. Now wait just outside for at least 15 minutes，then，I'll have a look at your reaction.

护士：有些病人有可能对不同批号的青霉素过敏，即使他以前使用过青霉素。虽然这种情况很少，但我们还是应该谨慎，因为青霉素过敏的后果很严重，甚至会有生命危险。现在你在外面等至少 15 分钟，然后我再看看你的反应。

（After fifteen minutes）

（15 分钟后）

Nurse：Please come in. Let me have a look at your arm.

护士：请进来，让我看看你的手臂。

Patient：Here. Nothing seems to have happened.

病人：好像没什么。

Nurse：No，there is no red or swelling. That's all right. The test shows you are not allergic to penicillin. Now I am going to give you the first injection.

护士：是的，没有红肿。皮试证明你对青霉素不过敏。现在我给你打第一针。

Patient：You know I am kind of nervous and I hate shots.

病人：我有点紧张，我讨厌打针。

Nurse：Take it easy. I will use this swab to sterilize first. Do you feel a pain where I am pressing? Bend your leg a little and relax your muscle，try to relax as much as possible.

护士：放松点，我先用棉球给你消毒。我按压的地方痛吗？把腿稍微蜷起来，肌肉放松，尽量放松。

Patient：Oh，it really hurts. How long will the pains last?

病人：哦，好痛。疼痛要持续多久？

Nurse：Don't worry. When you get home，put a warm towel onto the injection spot. But don't press too hard. Don't rub it. The pain will go away in a couple of hours.

护士：别担心，回家后，用热毛巾敷在打针的部位，但别用力按压，也别擦，疼痛会在几小时内消退。

### （4）

Patient：Excuse me. Is this the injection room?

病人：请问，这里是注射室吗？

Nurse：Yes，please show me your file. Are you Huang Lu?

护士：是的，请把你的病历给我。你叫黄路，是吗？

Patient：Yes.

病人：是的。

Nurse：You've got pneumonia. The doctor has prescribed penicillin.

护士：你得了肺炎，医生给你开了青霉素。

Patient: What is that?

病人：这是什么药？

Nurse: It is a kind of antibiotic. Have you used it before?

护士：是一种抗生素，你以前用过这种药吗？

Patient: Yes, about three or four years ago.

病人：三四年前用过。

Nurse: Are you allergic to it?

护士：你对这药过敏吗？

Patient: What do you mean?

病人：你指什么？

Nurse: Well. Did you feel any discomfort, such as: dizziness, sweating or chest distress after given it?

护士：就是说，打完针后是否有头晕、盗汗或胸闷的现象？

Patient: Well, let me see. Perhaps not.

病人：哦，我想想，好像没有。

Nurse: I wonder if anyone in your family has been allergic to it.

护士：你家里有人对这药过敏吗？

Patient: I don't think of anyone.

病人：没有。

Nurse: OK. Please roll up your sleeves and stretch out your hand. I'll give you an allergy test.

护士：好的，请把你的袖子卷起来，伸出手，我来给你做皮试。

Patient: I hate shots. It is really painful.

病人：我讨厌打针，好痛。

Nurse: Don't be nervous. It is just a small shot. Please sit down.

护士：别紧张，就是一个小小的皮试。请坐。

(Giving the patient an allergy test)

（护士给病人做皮试）

Patient: Ouch!

病人：哎哟！痛呀！

Nurse: You will fell a bit swollen. It will be all right soon. Please sit here for 20 minutes to get the result and don't scratch the injection spot. You can watch TV for a while. If you have any discomfort, please tell me in time, OK?

护士：有点胀，很快就会好。请在这等 20 分钟，别抓打针的地方，你可以看会儿电视。假如有什么地方不舒服，请立刻告诉我，好吗？

Patient: OK. Thank you.

病人：好的，谢谢。

(Twenty minutes later)

（20 分钟后）

Nurse: Let me have a look. There is no red and swelling. That's all for penicillin.

护士：让我看看，没有红肿现象，这说明你对青霉素不过敏。

# 10. Preoperative Preparation

# 术前准备

## A. Sentences Commonly Used（常用语）

1. You should sign the consent.
   你需要签署一份手术同意书。
2. I'll give you an enema tonight. After that please don't take any food or water before the operation.
   今晚我要给你灌一次肠，灌肠后直至手术前请不要吃东西或喝水。
3. We are going to do the operation on you tomorrow. I hope you won't worry.
   我们明天就要给你做手术，希望你不要紧张 / 担心。
4. The doctor who will operate on you is very experienced and considerate.
   给你做手术的医生很有经验，而且耐心细致。
5. We'll give you anesthesia. Please let me know if you feel any pain during the operation.
   我们会使用麻醉药，不过手术期间如果你感到疼痛，请告诉我。
6. If you have any discomfort during the operation, please don't hesitate to tell me.
   手术中有什么不舒服，请尽管告诉我，不要犹豫。
7. If you have any problems, please let me know.
   有什么不舒服尽管告诉我。
8. I'm afraid you're still too feeble to get up.
   恐怕你还太虚弱，还不能下床。
9. Ring any time you need help.
   需要帮助时请随时按铃。
10. If you need anything, just ring the bell.
    如果你有什么需要就按铃。
11. Are you in pain?
    你疼吗？
12. How are you feeling?
    你感觉怎么样？
13. The doctor needs to do some tests.
    医生需要做些检查。
14. You will need an X-ray.

你需要做X线检查。

15. Do you need any pain relief?
你需要些止痛药吗？
16. The doctor needs to do some blood tests.
医生需要做血液检测。
17. I need to have a specimen of urine/faeces.
我需要一些尿液/粪便样本。
18. The doctor will come to see you as he needs to examine you.
医生一会过来给你做检查。
19. Show me where the pain is.
指给我看哪里疼。
20. What are your symptoms?
你有什么症状吗？
21. How long have you had this pain?
这种疼痛持续多久了？
22. Have you been able to eat?
你能进食了吗？
23. Have you passed urine?
你排尿了吗？
24. The doctor has ordered a CT scan.
医生给你安排了CT扫描。
25. The doctor would like you to have an ECG test.
医生希望你做一下心电图检测。
26. When did you last have your bowels open，was it normal?
上次大便是什么时候，正常吗？
27. Do you have diarrhea?
你腹泻吗？
28. Is there anything you would like to ask me?
你还有什么需要问我的吗？
29. Has the doctor told you that you might need surgery?
医生告诉过你需要进行手术吗？
30. The doctor says you will need surgery.
医生说你需要接受手术。
31. The doctor has said that you need a lumbar puncture.
医生说你需要接受腰椎穿刺。
32. The doctor has said you are going to need an angioplasty（angiogram）.
医生说你需要做血管造影术。
33. You will have the results of your tests later today，the doctor will come and tell you.
化验结果今天晚些时候会出来，医生会过来告诉你结果。
34. When the doctor has the results，he will come and tell you.

医生知道结果后会过来告诉你。

35. A surgeon will come to see you before you have surgery.
在你开始手术之前，外科医生会过来看你。
36. An anesthesiologist will come to see you and examine you and ask you some questions.
麻醉师会过来检查并问你一些问题。
37. The doctor has prescribed a pre-med injection for you before you come to the Operating Boom，it will help you relax.
在你进手术室之前，医生给你开了些镇静剂，可以帮助你放松下来。
38. A nurse will come and prepare you for theatre when it is time.
到时间护士会过来准备手术的一切。
39. You will go to the Operating Room on a trolley（gurney）.
我们会用推车推着你进手术室。
40. After your surgery you will come back here.
手术过后你还是回来这里。
41. After your surgery you will have intravenous fluids.
手术过后你需要输液。
42. After surgery you will have a drain coming from your wound.
手术过后，你的伤口需要引流管接入。
43. After surgery you will have a urinary catheter to help you pass urine.
手术过后会用导尿管帮助你排尿。
44. You will be prescribed medication for pain relief，please tell me one of the nurses when you are in pain or discomfort.
当你疼痛或者不舒服的时候请告诉护士，我们会给你开止痛药。
45. You will be on fluids only for...（a couple of days/two days）.
你只能喝流质的东西……天（两天）。
46. The doctor will come and see you，to explain how your surgery went.
医生会过来看你并告诉你手术完成的情况。
47. The surgery will explain to you what surgery you will be having and you will need to sign the consent form.
外科医生会告诉你将要进行的手术，你需要签署手术同意书。
48. Because you are having an invasive procedure，you will need to sign a consent form.
因为你将要进行开刀手术，你需要签署手术同意书。
49. The doctor will explain exactly what he is going to do，the risks involved and what would happen if you did not have this surgery，you will then need to sign the consent form agreeing to the procedure.
医生会如实告知你他接下来将要做的事情，这样做涉及的风险以及你不进行手术会发生的后果。你需要签署手术同意书，同意进行手术。
50. The doctor will be unable to perform this procedure，if you do not sign the consent form agreeing to it.
如果你不签署手术同意书同意这么做，医生将没法给你动手术。

51. If you do not understand everything the doctor says, the hospital can get you an interpreter.
如果你听不懂医生说的话，医院可以给你找个翻译。

## B. Situational Conversation(情景会话)

### (1)

Nurse: Miss Li, your condition has been better and you are scheduled to have an operation next Thursday.

护士：王小姐，你的状况好一点了，因此下周四我们给你安排了手术。

Patient: Can you give me some advice?

病人：能给我些建议吗？

Nurse: You have such beautiful long hair, Miss Wang.

护士：你有一头漂亮的头发。

Patient: Thank you, nurse.

病人：谢谢你，护士。

Nurse: Would you mind having it cut?

护士：你介意把头发剪掉吗？

Patient: I don't want to lose it. But if it's necessary indeed, I think I will have to.

病人：我不想，但如果一定要剪，我也只能那样了。

Nurse: It is necessary for the operation. Someone will take care of that before the operation. Don't worry, you'll have it again just in a couple of months, I believe. Also I'll give you this polish remover and several cotton balls. So you can take off your finger nail polish.

护士：做手术必须剪掉头发，术前会有人为你剪的。不过别担心，在几个月内你又会有一头漂亮的头发的。我还会给你一瓶去甲油和一些棉球，用它来去掉你指甲油的颜色。

Patient: Could you tell me the reason for that?

病人：为什么？

Nurse: Because during the operation, we need to examine the color changes of your nail bed for assessing your condition. Also, it'll interfere with pulse oximeter readings. On Thursday morning, I'll give you a hospital gown to wear during surgery. Do remember to take off all your clothes including underwear.

护士：因为在手术中，我们要观察你甲床的颜色以便及时监控你的身体状况。同时，它也会影响血氧定量计的读数。下周四早上我会给你拿一套手术服，记住脱掉所有的衣服包括内衣，换上手术服。

Patient: Nurse, may I wear my wedding ring?

病人：护士，我可以戴结婚戒指吗？

Nurse: I'm afraid not. It could cut off the circulation if your fingers swell during the surgery. Have you any dentures?

护士： 恐怕不行。在手术中，手指发胀会影响血液循环。你戴了假牙吗？

Patient: Yes, I have.

病人： 是的。

Nurse: Well, you must remove them in the evening of next Wednesday, because they can slip during the surgery and block the airway. By the way, you must remove your contact lenses as well.

护士： 你必须在下周三晚上把它取下，否则在手术中它会滑落，导致呼吸道阻塞。顺便说一下，你还必须把隐形眼镜取出来。

### (2)

**Before Operation 在手术前**

Nurse: Good morning, Mr. Li. How are you feeling today?

护士： 早安，李先生，今天你好吗？

Patient: Not too bad. Did they tell you that Dr Zhang, head of the surgery department had decided to perform gastrectomy on me?

病人： 还不错。他们有没有告诉你外科张主任决定要给我做胃切除术？

Nurse: Yes. I took part in the discussion on your treatment. It was decided that you should undergo surgery. I was afraid that you would worry about it, so I'll come to put you at ease.

护士： 是的。我参加了有关你的治疗方案的讨论。已决定对你进行手术。我担心你会紧张，所以来解除你的顾虑。

Patient: Of course, I'm worried. I know it is a major operation.

病人： 的确有点紧张。因为我知道这是一个大手术。

Nurse: Please don't worry. I will explain everything to you.

护士： 请不要紧张。我可以详细对你讲讲。

Patient: That's fine.

病人： 太好啦。

Nurse: We know you have had gastric ulcer for many years and it is getting worse. According your X-ray pictures, we think it is wise to do a partial gastrectomy on you. This will relieve you from further stomach pain.

护士： 我们知道你得溃疡病已多年了，而且愈来愈严重。根据你的X线检查结果，我们认为你最好做胃部分切除术，这样你就不会再胃痛了。

Patient: I'm glad you have decided to do that because the pain has affected my life and work.

病人： 我很高兴你们这样做，因为胃痛已经影响了我的生活和工作。

Nurse: Now let me tell you something about what we should do before and after the operation. First of all, we must take care that you do not catch cold or run a fever. You should start using a bedpan now in order to accustom yourself to it.

护士： 现在让我给你讲讲手术前后应注意的问题。首先，在手术前别着凉，别感冒发烧。你现在要在床上练习使用便盆，免得术后不习惯。

Patient: Why do I have to use a bedpan?

病人： 我为什么要在床上用便盆？

Nurse： Because after the operation you will not be able to get up to go to the toilet.

护士： 因为手术后你不能下床到厕所去。

Nurse： The day before the operation the anesthetists will come to visit you and select the most suitable anesthetics for you. Then we'll let you have a good night's sleep.

护士： 手术前一天麻醉师会来看你。他们将为你选择最合适的麻醉药。到晚上让你睡个好觉。

Nurse： The next morning we will take you to the operation room and introduce you to the medical staff there.

护士： 第二天早上，我们送你到手术室，并把你介绍给那里的医务人员。

Nurse： While you are in the operation room, we will change your bed and make it warm and comfortable for you when you return. After the operation, an anesthetist will come back with you and observe you on the way. A nurse will then be responsible to look after you. She will come frequently to see about your condition and to take your blood pressure and pulse rate.

护士： 你在手术室时，我们要在病房给你准备一个温暖而舒适的床铺。手术结束后，会有麻醉师护送你到病房，并在路上观察你的情况。还有一位护士负责护理你。她将经常观察你的病情，给你测血压和脉搏。

Patient： Can I eat anything after the operation?

病人： 手术后我能吃东西吗？

Nurse： No. You will be give intravenous infusion not only after but even during the operation. We will put you on a liquid diet soon after your condition permits.

护士： 不能。在手术和手术后，都要给你静脉输液。以后根据你的病情，可以给你吃流质饮食。

Patient： Will I be allowed to move a little after the operation?

病人： 我手术后能动吗？

Nurse： You should try to turn over slightly. It will promote your bowel movement and eliminate the gas in the abdomen.

护士： 你可以轻轻地翻身。这样可以促使你的肠蠕动，对排便和排气都有帮助。

Patient： Will the wound be awfully painful?

病人： 伤口会痛吗？

Nurse： There may be slight pain which I am sure you can stand. If it distresses you too much, we will give you something for it.

护士： 可能有轻微疼痛，但是我可以肯定你会经受得住。如果实在痛得厉害，我们可以给你用点药。

Patient： Thank you for your explanation. When will I be able to leave the hospital?

病人： 谢谢你的说明，我什么时候可以出院？

Nurse： Your sutures may be removed seven days after the operation. Then you can go home if everything goes smoothly. Before you leave, I will tell you how to take care of yourself at home.

护士： 手术后7天可以拆线。如果一切顺利，你就可以出院了。在你出院前，我会告诉你在家里应注意的事情。

Patient： Thank you for your kindness.

病人： 多谢你。

Nurse： You are welcome.

护士： 不客气。

## （3）

**Ward Round Conversation after Admission 巡诊对话**

Nurse： Hello，Mrs. Smith，Dr. Wang is coming to ask you questions similar to the questions the doctor in outpatients asked you and also examine you，is that OK?

护士： 你好，史密斯夫人，王医生会过来询问一些门诊医生问过的类似问题并对你进行检查，这样可以吗？

Patient： Yes，sure，do you have any idea what may be wrong with me?

病人： 是的，当然。你觉得我有可能是什么问题？

Nurse： The doctor might have to do some more tests，before he has an answer.

护士： 医生可能需要做更多的检测才能得出结论。

Patient： What tests will he be doing?

病人： 他将会做哪些检测？

Nurse： I'm not sure until he examines you and asks you some more questions，but he might do some more blood tests，maybe take another X-ray of your chest and he might need a specimen of sputum.

护士： 这要等到他检查并问过你问题后才清楚，他可能会做一些血液检测、胸部X线检查和唾液检测。

Patient： How long do I need to stay in hospital?

病人： 我需要住院多久？

Nurse： As soon as the doctor knows what the problem is，he will treat you，and as soon as you're better you can go home.

护士： 医生一确诊就会马上治疗，只要你有了好转就可以出院。

Patient： Will I need any medication?

病人： 我需要吃什么药吗？

Nurse： You might need to take medication，if so the doctor will prescribe some for you.

护士： 如果医生给你开了药你就需要吃。

Patient： Do I need to have this oxygen mask on all the time?

病人： 我需要一直戴着这个氧气面罩吗？

Nurse： Yes，you do I'm afraid，because you are having trouble breathing，it will help you.

护士： 是的，恐怕是这样。你呼吸困难，它能帮助你。

Patient： When will you know what's wrong with me?

病人： 什么时候能确诊呢？

Nurse： As soon as the doctor has all the test results，he will let you know.

护士： 所有检查结果之后，医生会过来告诉你。

Patient: Can I get out of bed and walk around?

病人： 我能下床走走吗？

Nurse: I'm sorry you can't at the moment, as you need to have the oxygen. But you can sit next to the bed if you like, I will help you.

护士： 很抱歉，你现在不能，因为你需要戴着氧气面罩。不过你可以坐在床边，如果需要那样坐，我会帮助你。

**(4)**

**Ward Round Conversation 巡诊对话**

Nurse: Good morning, Mrs. Jones, did you sleep well?

护士： 早上好，琼斯夫人，你睡得好吗？

Patient: No, not very well, nurse.

病人： 不是很好，护士小姐。

Patient: When will I get the results from my tests? Where do I have to go to have the tests? I don't speak any Chinese.

病人： 检测结果什么时候出来？该去哪里做检查？我不懂中文。

Nurse: Please don't worry, I will go with you, and explain to you what is happening, the doctor will have the results later today and he will come and see you then.

护士： 请不要担心，我会带你过去给你解释接下来的事情。今天晚些时候医生就能拿到检测结果，到时他会过来看你。

Patient: What will happen if I need an operation (surgery)?

病人： 如果我需要动手术的话，该怎么做？

Nurse: It will be the same procedure as in your country, you will have to starve for at least eight hours before surgery. The surgeon and anesthesiologist will come and see you, the anesthesiologist will ask you a few questions about your general health, and prescribe any pre-med he might like you to have. The surgery will discuss with you the surgery he will perform, and ask you to sign a consent form. And a few hours before your surgery a nurse will prepare you for surgery, and escort you to the operating rooms when the time comes.

护士： 手术的程序步骤和你们国家的差不多，你手术前 8 小时不能进食，外科医生和麻醉师会先过来看你，麻醉师会问你一些身体健康情况，给你开一些药。外科医生会跟你讨论一下将要进行的手术，要求你签一份手术同意书。手术开始前几个小时，护士会开始准备，手术时间到的时候会护送你进入手术室。

Patient: Am I able to walk around if I want to?

病人： 我能下来走走吗？如果我想的话？

Nurse: Well, you will be having an intravenous drip, so you will need to be very careful if you want to walk around, you will need to ask me or one of the other nurses if they can help you.

护士： 你将要打点滴，如果你确实想要走走的话必须非常小心，最好是先问问我或者其他护士是不是能够帮你。

Patient: Can I have something to eat, something light?

病人: 我能吃点清淡的东西吗？

Nurse: No, I'm afraid not, just sips of water for now in case you need surgery.

护士: 不，恐怕不行。只能喝一点点水，因为你要动手术。

Patient: Oh OK, can I have visitors?

病人: 哦，好的，能探访吗？

Nurse: Yes, of course. Are there any other questions you would like to ask me?

护士: 当然可以，还有什么问题需要问我的吗？

Patient: No, not right now, thanks, maybe later.

病人: 没有了，现在没有，谢谢。

Nurse: If you have any problems please ask me or any of the nurses, if we can't help you, we will find someone who can.

护士: 如果你有什么问题，你可以问我或其他护士，如果我们不知道怎么办，我们可以找知道的人来帮助你。

Patient: OK, thanks very much.

病人: 好的，非常感谢。

Nurse: You're welcome, see you later.

护士: 不客气，一会见。

## (5)

**Telling a Patient Needing Surgery 告知病人动手术**

Nurse: Mrs. Jones, has the doctor discussed with you the results of your tests?

护士: 琼斯夫人，医生告诉过你检测结果吗？

Patient: Yes, he has. When am I going to have surgery?

病人: 是的，他说过。我什么时候动手术？

Nurse: Surgery has been scheduled for later on today about 16: 00.

护士: 手术已经预订在今天稍晚些时候，大约下午4点。

Patient: Is it OK to have surgery so soon, is it an emergency?

病人: 我这么快动手术合适吗？很紧急吗？

Nurse: Yes, the surgery needs to do it as soon as possible, you have only had intravenous fluids since you came to hospital, and so it will be safe to do it this afternoon.

护士: 是的，需要尽快进行手术。从你进医院我们就只给你静脉输液，因此在今天下午可以进行手术。

Patient: So what's going to happen now?

病人: 那现在该做什么？

Nurse: A surgery will come to see you before you have surgery and explain what he is going to do and ask you to sign a consent form.

护士: 一个外科医生将在手术之前过来看你并向你解释他将做的事情，同时会要求你签手术同意书。

Patient: Oh, OK. Does he understand English?

病人：哦，好的。他懂英文吗？

Nurse: If you do not understand, please say and we will arrange for a translator (interpreter).

护士：如果你听不懂他的话，请告诉我们以便安排翻译。

Patient: Will that be OK? The surgeon won't be offended, will he?

病人：那样行吗？外科医生不会生气？

Nurse: No, of course not, also an anesthesiologist will come to see you and examine you and ask you some questions.

护士：当然不会。麻醉师也会过来看你并做检查，同时问一些问题。

Patient: Will I have a pre-med (medication) injection before I go?

病人：在手术之前，我是否要注射镇静剂吗？

Nurse: If you think you need one, please ask the anesthesiologist and he can prescribe a pre-med injection before you come to the Operating Room.

护士：如果你觉得需要，请在来手术室之前叫麻醉师给开出镇静剂。

Patient: So what do I do now?

病人：那我现在做什么？

Nurse: A nurse will come and prepare you for theatre when it is time; and you will go to the Operating Room on a trolley and after your surgery you will come back here.

护士：时间一到，护士会过来为你做去手术室的准备。你将被用轮椅推进手术室，结束之后请回到这里。

Patient: How long will the operation take? What will happen?

病人：手术将持续多久？将会怎样？

Nurse: It is hard to say, the surgeon will explain when he comes to see you.

护士：很难说，外科医生过来时会给你解释。

Patient: Oh, OK.

病人：噢，好的！

Nurse: The doctor has prescribed medication for your abdominal pain. Please tell a nurse if you are in pain or discomfort. She will then give you an injection to help.

护士：医生已经为你的腹痛开药了。如果疼痛或不舒服，请告诉护士，她会给你注射。

Patient: OK, thanks very much.

病人：好的，谢谢！

Nurse: Please call me if you have any problems.

护士：如果有什么问题，请呼叫我。

Patient: OK, nurse, thanks.

病人：好的，谢谢你，护士小姐。

# 11. Postoperative Care

# 术后护理

## A. Sentences Commonly Used(常用语)

1. The operation went very well.
   手术很顺利/成功。
2. Please turn from side to side every two or three hours.
   请你每两三个小时翻一次身。
3. I'm going to empty the bedpan.
   我去把便盆倒掉。
4. You have to stay here for another two weeks.
   你还得再在医院住两周。
5. How are you feeling?
   你觉得怎么样?
6. Are you in any pain?
   你有什么地方疼吗?
7. The doctor will prescribe some stronger pain killers(pain relief).
   医生会给你开些强止痛药。
8. Your operation went well, no complications.
   你的手术很成功,没有并发症。
9. The histology results will be back tomorrow.
   组织检测结果明天出来。
10. You will be discharged in a few days.
    过几天你就可以出院了。
11. I'm going to look at your wound.
    我接下来要查看你的伤口。
12. Does your wound feel sore or uncomfortable?
    你的伤口感到疼或不舒服吗?
13. Is your wound painful if I touch it?
    我碰到伤口时,会觉得疼吗?
14. There is no blood or fluid in the drainage bag, the doctor has told us to take it out for you.
    引流袋里面没有血或液体,医生已经让我们倒出来了。

15. Have you passed urine?
你排尿了吗？
16. Have you had your bowels open?
你大便了吗？
17. Have you passed any wind/gas/flatulence?
你放屁了吗？
18. Are you drinking OK?
你现在喝东西怎么样？
19. If you are drinking OK，the intravenous drip will come down.
如果你能正常喝东西，就可以不输液了。
20. Have you had anything to eat?
你吃什么东西了吗？
21. You need to get out of bed and walk around for a little while，it will help your circulation.
你需要下床走走，这样有助于血液循环。
22. Do you have any questions?
你有什么疑问吗？

## B. Situational Conversation(情景会话)

### (1)

Nurse: You look a little better today.
护士：今天看来你精神好一些。
Patient: Yes，but lying in bed all day，I feel uncomfortable all over.
病人：是的，不过整天躺着我觉得全身不舒服。
Nurse: You can get out of bed today. First，sit on the edge of the bed and if you don't feel dizzy then you can get out of bed.
护士：你今天可以下床了，但在下床前先要在床边坐坐，不感到头晕才能下床。
Patient: But I feel distended in the abdomen.
病人：不过我感到腹胀得很。
Nurse: Did you pass any wind by rectum?
护士：有气从肛门排出吗？
Patient: No.
病人：没有。
Nurse: You can lie on your side more often，and if the wound does not hurt，you can get out of bed and walk around，that will help peristalsis of the intestine，which will help to pass gas，and lessens distension.
护士：你可以多翻身，如果伤口不疼可下床活动，那样有助于恢复肠蠕动，使气体排出减轻腹胀。
Patient: The wound is painful and the sputum is difficult to expectorate.

病人： 伤口疼，而且有痰又难咳出来。

Nurse： You should sit up. That will help your deep breathing, and help you to expectorate and prevent the sputum from accumulating in your lungs to cause pneumonia.

护士： 你应该坐起来，那样可以帮助你深呼吸，使痰较容易咳出，以防痰积在肺内引起肺炎。

Patient： All right.

病人： 好的。

Nurse： Did you drink any water?

护士： 你喝过水了吗？

Patient： Yes.

病人： 喝过了。

Nurse： Do you feel distended and nausea?

护士： 你感觉胃胀和恶心吗？

Patient： No.

病人： 没有。

Nurse： That's good. You can start on a fluid diet and porridge in two days.

护士： 那很好，你可以开始吃流质，过两天吃稀饭。

Patient： Thank you.

病人： 谢谢。

Patient： How long must I stay in hospital?

病人： 我住院还需多久？

Nurse： You can go home in about a week.

护士： 一周左右就可出院了。

Nurse： Good morning, doctor.

护士： 医生，早晨好。

Doctor： Good morning. How is the patient after surgery?

医生： 早晨好，病人手术后情况如何？

Nurse： The patient has a slight pain in the wound. Some blood has been oozing from the draining wound; the dressing has been changed once.

护士： 伤口有点疼。伤口引流有些渗血，换过一次敷料。

Doctor： That's good.

医生： 那很好。

Nurse： Does he still need intravenous infusion and penicillin?

护士： 是否继续静脉输液和青霉素？

Doctor： Yes.

医生： 继续。

**（2）**

**Post-operative Ward Round　术后巡诊**

Nurse： Hello, Mrs. Jones, how are you feeling?

护士： 你好，琼斯夫人，感觉怎么样？

Patient: Not too great, nurse.

病人：不是太好，护士小姐。

Nurse: Are you in any pain?

护士：你感到疼痛吗？

Patient: Yes, I'm in a lot of pain.

病人：是的，我很疼。

Nurse: I will ask the doctor to prescribe something stronger for you, and a nurse will come and give you an intramuscular injection.

护士：我会让医生给你开一些强止痛药，护士会给你进行肌内注射。

Patient: Thank you, I would really appreciate it.

病人：谢谢，我真的非常感谢。

Nurse: You operation went well, no complications, and the histology results will be back tomorrow.

护士：你的手术很成功，没有并发症。组织检测结果明天出来。

Patient: Oh, good.

病人：哦，真好！

Nurse: You will have intravenous fluids for more days, and I'm afraid you can only have sips of water today.

护士：你将要在未来几天内进行静脉输液，恐怕今天你只能喝少量水。

Patient: Is that all? I'm very thirsty.

病人：就这点水么？我很渴。

Nurse: Yes, I'm sorry, but you need to give your bowel a rest. Have you passed any wind/gas?

护士：是的，非常抱歉，但是得让你的肠胃休息。你放过屁了吗？

Patient: No, I don't think so. I've been in too much pain to notice.

病人：我觉得没有。我太疼了而无法关注这个。

Nurse: You also have a drain coming from your wound, and a urinary catheter to help you pass urine.

护士：我们会接个引流管在你的伤口处，还会接一条导尿管帮助你排尿。

Patient: Yes, I know. I don't like the catheter, it's very uncomfortable when you are going to take it out.

病人：是的，我知道。我不喜欢排尿管，因为当你将其取出来的时候很不舒服。

Nurse: A nurse will take it out in a couple of days, when you are feeling better and walking around. The drain will be removed tomorrow.

护士：两天后，当你感觉好点并能走动时护士会把它取出来。伤口处的引流管在明天被撤下。

Patient: I guess I'll have to wait then.

病人：我想我不得不等了。

Nurse: I'm going to look at your wound.

护士：我接着要检查一下你的伤口。

Patient: OK, be careful.

病人：好的，当心点。

Nurse: That looks OK, the doctor will be around later and he will put another dressing on it, do you have any questions for me.

护士：看起来不错，医生在附近，他一会过来给你放敷料，你还有什么问题吗？

Patient: When do you think I'll be able to go home?

病人：你认为我什么时候可以回家？

Nurse: You should be discharged in about seven days, it depends on your progress.

护士：你7天之后可以出院，这具体取决于康复的进展。

Patient: That long OK, what is that other bag of fluid that they are putting in my vein?

病人：好的，将给我输的另一包药液是什么？

Nurse: You are having intravenous antibiotics three times a day, you have been prescribed antibiotics for seven days, when you are eating and drinking you can take the antibiotics orally.

护士：你现在需要每天静脉注射3次抗生素。另外已经开了7天的抗生素，当你能吃饭、喝水时，可以用于口服。

Patient: OK, thanks, no more questions.

病人：好的，谢谢，没有其他的问题了。

Nurse: OK, Mrs. Jones, I'll see you later.

护士：好的，琼斯夫人，一会见。

# 12. Operation Nursing Procedures

# 手术护理过程

## A. Sentences Commonly Used(常用语)

**Urine　尿液**

1. Have you passed urine today?
   你今天排尿了吗？
2. Have you emptied your bladder?
   你排尿了吗？
3. Have you been to the toilet/ bathroom?
   你上过厕所了吗？
4. How many times have you passed urine today?
   你今天排了几次尿？
5. What color is your urine?
   你的尿液是什么颜色的？
6. I need a specimen of urine.
   我需要你的尿样。
7. I need to test your urine, please give me a specimen in this container.
   我需要检测你的尿样，请用这个容器装些给我。

**Urine Catheterization　导尿管插入**

8. I need to catheterize you.
   我要给你插入导尿管。
9. I need to put a tube into your bladder to help you pass urine.
   我要接一条管子到你的膀胱帮助你排尿。
10. The catheter will be attached to a bag, which will collect the urine, and it will be emptied when it becomes full.
    导尿管会连接到一个专门用来盛尿的袋子上，当袋子装满的时候会有人来倒掉。
11. Please lay down.
    请躺下。
12. Please open your legs.
    请张开腿。
13. I will clean you with some fluid.

我将用些液体给你擦洗。

14. It will feel cold/warm.
    会感觉有冷/热。
15. Please take a deep breath, and breathe out slowly through your mouth.
    请深吸一口气，然后慢慢地用嘴呼出来。
16. Please tell me if this feels uncomfortable.
    如果感到不舒服，请告诉我。
17. I have finished, I have attached a bag to your catheter.
    我完成了，我已经将一个袋子连接到你的导尿管上了。
18. Please do not worry about passing urine.
    请不要担心排尿问题。
19. It is a strange feeling, you will feel that you want to pass urine, but you will get used to it after a short time.
    感觉会有点怪，你会感觉有尿意，不过很快你就会适应它的。
20. If you walk around you need to take the bag with you.
    如果你要四处走动的话，请记着带上袋子。
21. If the bag becomes full, please ask a nurse to empty it.
    如果袋子盛满了，请通知护士过来倒掉。

**Removal of Catheter　导尿管移除**

22. I need to remove your catheter.
    我需要移除你的导尿管。
23. I need to do this over a period of time.
    移除过程可能会花一些时间。
24. I will clamp your catheter for two hours, and then come back and release it.
    我会夹住你的导尿管 2 小时左右，然后再松开它。
25. I will clamp your catheter for three hours/four hours and then release it.
    我会夹住你的导尿管 3/4 个小时左右，然后再松开它。
26. It is done slowly to help you get muscle tone back in your bladder sphincter muscle.
    操作这么慢是为了帮助你的膀胱括约肌恢复张力。
27. If you feel very uncomfortable or in pain, please tell me.
    如果你感到不舒服或者疼痛，请告诉我。
28. Please lay on the bed with your legs open.
    请张开腿躺在床上。
29. I will clean you with some fluid.
    我将用一些液体给你擦洗。
30. Please take a deep breath, and breathe out slowly through your mouth.
    请深吸一口气，然后慢慢地用嘴呼出来。
31. The catheter is out.
    导尿管取出来了。
32. Please tell me when you have passed urine normally.

你正常排过尿后请告诉我。

33. Please tell me if you can't pass urine and are in any discomfort or pain.
如果你不能排尿或者感到不舒服或者疼痛，请告诉我。

**Stools /Faeces 粪便**

34. Have you had your bowels open today?
你今天大便了吗？

35. How many times have you had your bowels open?
你大便了几次？

36. What did it look like?
粪便看起来什么颜色？

37. Have you passed any wind?
你放屁了吗？

38. Do you feel uncomfortable?
你感到不舒服吗？

39. Are you constipated?
你便秘吗？

40. When was the last time you had your bowels open?
你上次大便是什么时候？

41. I need a stool specimen.
我需要粪便的样本。

42. Please use the bedpan, here is the container, please let me know when you have a specimen.
请使用便盆，给你这个。取样之后请告诉我。

**Enema 灌肠**

43. You need a bowel prep.
你需要使用 bowel prep（一种强泻剂）。

44. You need an enema.
你需要进行灌肠。

45. I will give you medication to help you.
我会给你一些药帮助你。

46. I need to insert some suppositories.
我需要插入一些栓剂。

47. You need to insert these suppositories.
我需要插入这些栓剂。

48. Please lay down on you left side with your knees up as far as you can.
请左侧躺着，膝盖尽可能抬高。

49. I am going to insert a small tube into your rectum. Please take a deep breath and breathe out slowly.
我将插一条小管到你的直肠，请慢慢深呼吸。

50. You will feel pushing as the fluid enters.
药液进入的时候你会感觉有些紧。

51. Please keep as still as you can.
请尽量保持不动。
52. I have finished, please get up gently, and try and keep the fluid in your bowel as long as possible before you go to the bathroom/ toilet.
我完成了，请慢慢站起来。在上厕所前，尽量地让药液留在你的肠道里面。
53. Please tell me if you have any problems or concerns.
如果你有什么问题或忧虑，请告诉我。
54. Please tell me when you have emptied your bowels.
你大便之后请通知我。
55. Please tell me when you have been to the bathroom/ toilet.
你上过厕所之后请告诉我。
56. You will need to empty your bowels in a bedpan, please tell me when you are ready.
你需要在便盆里面大便，当你准备好的时候告诉我。

**Taking Blood Specimens( Sample ) 血液取样**

57. I need to take a specimen/sample of blood.
我需要取血样。
58. The blood tests are for...
血液检测是为了……。
59. I am going to take the specimen (sample) from your arm/ elbow /hand/ wrist/groin/ankle/neck.
我将从你的手臂 / 肘 / 手掌 / 手腕 / 腹股沟 / 脚踝 / 脖子处取血样。
60. I'm going to put a tourniquet around your arm/leg, it will feel tight.
我将给你的手臂 / 大腿绑止血带，会有点紧。
61. Please open and close your hand.
请握紧和放松你的手。
62. I'm just going to clean the skin.
我接下来给你清洁皮肤。
63. You will feel a slight prick.
你会感到有点刺痛。
64. Please stay still.
请保持不动。
65. Please bend your arm, and leave it like that for a few minutes.
请弯一下你的手臂，一直这样保持几分钟。
66. Please press hard on this dressing.
请用力压着敷料。
67. I need to press your groin for 10 minutes, please try and keep still.
我需要压着你的腹股沟十分钟，请尽量保持不动。
68. I will put a dressing on this, you can take the dressing off in a couple of hours.
我给你放敷料，你两个小时后可以取下来。
69. The doctor will tell you the results as soon as they are here.
医生一到这里就会告诉你结果。

70. The results will be back in a couple of hours please go to 2nd floor to collect them.
结果两个小时后出来，请到二楼去取。

71. The results will be back in a couple of hours，the doctor will come and tell you the results.
结果两个小时后出来，医生会过来告诉你结果。

**Cannulation 插管**

72. I need to insert a cannula /small tube into your vein.
我需要插一根管子到你的血管中。

73. It will be in your wrist /hand/elbow/foot/groin.
（插入的位置）在你的手腕 / 手掌 / 肘 / 脚 / 腹股沟。

74. I will put a tourniquet around your arm/lower leg，it will feel tight.
我将在你的手臂 / 小腿处绑止血带，会有点紧。

75. You will feel a small prick and some pressure，please try and keep still.
你会感到有点刺痛和紧，请尽量不要动。

76. I will secure this with a dressing，so it doesn't come out.
我会放敷料来防护，这样管子不会掉出来。

77. I am going to attach the intravenous tubing.
我接下来要给你接上静脉管。

**Intravenous Fluids 静脉输液**

78. The doctor has said you need to have intravenous fluids.
医生说你需要输液。

79. I will need to insert a cannula into your vein.
我需要插套管到你的血管中。

80. It will be in your wrist /hand/elbow.
（插入的位置）在你的手腕 / 手背 / 肘部。

81. I am going to attach the intravenous tubing to your cannula.
我接下来要把静脉管连接到你的套管中。

82. You will need intravenous fluids for...days.
你需要输液……天。

83. The doctor has prescribed intravenous fluids for...days.
医生开了……天的静脉输液。

84. Please can I check your cannula and dressing.
请让我检查一下你的套管和敷料。

85. The intravenous fluids are called...
输的液体为……。

86. You need intravenous fluids because you are dehydrated.
你需要输液，因为你现在脱水。

87. You need intravenous fluids to give you the antibiotics that the doctor has prescribed.
你需要通过输液注入医生给你开的抗生素。

**Electrocardiogram（ECG） 心电图**

88. The doctor would like you to have an ECG test.

医生希望你做心电图检测。

89. You need to have an ECG test.
你需要做心电图检测。

90. Please come with me，I need to do an ECG test.
请跟我来，我需要给你做心电图检测。

91. Please lay on the couch and wait for me.
请躺在床上等我。

92. Please take off your top/shirt/ bra.
请脱掉你的外衣 / 衬衣 / 胸罩。

93. I am going to put these little pads on your chest，they will feel cold.
我接下来要将这些电极片放到你的胸上，会感到有点凉。

94. Please try and keep still.
请尽量不要动。

95. I've finished now，you can get dressed.
我完成了，你可以穿衣服了。

**Cleaning，Dressing & Checking of Wounds　清理、敷料处理和检查伤口**

96. I need to check your dressing today.
我今天需要检查你的敷料。

97. Please can I see your dressing?
我能看一下你的敷料吗？

98. Does your dressing need changing?
你的敷料需要更换吗？

99. I need to change your dressing.
我需要更换你的敷料。

100. Please don't get your dressing /bandage/plaster wet.
请不要沾湿敷料 / 绷带 / 石膏。

101. I need to re-bandage this.
我需要重新包扎一下。

102. Please lay on the bed/examination couch.
请躺在床上 / 检查床上。

103. Please lift up your clothes.
请将衣服拉起来。

104. Let me see your dressing/wound.
让我看看你的敷料 / 伤口。

105. Does that feel comfortable?
舒不舒服？

106. Is that too tight?
会不会有点紧？

107. Does your wound feel sore or uncomfortable?
你的伤口感到疼或者不舒服吗？

108. Is your wound painful if I touch it?
我触碰的时候你的伤口会疼吗？
109. I need to remove your stitches/clips/sutures.
我需要给你拆线。
110. I am going to remove the dressing.
我接下来给你移除敷料。
111. I am going to clean your skin with...
我接下来用……给你清洁皮肤。
112. Please take a deep breath, and breathe out through your mouth.
请深吸一口气，然后慢慢地用嘴呼出来。
113. Please tell me if I am hurting you.
如果我弄疼你了，请告诉我。
114. Your wound looks OK.
你的伤口看起来没事了。
115. Your wound looks a bit red and sore.
你的伤口看起来有点红肿溃疡。
116. Your wound looks inflamed, does it hurt/ is it painful?
你的伤口看起来有点发炎，疼不疼？
117. Your wound is weeping a little bit.
你的伤口有点渗液。
118. I am going to remove your drainage tube.
我接下来移除你的引流管。
119. I am going to clean it with...
我接下来用……清理它。
120. Please take a deep breath.
请深呼吸。
121. I will just put a dry dressing on that.
我会放些干敷料在那上面。
122. Please let me know if it is weeping/ leaking.
如果有渗透，请告诉我。

**Assisting a Doctor in an Angioplasty　协助医生进行血管成形术**

123. You are here to have a catheter procedure, because the doctor in the Emergency Room has diagnosed a...
你来这里接受导管插入，因为急诊室的医生诊断出你患有……。
124. How are you feeling now?
你现在感觉怎么样？
125. This emergency procedure has to be done now.
这个紧急手术必须立刻进行。
126. Please can you sign this consent form giving us permission to perform the catheter procedure?

请问你能在手术同意书上面签字允许我们进行导管插入吗？

127. Please take off all your clothes and put on this gown, the ties need to be at the front.
请将所有衣服脱掉换上这件袍子，系带在前穿着。

128. Please give all your valuables to your friend/ husband for safe keeping.
为了安全起见，请将你所有值钱的东西交给你的朋友/丈夫。

129. Lay down on this couch and try to relax.
请躺在这张床上，尽量放松。

130. Roll up your sleeve, I need to take your pulse, blood pressure and take an ECG, I will put these pads on your chest.
请将袖子卷起来，我需要量你的脉搏、血压和做心电图检测。我接下来将把这些电极片放在你的胸上。

131. I am going to put this peg on your finger, this takes your pulse, it is not heavy and it doesn't hurt.
我把这个指套放在你的手指上，这是用来量脉搏的。指套不会太重，也不疼。

132. The operation takes about half an hour.
手术大概需要持续半小时。

133. I need to give you intravenous fluids, so I need to put a cannula into your hand.
我需要给你输液，所以我需要将套管连接到你的手上。

134. I am going to give you some oxygen, please put this oxygen mask over your face.
我接下来给你供氧，请将这个氧气罩戴上。

135. This is Dr..., he is going to do your catheterization, he is just getting the equipment ready.
这是……医生，他是来给你做导管插入术的，他现在在准备所用的仪器。

136. The doctor is going to give you a local anesthetic.
医生接下来给你做局部麻醉。

137. The doctor will insert a catheter into your artery, and send it to your heart.
医生将插一根管子到你的动脉，并送到你的心脏处。

138. The equipment is needed, so he can see what is happening.
这仪器很必要，只有这样他才能看到正在发生的事情。

139. If you feel any pain, please tell us, and the doctor can give you some more local anesthetic.
如果你感到疼痛请告诉我，医生会给你更多的局部麻醉。

140. The doctor has finished now.
医生完成了。

141. He is now putting pressure onto your wound to stop the bleeding, this will be for about fifteen minutes.
他现在要压着你的伤口以止血，这个过程大概需要 15 分钟。

142. You will have to stay for about three days for anti-coagulation treatment, IV antibiotics, chest X-ray and an ECG check.
你需要留院 3 天接受抗凝结治疗、静脉抗生素输液、胸部 X 线检查和心电图检测等。

**Assisting a Doctor in a Lumbar Puncture Procedure 协助医生进行腰椎穿刺术**

143. The doctor needs to do a lumbar puncture to get some spinal fluid for tests.
医生需要进行腰椎穿刺手术来采取一些脊髓液进行检测。
144. Please turn onto your left side.
请左侧躺下。
145. Can you bend your knees as far as you can.
请将膝盖尽量弯曲。
146. Can you bend your head to touch your chest as far as you can.
请尽量地低头触碰你的胸部。
147. I need your back curved as much as possible.
我需要你背部尽量地弯曲。
148. The doctor is going to clean your skin with an antiseptic，it will feel very cold.
医生接下来会用杀菌剂清洗你的皮肤，会感觉很凉。
149. He is going to put a clean towel on your back，please do not touch it.
他接下来会放一条毛巾在你的背部，请不要碰它。
150. The doctor is going to start the procedure now.
医生接下来开始动手术了。
151. He is going to give you a local anesthetic，you will feel a sharp prick，please try not to move.
他接下来要给你进行局部麻醉，你会感觉突然刺痛，请不要动。
152. You will feel pushing and pressure on your back.
你会感到背部有压力。
153. If you feel any pain，please tell me，and I will ask the doctor to give you some more local anesthetic.
如果你感到任何程度的疼，请告诉我。我会告诉医生给你进行更多的局部麻醉。
154. The doctor has finished now and is putting a dressing on your back.
医生处理完了，他现在给你背部敷料。
155. Please roll back onto your back.
请转过来平躺着。
156. You will need to stay in bed for twelve hours with no pillow.
你需要不枕枕头地平躺着 12 个小时。
157. Please do not sit up，if you try to sit up you will have a very severe headache.
请不要坐起来，如果你尝试坐起来，你会感到严重的头痛。
158. If you need anything，please ring for a nurse.
如果你需要什么东西，请呼叫护士。
159. Your test will be back in...days.
你的化验结果……天后出来。
160. The doctor will come and see you and tell you the results.
医生会过来看你并告诉你结果。

## B. Situational Conversation(情景会话)

### (1)

**Urine Catheterization** 导尿管手术

Nurse: Hello, Mrs. Jones, the doctor says you need to have a urine catheter, so I need to catheterize you.

护士：你好，琼斯夫人，医生说你需要导尿，所以我需要给你插入导尿管。

Patient: Oh, OK, what does that mean, what are you going to do?

病人：哦，好的。你所谓的插入导尿管指什么？你接下来要做什么？

Nurse: I am going to put a tube into your bladder, to help you pass urine.

护士：我接下来要连接一根管子到你的膀胱以帮助你排尿。

Patient: What happens when I want to go to the toilet?

病人：当我想上厕所的时候会怎么样？

Nurse: The catheter will be attached to a bag, which will collect the urine, and it will be emptied when it becomes full.

护士：导管会接连到一个用来收集尿的袋子上，当袋子盛满的时候，会有人过来倒掉。

Patient: Does the doctor really think I need to have this?

病人：医生确实需要我这样做吗？

Nurse: Yes, he does. Please will you lay down for me and open your legs?

护士：是的，他确定。请问你能躺下并把腿张开吗？

Patient: Yes, OK.

病人：是的，可以。

Nurse: I am going to clean you with some fluid, it might feel cold.

护士：我接下来用一些液体给你清洗，会感觉有点凉。

Patient: Oh, yes, that is a bit cold.

病人：哦，是的，确实有点凉。

Nurse: Please take deep breaths, and breathe out slowly through your mouth.

护士：请深吸一口气，并慢慢地用嘴呼出来。

Nurse: Please tell me if this feels uncomfortable.

护士：如果你感到不舒服，请告诉我。

Patient: It feels a bit uncomfortable, but it's OK.

病人：是感觉有点不舒服，不过没有问题。

Nurse: OK, I've finished, and I have attached a bag to your catheter, so please do not worry about passing urine.

护士：好的，我完成了。我已经将导管连接到袋子，请不要担心排尿问题。

Patient: It feels very strange, it feels as if I want to pass urine.

病人：我感觉很怪，就像我时刻有尿意似的。

Nurse: It is a strange feeling, you will feel that you want to pass urine, but the feeling will go

after a while and you will get uses to it.
护士：是这种奇怪的感觉。你会感觉你想排尿，但过一会儿就会消失，你会习惯的。
Patient：OK，what happens if I want to walk around?
病人：好的。如果我想到处走走呢，怎么办？
Nurse：If you walk around，you need to take the bag with you.
护士：如果你想走动，你需要带着那个袋子。
Patient：What do I do if the bag feels up with urine?
病人：如果袋子盛满了怎么办？
Nurse：If the bag becomes full，please ask me or another nurse to empty it.
护士：如果袋子满了，请告诉我或其他护士过来倒掉。
Patient：OK，nurse，thanks very much.
病人：好的，护士小姐，非常感谢。
Nurse：If you have any problems or worries，please come and tell me.
护士：如果你有什么问题或忧虑，请过来告诉我。
Patient：OK，I will. Thanks!
病人：好的，我会的。谢谢！

**（2）**

**Removal of Catheter　导尿管移除**

Nurse：Hello，Mrs. Jones，how are you? I'm here as I need to remove your urine catheter.
护士：你好，琼斯夫人。你感觉怎么样？我来移除你的导尿管。
Patient：Oh，that's great，how are you going to do this，just take it out?
病人：哦，太好了。你怎么办，只是拔出来吗？
Nurse：I shall need to do this over a period of time as you have had the catheter in for a few days.
护士：由于这导尿管已经插了几天了，所以我需要花一段时间才能将它取出来。
Patient：Oh，really? So what are you going to do?
病人：哦，真的？那你将怎么做？
Nurse：I will clamp your catheter for two hours，and then come back and release it.
护士：我将夹着导管 2 个小时，然后再松开。
Nurse：I will clamp your catheter for three hours，and then come back and release it.
护士：我将夹着导管 3 个小时，然后再松开它。
Patient：Oh，why do you have to do that，and not just take it out?
病人：哦，为什么你需要这么做而不是直接取出来？
Nurse：It is done slowly to help you get muscle tone back in your bladder sphincter muscle.
护士：操作这么慢是为了帮助你的膀胱括约肌恢复张力。
Patient：Oh，OK，that makes sense I guess.
病人：哦，好的，我想我懂了。
Nurse：If you feel very uncomfortable or in pain，please tell me.
护士：如果你感到非常不舒服或者疼痛，请告诉我。

Patient: Oh, right. I will. How many times do you need to do this for before you take the catheter out?

病人：哦，好的。在导管取出来之前，你需要这样操作多少次？

Nurse: Two or three times.

护士：2次或3次。

Patient: OK.

病人：好的。

Nurse: Mrs. Smith, I've come to take your catheter out, please can you lay on the bed with your legs open.

护士：史密斯夫人，我过来移除导管，请问你能躺在床上并将腿张开吗？

Patient: OK.

病人：好的。

Nurse: I'm going to clean you with some fluid, it might feel a bit cold.

护士：我接下来会用一些液体给你清洗，会感觉有点凉。

Nurse: Please take deep breaths, and breathe out slowly through your mouth.

护士：请深吸一口气，然后慢慢地用嘴呼出来。

Nurse: OK, the catheter is out.

护士：好的。导管取出来了。

Patient: OK, that's a relief!

病人：好了，解放了！

Nurse: Please tell me when you have passed urine normally.

护士：你正常排尿之后请告诉我。

Patient: Shall I just carry on normally or drink lots of water?

病人：我是正常喝水还是要喝很多？

Nurse: Drink some water, but you don't have to drink too much, and please tell me if you can't pass urine and if you are in any discomfort or pain.

护士：喝一些水，但你不需要喝很多。如果你不能正常排尿或者感到不舒服和疼痛，请告诉我。

Patient: How long should I wait to tell you if I don't pass urine?

病人：我多长时间不排尿需要通知你？

Nurse: The normal length of time is about two to three hours.

护士：正常的时间间隔是2～3小时。

Patient: OK, thanks.

病人：好的，谢谢。

**(3)**

**Enema 灌肠**

Nurse: Hello, Miss Smith, you are having your surgery this afternoon, so you will need a bowel prep.

护士：你好，史密斯小姐。你今天下午要进行手术，所以你需要用bowel prep（一种强泻剂）。

Patient: What do you mean by that?

病人: 你什么意思?

Nurse: It means you need to empty your bowels of faeces.

护士: 我指的是你需要将肠里面的粪便排干净。

Patient: How are you going to do that?

病人: 你们打算怎么做?

Nurse: I am going to give you an enema.

护士: 我将对你使用一种灌肠剂。

Patient: Oh, that's not going to be very pleasant.

病人: 哦,感觉很糟糕。

Nurse: Please come with me to the Treatment Room.

护士: 请跟我过来到治疗室。

Patient: OK.

病人: 好的。

Nurse: Miss Smith, please lay down onto your left side with your knees up as far as you can.

护士: 史密斯小姐,请朝左侧躺着,尽量将膝盖抬高。

Patient: This doesn't feel very comfortable.

病人: 这样感觉很不舒服。

Nurse: I am going to insert a small tube into your rectum. Please take a deep breath and breathe out slowly; you might feel some pushing as the fluid enters.

护士: 我将插一根管子到你的直肠。请深呼吸。当液体进入的时候,你会有一定程度的紧压感。

Patient: That feels very uncomfortable.

病人: 感觉太糟糕了。

Nurse: Yes, I know, I'm sorry, but please keep as still as you can.

护士: 我知道,很抱歉,不过请尽量保持别动。

Patient: Well, I'll try, but I don't like it at all.

病人: 好吧,我尽量,不过我真的很不喜欢这样。

Nurse: I have finished, please get up gently, and try and keep the fluid in your bowel as long as possible before you go to the bathroom (toilet).

护士: 我完成了,请慢慢起来。在上厕所前,尽量地让这些药液在你的肠道里停留更多的时间。

Patient: How long do I try to keep it inside before I can go to the toilet?

病人: 我需要让这些药液在身体里停留多久才能上厕所?

Nurse: There is no time, but the longer you can hold the fluid the better the result, but please don't make yourself very uncomfortable.

护士: 没有确定的时间,你让药液在体内停留的时间越长效果越好,当然不要因此太为难自己。

Patient: OK, I'll try to keep it as long as I can, do you want me to tell you when I have been to the toilet?

病人：好的，我会让药液保留的时间尽量的久，当我去完厕所的时候需要告诉你吗？

Nurse：Yes，please tell me when you have emptied your bowels.

护士：是的，你上完厕所之后请告诉我。

Patient：OK，nurse，thanks.

病人：好的，谢谢你，护士小姐。

※ ※ ※

Nurse：We are going to give you an enema. Do you mind?

护士：我们准备给你灌肠，有问题吗？

Patient：No. But I am not constipated. Why do I need it?

病人：没有。不过我并不便秘。为什么给我灌肠？

Nurse：From your chart I know your bowel movement is normal. But we must do it to prepare for your operation.

护士：从你的病历上我知道你排便正常，但这是手术前必须要做的准备工作。

Patient：Why do I need enema before the operation?

病人：手术前为什么要做灌肠呢？

Nurse：It is necessary to flush out intestine in order to keep your bowel clean for the operation.

护士：为了在手术时保持你的肠道清洁，你必须先冲洗一下。

Patient：I see. Where shall we do it?

病人：好。在什么地方做？

Nurse：If you can get up，it is better to have it done in the Treatment Room.

护士：如果你能起床，最好是在治疗室做。

Patient：OK. I'll go with you now.

病人：可以。我现在跟你去。

Nurse：May I help you to put on your clothes?

护士：我帮你穿上衣服好吗？

Patient：Yes. Thank you.

病人：好的。谢谢。

Nurse：But wait. I'll first have to go and get the enema tray and everything else ready. Then I'll come back for you.

护士：但是等一下。我必须先去准备好所有的灌肠用品，再来找你。

(In the Treatment Room)

(在治疗室)

Nurse：Now we are ready. Please lie on your left side.

护士：现在已经准备好。请你左侧位躺下。

Patient：What kind of solution are you using?

病人：你用什么水灌肠？

Nurse：This is soap water. But we often use saline solution，too.

护士：这是肥皂水。但我们也经常用盐水。

Patient：Is the saline enema more comfortable?

病人：盐水灌肠是不是更舒服一些？

Nurse: Yes, it is. But we believe soap water is more effective in your case. However, the relative comfort of an enema depends mainly upon the temperature of the solution and how fast it flows from the bottle. I'll try to hold the bottle in such a way as to keep it from going too fast. Let me know if you feel any discomfort.

护士：是的，但是我们认为肥皂水灌肠对你更适宜。而灌肠是否舒服主要与液体的温度和流入的速度有关。我尽量使液体灌入得慢一些。如果你觉得不舒服就告诉我。

Patient: How much solution is there still left in the bottle? I can't hold much longer.

病人：还有多少液体？我坚持不住了？

Nurse: It will be finished soon. Please take a deep breath with your mouth open. This will help you to hold a little longer.

护士：快要完了。请你张口深呼吸，这样可以使你多坚持一会儿。

Nurse: Now we are through. Try to lie on your back or on the right side for a few minutes. I'll then help you to the toilet.

护士：现在灌肠完毕。你要平卧或右侧卧几分钟，然后我扶你去厕所。

Patient: Thank you. I don't feel so uncomfortable now. So I can go there by myself.

病人：谢谢你。我并没有感到很难受。我可以自己去厕所。

(On the way back to his ward)

(在回病房路上)

Patient: It seems that the enema worked well. It is much better than taking a purge.

病人：灌肠效果很好。比吃泻药好多了。

Nurse: Right. Enema is always better than medicine. It is often given also to relieve constipation caused by long bed rest. Have you ever had your stool examined for parasites?

护士：对。一般来讲，灌肠是比吃药好。长期卧床的便秘病人也常用灌肠法。你查过大便内寄生虫吗？

Patient: Yes. But they didn't find anything.

病人：查过。但是，没发现什么。

Nurse: Fine. Now you can lie down and take a rest. Please call if you need me.

护士：好，现在你可以上床休息了。需要时请叫我。

Patient: Thank you ever so much.

病人：多谢你了。

## (4)

**Taking Blood Specimens 取血样**

Nurse: Mrs. Smith, the doctor needs you to have some blood tests, so I will need to take some blood from you.

护士：史密斯夫人，医生需要做些血液检测，所以我过来取些血样。

Patient: Why does the doctor need more tests, what are they for?

病人：为什么医生又需要做血液检测？检测什么？

Nurse: The doctor would like a blood sugar and liver function test to help him in his diagnosis.

护士：医生想做一下血糖和肝功能检测以帮助诊断。

Patient: Oh, OK, I guess.

病人：哦，我想可以吧。

Nurse: Please come with me to the Treatment Room.

护士：请跟我来治疗室。

Nurse: I am going to take the specimen (sample) from your arm, I'm going to put a tourniquet around your upper arm it will feel tight.

护士：我将从你的手臂部取些血样，我接下来要在你的上臂放压脉器，会感觉有点紧。

Patient: OK.

病人：好的。

Nurse: Please open and close your hand for me, I'm just going to clean the skin, you will feel a slight prick, please try and stay still.

护士：请松开然后握紧你的手。我接下来给你清洁皮肤，(针管插入时)你会感觉有点刺痛，请尽量不要动。

Nurse: Please bend your arm for me and leave it like that for a few minutes.

护士：请弯着你的手臂，保持这个姿势几分钟。

Patient: When will you get the results?

病人：结果什么时候能出来？

Nurse: The results will be back in a couple of hours, the doctor will tell you the results as soon as they are here.

护士：结果两个小时后出来，结果一出来医生就会告诉你。

Patient: OK, thanks very much!

病人：好的，非常感谢！

## (5)

**Intravenous Fluids 静脉输液**

Nurse: Miss Smith, the doctor has said you need to have intravenous fluids.

护士：史密斯小姐，医生说你需要输液。

Patient: Yes, he told me, he said you would put a cannula in my arm and give me intravenous fluids.

病人：是的，他告诉过我。他说你需要接一个套管到我的手臂处给我输液。

Nurse: Yes, I have come to insert cannula into your vein and give you some fluids.

护士：是的，我过来给你的血管插入套管进行输液。

Patient: Are you going to do it here?

病人：你是在这里进行吗？

Nurse: No, please come with me to the Treatment Room.

护士：不，请跟我到治疗室。

Patient: Where are you going to put the cannula?

病人： 你将要把套管接到什么地方？

Nurse： I will put it in your wrist.

护士： 我会接到你的手腕处。

Patient： OK.

病人： 好的。

Nurse： I am going to put a tourniquet around your arm it will feel tight，you will feel a small prick and some pressure，please try and keep still.

护士： 我接下来要绑一个止血带到你的手臂处。你会感觉有点紧、有点疼和压迫感，请尽量保持不要动。

Nurse： OK，I've finished，I will secure this with a dressing so it doesn't come out and I am going to attach the intravenous tubing.

护士： 好的，我完成了。我会放敷料来防止它掉出来。接下来我要将它连接到输液管上。

Patient： OK，nurse，thanks，how long do I need to have intravenous fluids for?

病人： 好的，谢谢你，护士小姐。我需要输液多长时间？

Nurse： The doctor has prescribed intravenous fluids for the next 3 days.

护士： 医生给你开的是三天的量。

Patient： Can I still walk around?

病人： 我还能到处走动吗？

Nurse： Yes，you can walk around with a drip stand.

护士： 可以。你可以举着输液架走动。

Patient： What fluid has the doctor prescribed?

病人： 医生给开的是什么药液？

Nurse： The intravenous fluids the doctor has prescribed is called dextrose & saline（glucose & saline）.

护士： 医生给你开静脉滴注液是"葡萄糖盐水"。

Patient： OK，nurse，thanks.

病人： 好的，谢谢你，护士小姐。

## （6）

**Cleaning，Dressing & Checking of Wounds　清洗、敷料处理和检查伤口**

Nurse： Good morning，Mrs. Jones，I need to check your dressing today.

护士： 早上好，琼斯夫人。我今天需要检查你的敷料。

Patient： OK，nurse.

病人： 好的，护士小姐。

Nurse： Please can I see your dressing，does it need changing?

护士： 请问我能看看你的敷料需要更换吗？

Patient： No，it seems OK.

病人： 不用，看起来还行。

Nurse： Please come to the Treatment Room with me.

护士：　请跟我来治疗室。

Nurse：　Please lay on the examination couch and lift up your clothes.

护士：　请躺在检查床上，把衣服往上拉起来。

Nurse：　Does your wound feel comfortable?

护士：　你的伤口感觉舒服吗？

Patient：　Yes，it feels fine.

病人：　是的，感觉很好。

Nurse：　Your wound looks OK，I will just put a dry dressing on that，the doctor will come and have a look at your wound later today.

护士：　你的伤口看起来还行。我会放些干敷料在上面，医生今天过些时候会过来看你。

Patient：　OK，nurse，thanks.

病人：　好的，谢谢你，护士小姐。

Nurse：　Please don't get your dressing wet.

护士：　请不要弄湿你的敷料。

Patient：　No，I make sure I don't.

病人：　不会，我保证不会。

（7）

**Removal of Drainage Tube　引流管移除**

Nurse：　Hello，Mrs. Jones，I am going to remove your drainage tube today.

护士：　你好，琼斯夫人。我今天将移除你的引流管。

Patient：　OK，do I need to go to the Treatment Room with you?

病人：　好的，我需要跟你到治疗室吗？

Nurse：　Yes，please，come with me.

护士：　是的，请跟我来。

Nurse：　Please lay on the examination couch，and lift up your clothes，I am going to clean the area with disinfectant，it might feel cold.

护士：　请躺在检查床上，将衣服撩起来。我接下来要用消毒剂给你清洗，会感觉有点凉。

Patient：　Oh，yes，that's cold.

哦，是的，很凉。

Nurse：　OK，please take a deep breath and breathe out slowly as I take the tube out.

护士：　好了。当我移除的时候请深呼吸。

Patient：　That feels really uncomfortable.

病人：　感觉很不舒服。

Nurse：　OK，I've finished now，I will just put a dry dressing on that. Please let me know if starts leaking.

护士：　好的，我完成了。我会给你放些敷料。如果有渗透，请告诉我。

Patient：　OK，thanks nurse.

病人：　好的，谢谢你，护士小姐。

## （8）

**Assisting a Doctor in an Angioplasty 协助医生进行血管成形术**

Nurse: Hello, my name is Nurse Li DeHong, please call me Linda. What is your name?

护士：你好，我是李德红护士，请叫我琳达护士，你怎么称呼？

Patient: Hello, my name is Mary Smith.

病人：我叫玛丽.史密斯。

Nurse: Hello, Mary, you are here to have a Catheter procedure, because the doctor in the Emergency Room has diagnosed a problem with the veins to your heart. How are you feeling now?

护士：你好，玛丽。你来这里接受导管插入，因为急诊室的医生诊断出连接你的心脏的血管有问题。你现在感觉怎么样？

Patient: I feel dizzy, tired and have chest pain, And I'm feeling a little nervous.

病人：我感觉眩晕、疲惫、胸口痛，除此之外，我还感觉紧张。

Nurse: How long have you had the chest pain?

护士：你胸痛多长时间了？

Patient: About ten minutes.

病人：大约10分钟。

Nurse: Is the pain radiating to your shoulder? Is the pain in your shoulder or down your arm?

护士：疼痛辐射到你的肩膀处吗？肩膀还是腋下？

Patient: Yes, in my shoulder.

病人：是啊，在肩膀。

Nurse: This emergency procedure has to be done now. Please can you sign this consent form giving us permission to perform the catheter procedure.

护士：这个紧急手术必须现在进行。请问你能在手术同意书上面签字允许我们进行导管插入吗？

Patient: Yes, OK, what happens now?

病人：是的，可以。接下来会发生什么？

Nurse: Please take off all your clothes and put on this gown, the ties need to be at the front.

护士：请将所有衣服脱掉换上这件袍子，朝前系带。

Nurse: Please give all your valuables to your husband for safe keeping.

护士：请将你值钱的东西交给丈夫保管。

Then lay down on this couch and try to relax.

然后躺在床上，尽量地放松。

Roll up your sleeve, I need to take your pulse, blood pressure and take an ECG. I will put these pads on your chest.

请将袖子卷起来，我需要量一下你的脉搏、血压和做心电图检测。我接下来将把这些电极片放在你胸上。

I am going to put this peg on your finger, this takes your pulse, it is not heavy and it doesn't hurt.

我把这个指套放在你的手指上，这是用来量脉搏的。指套不会太重，也不疼。

Patient: How long will this procedure take?

病人：手术要持续多久？

Nurse: The operation takes about half an hour.

护士：手术大概需要持续半小时。

I need to give you intravenous fluids, so I need to put a cannula into your hand.

我需要给你输液，所以我需要将套管连接到你的手上。

I'm going to put a tourniquet on your arm, it will feel tight.

我接下来给你绑止血带，会感觉有点紧。

Please open and close your hand.

请松开然后握紧你的手。

You will feel a slight prick.

你会感觉稍微有点疼。

Please stay still.

请不要动。

I will put a dressing on this.

我会在上面放敷料。

I am going to attach some intravenous fluids now and give you some oxygen, please put this oxygen mask over your face. Does that feel comfortable?

我接下来要给你输液和供氧，请将这个氧气罩戴上。感觉舒服吗？

Patient: Yes, thank you. What is the intravenous fluid that you are giving me?

病人：是的，谢谢。你给我的静脉滴注什么液？

Nurse: Glucose Saline.

护士：葡萄糖盐水。

Nurse: This is Dr. Wang, he is going to do your catheterization, he is just getting the equipment ready.

护士：这是王医生，他是来给你做导管插入术的，他现在在准备所用的仪器。

Nurse: The Emergency Room nurse has already shaved you.

护士：急诊室的护士已经给你刮过毛了。

The doctor is going to clean your skin, the fluid is very cold.

医生接下来要清洗你的皮肤，会有点凉。

He is going to give you a local anesthetic, you will feel a sharp prick, but it will go away very quickly.

他接下来给你进行局部麻醉，你会感觉到有些刺痛，但是很快就会消失。

He will then insert a catheter into your artery, and send it to your heart.

他会插入一根管子到你的动脉，并送到你的心脏处。

The equipment is needed, so he can see what is happening.

这仪器很必要，这样他可以清楚看到发生的事情。

If you feel any sharp pain tell us, and the doctor can give you some more local anesthetic.

如果你感到疼痛请告诉我，医生会给你更多的局部麻醉。

The doctor has finished now. He is now putting pressure onto your wound to stop the bleeding, this will be for about fifteen minutes.

医生已经完成了。他现在要压着你的伤口以阻止流血，这个过程大概需要 15 分钟。

Are you OK?

你还好吗？

Patient: Yes, thank you.

病人：是的，谢谢。

Nurse: I will put a dressing on this for you.

护士：我在这上面放些敷料。

We will help you to get onto a bed.

我们会帮助你回到床上。

And we will take you to get you to the ward.

我们会带你回到病房。

Patient: How long will I be in hospital?

病人：我需要住院多久？

Nurse: You will have to stay for about three days for anti-coagulation treatment, IV antibiotics, chest X-ray and an ECG check.

护士：你需要留院 3 天接受抗凝结治疗、静脉抗生素输液、胸部 X 线检查和心电图检测等。

Patient: OK, thanks very much for all your help and kindness.

病人：好的，非常感谢你的热心帮助。

Nurse: Please, it was no problem. I hope you get better soon.

护士：不客气。我希望你尽快康复。

**(9)**

**Lumbar Puncture 腰椎穿刺**

Nurse: Mrs. Smith, the doctor needs to do a lumbar puncture procedure to get some spinal fluid for tests.

护士：史密斯夫人，医生需要对你进行腰椎穿刺手术来取一些脊髓液进行检测。

Patient: Oh, when does he want to do the test?

病人：哦，他想什么时候进行检测？

Nurse: He is going to do it now, please come with me to the Treatment Room.

护士：他想现在做。请跟着我到治疗室。

Patient: OK.

病人：好的。

Nurse: Mrs. Smith, please lay on the couch, and will you turn onto your left side and bend your knees as far as you can.

护士：史密斯夫人，请左侧位躺在床上，膝盖尽可能地弯曲。

Patient: This feels uncomfortable.

病人：这样感觉很不舒服。

Nurse: Please will you bend you head to touch your chest as far as you can? I will put a pillow under your head, so it is more comfortable.

护士：请问你能尽量地低头碰你的胸部吗？我会在你的头下面垫个枕头，这样会舒服很多。

Patient: Nurse, this really does feel very uncomfortable.

病人：护士小姐，这样真的很不舒服。

Nurse: Yes, I know. I'm very sorry, but the doctor needs your back curved as much as possible.

护士：是的，我知道。很抱歉，不过医生需要你的背尽量地弯曲。

Patient: Yes, I do understand. But it is difficult to stay like this.

病人：是的，我明白。但是这样很难保持。

Nurse: The doctor is going to clean your skin with an antiseptic, it will feel very cold.

护士：医生接下来会用杀菌剂清洁你的皮肤，会感觉很凉。

He is putting a clean towel on your back, please do not touch it.

他接下来会放一条毛巾在你的背部，请不要碰它。

He is going to start the procedure now, he is going to give you a local anesthetic, you will feel a sharp prick, please try not to move.

他接下来要给你进行局部麻醉，你会感觉很疼，请不要动。

You will feel the doctor pushing and putting pressure on your back, if you feel any pain please tell me and I will ask the doctor to give you some more local anesthetic.

你会感觉到医生在用力地压着你的背，如果你感到任何程度的疼痛，请告诉我。我会告诉医生给你进行更多的局部麻醉。

Patient: Has he finished now? I don't think I can stay like this for much longer.

病人：他完成了吗？我想这个姿势我坚持不下去了。

Nurse: The doctor has finished now, he is just going to put a dressing on your back.

护士：医生完成了，他现在给你背部放敷料。

Patient: Thank goodness.

病人：谢天谢地。

Nurse: Please roll back onto your back.

护士：请转过来平躺着。

Nurse: You will need to stay in bed for twelve hours with no pillow, if you try to sit up, you will have a very severe headache.

护士：你需要不枕枕头地平躺 12 个小时，请不要坐起来，如果你尝试坐起来，你会有严重的头疼。

Patient: What happens if I need to go to the toilet or need a drink or something?

病人：如果我要上厕所或者喝东西要怎么办？

Nurse: If you need anything, please ring for a nurse.

护士：如果你需要什么东西，请呼叫护士。

Patient：When will you know the results?

病人：结果什么时候出来？

Nurse：Your test will be back later today，the doctor will come and tell you the result.

护士：你的化验结果今天晚些时候出来，医生会过来告诉你结果。

Patient：OK，thanks very much.

病人：好的，非常感谢。

## （10）

**Intensive Care Unit　监护室**

Nurse：Dr. Wang，the condition of that patient is very poor. He's so excited，I can't quiet him down.

护士：王医生，那个病人情况不好。他躁动得厉害。我不能使他安静下来。

Doctor：I'm afraid he will be in a state of shock. It's necessary to take his pulse，respiratory rate and blood pressure regularly.

医生：恐怕他进入早期休克了，要定期测量他的脉搏、呼吸和血压。

Nurse：All right. I'll take them every hour.

护士：好，我每小时测一次。

Doctor：No，you'd better take them half an hour.

医生：不，最好半小时测一次。

Nurse：His blood pressure is eighty six over fifty mmHg and he has rapid pulse and respiratory rate.

护士：他的血压86/50 mmHg，脉搏及呼吸加速。

Doctor：Place the patient in the head-low position. Elevate the foot of the bed. Put hot water bottles around him. Telephone to the blood bank to ask whether there is blood available for this patient. His blood is type O. I'll give him a blood transfusion.

医生：将病人置于头低位，抬高床腿。患者身旁放些热水袋。电话问一下有没有合适的血，他是O型血。我准备给他输血。

Nurse：What if there is no type O blood available for him?

护士：如果没有O型血怎么办？

Doctor：In that case，please tell the patient's relatives to donate blood to him.

医生：若那样，就通知病人亲属给他献血。

Nurse：Is oxygen given?

护士：吸氧吗？

Doctor：Yes，of course. The patient's condition is very critical and his life is in danger，but we'll do everything possible to save him. Head nurse，please get the emergency drugs ready as soon as possible.

医生：当然要吸氧。患者病情危重，有死亡的危险。我们要尽一切努力抢救他。护士长，请尽快把急救药品准备好。

Head Nurse：All right，I'll do so. What else?

护士长： 好，我会照办的。还有其他吩咐吗？

Doctor： You'd better arrange special nursing care for him.

医生： 最好给他安排个特护。

Head Nurse： It is what I want to say.

护士长： 我也是这个意思。

Doctor： You should notice whether the patient is conscious or not and differentiation of his pupils，recording the volume of urine and other fluid in or out of his body accurately.

医生： 你们要注意观察病人的意识状态和瞳孔变化，准确记录尿量及其他液体出入量。

Nurse： I'll do it well.

护士： 我会干好的。

Doctor： Keeping his respiratory tract through，abstracting sputa from air way regularly，measuring his blood pressure in time，especially after noradrenaline or dopamine is given.

医生： 保持呼吸道通畅，定时吸痰，及时测量血压，特别是在用去甲肾上腺素或多巴胺后要注意监测。

Head Nurse： We'll clean his oral cavity twice a day and his eyes once a day.

护士长： 我们每天得做两次口腔清洁护理和一次眼部护理。

Doctor： It is skin that is the most important thing. You manage to protect him from bedsore occurring. Besides these，we should maintain the balance of three kinds of nourishing elements，water and electrolytes in his body. There are a lot of things for us to do.

医生： 最重要的是皮肤，你们要设法防止发生褥疮。此外，要维持病人体内的三大营养素和水电解质平衡。要做的事很多。

Nurse： Hope he would come to soon.

护士： 希望他会很快醒来。

## (11)

**Oxygen Delivery 给氧**

Prof. Chang： ...In short，oxygen is one of the most frequently ordered drugs for patients with a variety of disorders. Therefore，oxygen delivery is worth your much attention. Is there any question?

常教授： ……总之，对多种疾病的病人来说，氧气是最常用的药物之一。所以你们对给氧应给予足够的重视。有什么问题吗？

Student A： What should low-flow oxygen administration be applied to patients with chronic lung disease?

学生甲： 为什么治疗慢性肺疾病患者必须用低流量给氧？

Prof. Chang： A good question! Those patients usually have chronic $CO_2$ retention，they rely more on the hypoxemia stimulus to breathe whereas normal people utilize the

$CO_2$ mediated one. Too much oxygen may remove the hypoxic drive.

常教授：问得好！这些病人通常都有 $CO_2$ 滞留，正常人靠 $CO_2$ 刺激呼吸，而他们则更多地靠低氧血症来刺激呼吸，过多地给氧可能会消除这种低氧刺激。

Student B：It seems that all drugs have some kind of side effects. Does oxygen follow the same rule?

学生乙：所有的药物似乎都有副作用，氧气也有吗？

Prof. Chang：Certainly. Abuse of oxygen may cause hypoventilation and absorption atelectasis. So you should keep in your mind the dictum"Use the least oxygen to gain acceptable goal".

常教授：当然。氧气滥用有可能导致肺换气不足与吸收性肺不张，所以请记住这句格言"用最少的氧气达到可接受的目标"。

Student C：Then，how should oxygen administration be monitored?

学生丙：那么，给氧该如何监测呢？

Prof. Chang：Thanks to the advances in medical sciences，oxygen delivery is no longer empirical. Arterial blood gas analysis helps doctors to be more scientific in oxygen delivery.

常教授：由于医学科学的进步，给氧已不再是经验性的，动脉血气分析使得医生在氧疗中能做得更科学。

Prof. Chang：Any more question? Now Sister Li is going to give you a demonstration of oxygen administration.

常教授：还有问题吗？下面李护士长将为大家做给氧示范。

（Sister Li demonstrated the procedures for oxygen delivery.）

（李护士长演示了给氧方法。）

Student D：Sister Li. How shall we decide the proper depth a nasal cannula is to be inserted?

学生丁：李护士长，鼻导管进入的深度怎么确定呢？

Sister Li：The distance from nose to ear is usually considered as a proper indication of depth a nasal cannula should enter.

李护士：通常认为耳鼻间距是鼻导管插入深度的一适宜指标。

# 13. Collecting Medical History

# 采集病史

## A. Sentences Commonly Used 常用语

1. Do you have any existing medical health problems?
   你现在有什么已经确诊的病？
2. Are you on any medication for existing health problems?
   针对身体健康情况，你现在是否在吃什么药？
3. How often do you have to take it?
   多久吃一次药？
4. How long have you been taking your medication for these problems?
   你吃这药有多久了？
5. Are you taking any other medication for any reason?（e.g. birth control/ vitamins）
   除此之外，你还因为别的原因吃其他的药吗？（例如：避孕药、维生素之类）
6. Have you had any illnesses or physical problems recently（in the last year）?
   最近（过去一年）你得过什么病或身体有什么问题吗？
7. Have you had any infections or viruses recently?
   你最近是否受过什么感染或病毒侵袭？
8. Do you have a family history of diabetes / heart problems/ canner / lung complains?
   家庭中是否有糖尿病、心脏病、癌症或呼吸疾病的病史？
9. Are your vaccinations current?
   你在疫苗有效期内吗？
10. Have you ever had any surgery? What for?
    你进行过什么手术吗？因为什么原因动手术？
11. Do you have any allergies?
    你对什么过敏？
12. Have you had any medical tests recently?
    你最近是否进行过什么化验检查？
13. Is there anything you need to tell me，that you think will be useful?
    你觉得还有哪些对病情有用的信息可以提供给我？
14. Have you had any children? Were there any complication?
    你有孩子吗？怀孕期间有什么并发症？

15. I need to take your temperature, blood pressure, pulse, your weight and height.
    我需要量你的体温、血压、脉搏、体重和身高。
16. Have you had any fever?
    你发热了吗？
17. Was your temperature been taken?
    你量过体温了吗？
18. Do you have your blood pressure checked regularly?
    你是否经常量血压？
19. How much do you weigh? What is your weight?
    你的体重是多少？
20. Has your weight changed recently?
    最近你的体重有没有变化？
21. Have you gained any weight lately?
    你近来体重增加了吗？
22. How much did you weight last year?
    你去年的体重是多少？
23. How frequently do you have influenza?
    你多久患一次流感？
24. Have you been with anyone who has a cold?
    你与患感冒的人接触过吗？
25. Have you had a cold recently?
    你最近患过感冒吗？
26. Have you noticed any hair loss?
    你注意到有没有脱发现象？
27. How often do you have headaches?
    你多久头痛一次？
28. Have you ever had a head injury?
    你的头部受过外伤吗？
29. Have you ever been unconscious from an injury?
    你有过外伤所致的意识丧失吗？
30. Have you ever fainted?
    你晕过吗？
31. Have you ever been paralyzed?
    你曾经瘫痪过吗？
32. Have you ever passed out?
    你曾有过不省人事的现象吗？
33. Have you had any trouble (problems) with your eyes?
    你得过什么眼病没有？
34. Do you have any vision problems?
    你有什么视力问题吗？

35. Are you near-sighted or far–sighted?
你近视还是远视？
36. Do you wear glasses or contact lenses?
你戴眼镜或隐形眼镜吗？
37. Do you have trouble seeing at night?
夜里你的视力有问题吗？
38. Is your mouth dry?
你口干吗？
39. Do you have a stuffy nose?
你鼻子不通气吗？
40. Do you have nosebleed?
你流鼻血吗？
41. How are your teeth?
你的牙齿好吗？
42. Do your gums bleed when you brush?
你刷牙的时候牙龈出血吗？
43. Do you have any loosen teeth?
你有松动的牙齿吗？
44. Do you have wisdom teeth?
你长智齿了吗？
45. Do you wear dentures?
你戴假牙 / 义齿吗？
46. How often do you see the dentist?
你多长时间去看一次牙医？
47. When did you last see a dentist?
你上次去看牙医是什么时候？
48. How is your hearing?
你的听力好吗？
49. Do you have a rough throat?
你嗓音粗哑吗？
50. How long have you had hoarseness?
你声音嘶哑有多长时间了？
51. Do you have pain or stiffness in your neck?
你有颈项痛或颈项强直吗？
52. Have you ever had any heart trouble?
你得过心脏病吗？
53. Have you ever had a murmur?
你有过心脏杂音吗？
54. Do you want another pillow at night?
你睡觉时要垫高枕头吗？

55. Have you ever needed to sit up to breathe at night?
你曾经有过夜里需要端坐才能呼吸的情况吗？
56. Have you ever had asthma?
你得过哮喘吗？
57. Do you have shortness of breath?
你气短吗？
58. Do you have trouble breathing?
你的呼吸有问题吗？
59. Do you have any trouble with your chest?
你胸部有毛病吗？
60. Have you been coughing lately?
最近你咳嗽吗？
61. Have you ever coughed up blood?
你咳出过血吗？
62. Do you bleed easily?
你是否容易出血？
63. Have you ever had a blood transfusion?
你曾经输过血吗？
64. Do you have any trouble with urinating?
你排尿有什么困难吗？
65. Do you often wake up in the middle of the night to urinate?
你经常半夜起来小便吗？
66. How many times do you get up to urinate at night?
夜里你要起来排几次小便？
67. How often do you have a bowel movement?
你多久排一次大便？
68. When did you last have your bowels opened?
你最近一次排便是什么时侯？
69. Do you have difficult with passage of stools?
你解大便有困难吗？
70. Has there been a change in your bowels?
你的大便有异常吗？
71. Does your motion have any blood in it?
大便有血吗？
72. Have you ever had blood in your stools?
你曾有过大便带血的现象吗？
73. Is there any blood or mucus in the stool?
大便里有血或者黏液吗？
74. Have you ever had a fracture?
你曾经骨折过吗？

75. Do your hands shake?
    你的手抖吗？
76. Do your feet swell?
    你的脚肿吗？
77. Is your menstrual period regular?
    你的月经有规律吗？
78. At what age did you start having periods?
    你初潮时是在什么年龄？

**Cough 咳嗽**

79. How long have you had this cough?
    你咳嗽多久了？
80. Does it hurt your chest when you cough?
    当你咳嗽的时候，胸口疼吗？
81. Does your chest hurt when you breathe in and out（inspire，expire）?
    当你吸气和呼气的时候，胸口疼吗？
82. Do you have any sputum when you cough?
    你咳嗽的时候有痰吗？
83. What is it like，what color is it?
    是怎么样的？什么颜色的？
84. I need to take your temperature，pulse and B/P.
    我需要量一下你的体温、脉搏和血压。
85. The doctor says you need to have an X-ray of your chest and some blood tests.
    医生说你需要做胸透和血液检测。
86. The doctor has prescribed some medication for you.
    医生给你开了处方。
87. You need to take this medication for...days.
    你需要吃一个疗程……天。

**Diarrhea 腹泻**

88. How long have you had diarrhea?
    你腹泻多久了？
89. How many times have you had diarrhea today?
    你今天拉几次？
90. Is there any blood in your stools?
    粪便中带血吗？
91. What do your stools look like?
    你的粪便是什么形状的？
92. Do they smell?
    发臭吗？
93. Do you have any pain when you have diarrhea?
    你拉肚子的时候痛吗？

94. What kind of pain do you have?
是什么样的痛?
95. Where do you have the pain?
在什么地方痛?
96. Have you vomited?
你呕吐了吗?
97. How many times have you vomited?
你呕吐了几次?
98. Are you able to eat anything?
你现在能吃东西吗?
99. Are you able to drink fluids?
你现在能喝东西吗?
100. Do you feel weak and dizzy?
你感到虚弱和头晕吗?
101. Do you feel as if you have a fever or a headache?
你感觉好像是发烧或头痛吗?
102. Do you feel dehydrated?
你有脱水的感觉吗?
103. I need to examine you.
让我检查一下。
104. The doctor needs a specimen of your stools. Here is a specimen bottle.
医生需要你的粪便样本。给你标本瓶。
105. The doctor says you will need some blood tests.
医生说你需要做一下血液检测。
106. I need to take you to the X-ray department/ the Ultra-scan Department.
我要带你去放射科 / 超声波扫描室。
107. When the Doctor has the results, he will come and see you.
结果出来后,医生会过来看你。
108. The doctor says you will need intravenous fluids, I will show you where to go.
医生说你需要进行静脉输液,我带你过去。
109. The doctor says you must take fluids, and just have a light diet until you feel better.
医生说你需要吃流食,在好之前都要吃容易消化的食物。

**Abdominal Pain 腹痛**

110. How long have you had abdominal pain?
你腹痛多长时间了?
111. Where is it, can you show me?
是什么位置,你能指给我看吗?
112. How painful is it?
有多痛?
113. Did the pain start there or somewhere else?

是这里开始痛还是别的什么地方？

114. Does it hurt more if you move?
你动的时候疼痛加剧吗？
115. Do you feel that you have a fever?
你觉得发烧吗？
116. I need to take your temperature, pulse and B/P.
我要量一下你的体温、脉搏和血压。
117. Are you passing urine OK?
你排尿正常吗？
118. What does your urine look like?
你的尿液是怎样的？
119. Have you had your bowels open?
你大便了吗？
120. Are you menstruating (bleeding/ having a period)? Is it normal? (female only)
你是在月经期间吗？你的月经正常吗？(专指女性)
121. Have you vomited?
你呕吐吗？
122. What does it look like?
呕吐物怎么样的？
123. Have you been able to eat and drink anything?
你能正常进食吗？
124. Do you get the pain after eating or drinking?
吃饭或喝东西后都会痛吗？
125. Show me where it hurts?
请指给我看哪里痛。
126. I will tell the doctor, he will come and see you.
我会告诉医生，一会他会过来看你。

**Headache 头痛**

127. How long have you had your headache?
你头痛多长时间了？
128. Where does it hurt?
什么时候痛？
129. What does the pain feel like?
是怎样的一种痛？
130. Does your neck feel stiff?
你脖子感到僵硬吗？
131. Can you move and bend your neck?
你能转动和低头吗？
132. Can you touch your chest with your chin?
你能用下巴碰你的胸吗？

133. Does bright lights (photophobia) hurt your eyes and make your headache worse?
明亮的光线会让你眼睛疼痛并使头痛加剧吗？（畏光症）
134. Do you have a rash on your arms, legs or body?
你的手臂、腿部和身体有没有皮疹？
135. Do you have a fever?
你发烧吗？
136. Do you have any other symptoms?
你还有其他症状吗？
137. Do you suffer from migraines?
你是否有偏头痛？
138. Are you upset or stressed in any way?
你感到某种程度的烦恼或者压抑吗？
139. Have you vomited?
你呕吐了吗？
140. I need to take your temperature, pulse and B/P.
我要量一下你的体温、脉搏和血压。
141. I will tell the doctor you have a headache.
我会告诉医生你有头痛。
142. The doctor has prescribed some pain relief for you.
医生给你开了些止痛药。
143. If the pain doesn't go away, please let me know.
如果疼痛没有消失请告诉我。

**Eczema 湿疹**

144. How long has this been a problem?
问题出现有多久了？
145. Where did it start, on which part of the body?
从哪里开始的，身体的哪个部位？
146. Has it spread?
是否扩散？
147. Where did it spread to?
蔓延到什么地方了？
148. What does it look like when it is at its worse?
严重的时候看起来是怎样的？
149. Is it very itchy and sore?
痒和痛吗？
150. Do you take any medication or use any creams or ointments?
你吃过什么药和擦过什么药膏吗？
151. What diet are you on?
你平时饮食吃些什么？
152. The doctor has asked me to take a swab specimen from your skin. It won't hurt.

医生告诉我要取一些你的皮肤拭子样本。这样做不痛。

153. The doctor needs a blood and urine sample.
医生需要做血液和尿液检测。

154. The doctor will come and tell you the results.
医生会过来告诉你结果。

155. The doctor will prescribe medication for you.
医生会给你开处方药。

**Sprains and Fracture 扭伤和骨折**

156. Show me where it hurts.
指给我看哪里痛。

157. How did you do this?
你怎么弄成这样的？

158. How painful is it?
有多痛？

159. Can you move it?
你能移动那个部位吗？

160. Is your foot swollen?
你的脚肿吗？

161. Are your fingers swollen?
你的手指肿吗？

162. Can you feel your toes?
你的脚趾有知觉吗？

163. Can you feel your fingers?
你的手指有知觉吗？

164. Do you have any pins and needles or tingling?
你是否感到刺痛或麻痹？

165. You need to have a bandage.
你需要绑绷带。

166. You need to have a plaster cast.
你需要绑石膏绷带。

167. Your arm needs to be in a sling; you must keep it on for...days.
你的手臂需要用三角绷带固定……天。

168. You need an operation on your...
你需要做……手术。

169. The doctor will need to admit you into hospital.
医生需要你住院。

170. Here is the form, I will show you where you have to go.
这是(住院)表，我会带你过去办理。

171. You will need crutches to walk.
你要用拐杖帮助走路。

172. You must rest as much as you can.
你必须尽可能多的休息。
173. Do not walk on your foot，keep it elevated as much as you can.
不要让脚碰地走路，尽可能保持脚抬着。
174. The doctor has prescribed medication for your pain.
医生给你开了止痛药。
175. You need to come back here in...days.
……天后你需要回来复查。

**Health History 既往史**

176. Are your usually in good health?
你一向健康吗？
177. What disease have you had before?
你过去患过什么病吗？
178. Do you have any medical problems?
你有什么健康问题吗？
179. Please tell me something of your past illness.
请告诉我你过去生病的一些情况。
180. Did you have any childhood diseases?
你以前得过什么儿童疾病吗？
181. What kind of treatment did you have in the past?
你以前曾做过什么治疗吗？
182. Did you have any operation before?
你过去做过手术没有？
183. Have you ever been hospitalized before?
你以前住过院吗？

**Medicine Taken 服药史**

184. Are you taking any medicine now?
你现在服什么药吗？
185. What kind of medicine are you taking for the problem?
你在服什么药治疗这种病？
186. Did you take any medicine?
你吃过什么药没有？
187. Do you remember to take your medicine?
你记得吃药吗？
188. What kind of vaccination did you receive?
你打过什么预防针吗？
189. What medicines have you been using (taking)?
你一直在用/吃什么药？
190. Have you been taking the tables regularly?
你是按时服这种药片的吗？

191. To what medicine are you allergic?
你对什么药物过敏吗？
192. Are you allergic to any medicine?
你对什么药过敏吗？
193. Do you take aspirin?
你服阿司匹林吗？
194. Do you take sleeping pills?
你吃安眠药吗？
195. Have you taken any medicine for the pain?
你服过什么止痛药吗？
196. Do you use laxatives?
你吃泻药吗？
197. When did you stop taking the medicine?
你什么时候停服这种药的？

**Family History 家族史**

198. Now, I wound like to ask you some questions about your family.
现在，我想问一些有关你的家庭的问题。
199. Tell me something about your family, please.
请告诉我一些有关你的家庭的事情。
200. What sort of problems is your father having?
你父亲有什么病吗？
201. Are your parents still living?
你的父母还健在吗？
202. Is you father / mother living? How is his /her health?
你的父亲 / 母亲还在吗？他 / 她的健康如何？
203. How old was your father when he died?
你父亲去世的时候多大年纪了？
204. What was the cause of his death?
他是因为什么去世的？
205. Are there illnesses that seem to run in your family?
你的家里有什么遗传疾病吗？
206. Were your mother /father and their parents related by blood?
你的父母和祖父母是近亲结婚吗？
207. Does anyone in your family smoke?
你家里有人抽烟吗？
208. Does anyone in your family suffer from asthma?
你家里有人患哮喘病吗？
209. Has anyone in your family been seriously ill?
你的家人中有人得过重病吗？
210. Has anyone in your family had breast cancer?
你的家人中有没有人得过乳腺癌？

211. Has anyone in your family had the same trouble?
你家里有人得过这种病吗？
212. Is there any relative who has an unusual disease?
你有没有什么亲戚得了罕见的疾病？
213. Is there any relative who died from any unusual condition?
你有没有什么亲戚非正常死亡？

## B. Situational Conversation（情景会话）

### （1）

**Cough　咳嗽**

Nurse： How long have you had this cough?
护士： 你咳嗽多长时间了？
Patient： It started this morning.
病人： 今天早上开始的。
Nurse： What does your cough sound like?
护士： 你咳嗽起来声音是什么样的？
Patient： It sounds chesty.
病人： 呼吸音粗糙。
Nurse： Does it hurt your chest when you cough?
护士： 你咳嗽的时候胸口痛吗？
Patient： Yes，it does.
病人： 是的。
Nurse： Does your chest hurt when you breathe in and out（inspire，expire）?
护士： 当你吸气或呼气的时候痛吗？
Patient： It hurts when I breathe in.
病人： 当我吸气的时候会痛。
Nurse： Do you have any sputum when you cough?
护士： 你咳嗽的时候有痰吗？
Patient： No，not really just a little bit.
病人： 没有，仅仅是一点点。
Nurse： I need to take your temperature，pulse and B/P.
护士： 我需要量一下你的体温、脉搏和血压。
Nurse： I will tell the doctor how you are feeling.
护士： 我会告诉医生你的情况。

### （2）

**Diarrhea　腹泻**

Patient： Nurse，I have had diarrhea this morning.

病人：护士小姐，我早上拉肚子。
Nurse：How long have you had diarrhea?
护士：拉肚子有多长时间了？
Patient：Since I woke up this morning.
病人：早晨起来开始。
Nurse：How many times have you had diarrhea?
护士：你拉了多少次？
Patient：About three times.
病人：有3次了。
Nurse：Is there any blood in your stools?
护士：你的粪便带血吗？
Patient：No.
病人：没有。
Nurse：What do your stools look like?
护士：你的粪便是怎么样的？
Patient：Light brown and runny.
病人：浅棕色的，有点松软。
Nurse：Do they smell?
护士：发臭吗？
Patient：Just a bit.
病人：有一点点。
Nurse：Do you have any pain when you have diarrhea?
护士：当你拉肚子的时候伴随疼痛吗？
Patient：Yes，just before I want to go to the toilet.
病人：是的，上厕所之前感到痛。
Nurse：What kind of pain do you have?
护士：是怎样的一种痛？
Patient：It's a kind of griping pain.
病人：是一种夹痛。
Nurse：OK. I'll tell the doctor，he will come and see you.
护士：好的，我会告诉医生，他一会过来看你。

※ ※ ※

Nurse：When did your diarrhea start?
护士：你什么时候开始腹泻？
Patient：It started last night.
病人：昨天夜里开始。
Nurse：Do you remember how many times you went to the toilet?
护士：你记得去了多少次厕所吗？
Patient：I can't remember exactly. It must have been over ten times.
病人：记不准。要超过10次。

Nurse：What kind of stool did you notice，watery or mucous?

护士：你注意大便的样子了吗？是水样还是黏液样？

Patient：At first it was watery，but now I notice some mucous.

病人：开始是水样，现在有黏液。

Nurse：Do you feel abdominal pain when you go to the toilet?

护士：你上厕所时有腹痛感吗？

Patient：Yes.

病人：有。

Nurse：Have you vomited?

护士：吐没吐？

Patient：No，but I feel nauseated.

病人：没有，但我感到恶心。

Nurse：We will take a sample of your stool for examination. What did you eat last night for supper?

护士：我们要取点你的大便标本做检查。昨天晚饭你吃了些什么？

Patient：I had rice，some vegetables，a little meat and a glass of orange juice.

病人：我吃了些米饭、蔬菜、一点儿肉并且饮了一杯橘汁。

Nurse：Was the orange juice fresh?

护士：橘汁新鲜吗？

Patient：It tasted fresh.

病人：味道新鲜。

Nurse：Your condition doesn't seem serious，but we must give you intravenous infusion to prevent dehydration. We will also give you some antibiotics. You should drink plenty of water and follow a liquid diet. If your diarrhea stops tomorrow，you can take some semi-liquid food. I think you will recover in no time.

护士：看来你的病不重，但为了防止你脱水，我们必须给你静脉补液。我们还要给你用点抗生素。你要多喝水，进流质饮食。如果你明天不泻了，可以进半流质饮食。我想你将很快恢复健康。

## (3)

**Abdominal Pain　腹痛**

Patient：Nurse，I have a pain in my stomach（abdomen），it is quite painful.

病人：护士小姐，我肚子痛，非常的痛苦。

Nurse：How long have you had this abdominal pain?

护士：你肚子痛多久了？

Patient：It started last night，but it just felt uncomfortable then.

病人：昨天晚上开始的，一开始只是觉得不舒服而已。

Nurse：Where is it，can you show me?

护士：哪里痛，你可以指给我看吗？

Patient：It's just here.

病人：就这里。

Nurse：Did the pain start there or somewhere else?

护士：是这里开始痛，还是别的什么地方？

Patient：No，it's always in the same place.

病人：没有，总是一个地方痛。

Nurse：Does it hurt more if you move?

护士：你动的时候会痛得更厉害吗？

Patient：No.

病人：不会。

Nurse：Do you feel that you have a fever?

护士：你感到发烧吗？

Patient：No，I don't think so.

病人：没有，我不这么认为。

Nurse：I need to take your temperature，pulse and B/P.

护士：我需要量一下你的体温、脉搏和血压。

Patient：OK.

病人：好的。

Nurse：Are you passing urine OK?

护士：你小便正常吗？

Patient：Yes.

病人：是的。

Nurse：What does your urine look like?

护士：你的尿液是怎样的？

Patient：Normal color.

病人：正常的颜色。

Nurse：Have you had your bowels open today?

护士：今天大便了吗？

Patient：No.

病人：没有。

Nurse：Are you menstruating（bleeding）（having a period）? Is it normal?（female only）

护士：你是在月经期间吗？月经是否正常？（仅限女性）

Patient：No.

病人：没有。

Nurse：Have you vomited?

护士：你呕吐了吗？

Patient：No.

病人：没有。

Nurse：Have you had anything to eat or drink?

护士：你吃过喝过什么没？

Patient：Yes，I've had something to drink.

病人：是的，我喝了些东西。

Nurse：OK，I'll tell the doctor about your problem，and he will come and see you.

护士：好的，我会告诉医生你的情况，他一会过来看你。

Patient：Thanks very much.

病人：非常感谢。

## (4)

**Headache　头痛**

Nurse：How are you feeling?

护士：你感到怎样？

Patient：Not very well. I have a headache，severe dizziness，ringing noise in my ears，sleeplessness and poor memory. And，when I walk too fast，I get short of breath.

病人：我觉得不太舒服。我头痛、头晕得厉害，耳鸣，失眠和记忆力差，而且走路急时就气喘。

Nurse：How long have you suffered from all these?

护士：你有这些不适多久了？

Patient：Maybe eight years as far as I can remember. At first，I didn't pay any attention to them. Then，when my headache got worse，I went to see a doctor. He told me I had hypertension.

病人：我记得大约有八年了。开始我没注意，以后当头痛加重时，我就去看病。医生说我有高血压。

Nurse：Let me take your blood pressure.

护士：让我给你量血压。

（After taking blood pressure）

（量血压以后）

Nurse：It is a little high. Is there any member in your family who also suffers from hypertension.

护士：是高一点。你家里还有人患高血压吗？

Patient：Yes. My father has it. My grandfather died of apoplexy ten year ago，probably also due to hypertension.

病人：有的。我父亲也有高血压。我祖父10年前死于中风，可能也是高血压引起的。

Nurse：What kind of treatment have you had?

护士：你过去采取过什么治疗？

Patient：I have been given some antihypertensive drugs. They lowered my blood pressure somewhat; but it would go up again whenever I felt tired or worried.

病人：我曾用过降压药。使用后我的血压降低了一点，但是在疲劳或烦恼后，却又高了起来。

Nurse：It is very clear that you must rest more and stop worrying. You should follow a low-salt diet and eat lots of vegetables and fruit，but little meat. Do you smoke?

护士：这很清楚，你应该好好休息，不要烦恼。必须吃低盐食物，多吃蔬菜和水果，少吃肉。你吸烟吗？

Patient: Yes. But I'm smoking much less now.

病人：吸的，但现在吸得不多了。

※ ※ ※

Patient: Nurse, I have a headache.

病人：护士小姐，我头痛。

Nurse: How long have you had your headache?

护士：你头痛多长时间了？

Patient: About 4 hours now.

病人：大约4个小时了。

Nurse: Where does it hurt?

护士：你哪里痛？

Patient: Everywhere.

病人：整个头都痛。

Nurse: What does the pain feel like?

护士：痛起来是怎样的？

Patient: It feels like a tight band around my head.

病人：感觉整个头部被绷得紧紧的。

Nurse: Does your neck feel stiff?

护士：你脖子感到僵硬吗？

Patient: Yes, it does a little.

病人：是的，有一点。

Nurse: Can you move and bend your neck?

护士：你能转动和低头吗？

Patient: Yes.

病人：可以。

Nurse: Can you touch your chest with your chin?

护士：你能用下巴碰到你的胸吗？

Patient: Yes.

病人：可以。

Nurse: Does bright lights (photophobia) hurt your eyes and make your headache worse?

护士：明亮的光线会让你眼睛疼痛并使头痛加剧吗？

Patient: Yes, I feel it's too bright here for my eyes.

病人：是的，我觉得这里对我的眼睛来说就太明亮了。

Nurse: Do you have a rash on your arms, legs or body?

护士：你的手臂、腿部和身体有没有皮疹？

Patient: No, not that I have seen.

病人：没有，我看过了。

Nurse: Do you have a fever?

护士：你发烧吗？

Patient： I don't think so.
病人： 我认为没有。
Nurse： Do you have any other symptoms?
护士： 你还有其他症状吗？
Patient： I feel slightly sick.
病人： 我感到轻微的恶心。
Nurse： Do you suffer from migraines?
护士： 你是否有偏头痛？
Patient： No，not usually.
病人： 不是经常有。
Nurse： Are you upset or stressed in any way?
护士： 你感到某种程度的心烦或者压抑吗？
Patient： Not that I can think of.
病人： 我没有这种感觉。
Nurse： Have you been drinking fluids regularly?
护士： 你经常喝水吗？
Patient： Yes，I'm drinking normally.
病人： 是的，我经常喝。
Nurse： I need to take your temperature，pulse and B/P.
护士： 我需要量一下你的体温、脉搏和血压。
Nurse： OK，I'll tell the doctor about your headache，he will come and see you and prescribe some pain relief for you.
护士： 好的，我会告诉医生你头痛的情况，他一会过来看你，他会给你开些止痛药。
Patient： Thanks very much，nurse.
病人： 护士小姐，非常感谢。

## （5）

**Eczema 湿疹**

Nurse： How long has this been a problem?
护士： 这情况出现多久了？
Patient： About a week.
病人： 大约一周。
Nurse： Where did it start，on which part of the body?
护士： 从哪里开始的，身体的哪个部位？
Patient： Just here on my elbow.
病人： 肘部关节处。
Nurse： Is it very itchy and sore?
护士： 瘙痒疼痛吗？
Patient： Yes，it is.
病人： 是的。

Nurse： Do you take any medication or use any creams or ointments?

护士： 你吃过什么药和擦过什么药膏吗？

Patient： I have some cream that my doctor prescribed.

病人： 我擦了些医生给开的药膏。

Nurse： What diet are you on?

护士： 你现在进行什么特殊饮食吗？

Patient： Just normal diet.

病人： 正常的饮食。

Nurse： The doctor has asked me to take a swab specimen from your skin，it won't hurt.

护士： 医生让我从你的皮肤里取些拭子样本，一点都不痛。

Nurse： And he needs a blood and urine sample.

护士： 同时，他还需要一些血液和尿液样本。

## （6）

**Sprains & Fractures 扭伤骨折**

Nurse： Show me where it hurts.

护士： 指给我看哪里痛。

Patient： Just here on my ankle.

病人： 脚踝处，就这里。

Nurse： How did you do this?

护士： 你怎么弄成这样的？

Patient： Slipped off a step in the subway.

病人： 在地铁的楼梯处滑了一下。

Nurse： How painful is it?

护士： 有多痛？

Patient： Very.

病人： 非常痛。

Nurse： Can you move it?

护士： 你能移动吗？

Patient： No，it's too painful.

病人： 不能，太痛了。

Nurse： Is your foot swollen?

护士： 你的脚肿了吗？

Patient： Just a little.

病人： 有一点点。

Nurse： Can you feel your toes?

护士： 你的脚趾有知觉吗？

Patient： Yes.

病人： 有。

Nurse： Do you have any pins and needles or tingling?

护士：你是否感觉到刺痛或者麻痹？

Patient：No.

病人：没有。

Nurse：The doctor has written you a form for an X-ray，I will get you a wheelchair and take you to the X-ray Department.

护士：医生给你开了X线检查，我等一会儿用轮椅送你去放射科。

Patient：OK，thanks，that'll be great.

病人：好的，谢谢，那太好了。

Nurse：The doctor says you have a sprain，and you will need to have your ankle bandaged.

护士：医生说你扭伤了，你需要给脚踝绑绷带。

Nurse：You will need crutches to walk，I will show you where to get them.

护士：你需要拐杖帮助走路，我带你过去拿。

Nurse：You must rest as much as you can.

护士：你必须尽可能多休息。

Nurse：Do not walk on your foot，keep it elevated as much as you can.

护士：走路的时候，脚不要着地，尽量地保持抬着。

Nurse：The doctor has prescribed medication for your pain.

护士：医生给你开了些止痛的药。

Nurse：You will need to come back in three days，but you must register again first.

护士：你3天后过来复查，不过你需要重新挂号。

※ ※ ※

Nurse：How did it happen?

护士：你怎么受伤的？

Patient：When I was riding my bike to my office，a bus came from behind and struck me. I feel down and felt a severe pain in my left leg.

病人：我骑车上班，一辆汽车从后面撞了上来。我立即跌倒。感到左腿剧痛。

Nurse：When did it happen?

护士：这在什么时候发生的？

Patient：An hour ago.

病人：1小时前。

Nurse：Did you faint?

护士：你晕倒了吗？

Patient：I think I did for a little while.

病人：是的，但时间很短。

Nurse：Could you stand on your legs and walk after the accident?

护士：出事以后你能站起来走路吗？

Patient：No，I couldn't stand up at all.

病人：不行。我一点也站不起来了。

Nurse：Can you bend your knees?

护士：膝盖能弯吗？

Patient: I cannot bend my left knee.

病人：左膝不能弯。

Nurse: Did you receive any treatment before you came to the hospital?

护士：来医院前做过什么治疗吗？

Patient: No. I was brought straight here immediately after the accident.

病人：没有。出事后我被立即送到了这里。

Nurse: Please point out where it hurts the most.

护士：请告诉我哪里最痛？

Patient: Here. In my left lower leg.

病人：这里。就在左小腿。

Nurse: I see. It looks swollen. Let us send you to the X-ray Department. We'll see if there is a fracture in your leg.

护士：唔，你的小腿已经肿了。我们送你到放射科去检查一下你的小腿是否有骨折。

(After the X-ray)

（X线检查后）

Nurse: The X-ray shows that the bone in your leg is broken. But don't worry. Dr. Zhang will make a cast for you. I think the bone will knit in ten weeks if there is no complication.

护士：X线表明你的小腿有骨折。但不要紧张。张医生会给你上石膏的。我想，如果没有并发症，10周后断骨将接上。

Patient: Is there anything I should pay attention to when I go home?

病人：我回家后应注意些什么？

Nurse: Yes. There are two things you must remember. First, you should move all the joints in your foot from time to time, and check the color of the toes. And second, if you feel any pain or numbness in your toes, please immediately notify me or Dr Zhang.

护士：你应该注意两件事。第一，经常活动趾关节，并注意脚趾的颜色。其次，若足趾感到痛或麻木，立即找我或医生。

Patient: I'll try to remember. Thank you.

病人：我一定记住。谢谢你。

Nurse: You are welcome.

护士：别客气。

# 14. Comforting

# 安慰

## A. Sentences Commonly Used(常用语)

1. Please relax.
   请放松。
2. Try to relax and keep calm.
   尽量放松，保持镇静。
3. It doesn't matter.
   没关系。
4. Never mind.
   没关系。
5. Don't be nervous.
   别紧张。
6. Take it easy.
   别着急，放心好了。
7. Don't let it worry you.
   请别担心。
8. There is nothing to worry about.
   没什么可担心。
9. Don't worry. There is not any danger.
   别担心，没有任何危险。
10. Don't worry about it.
    别为这事担心。
11. Don't take it so much to your heart.
    别把那件事放在心上。
12. It can't be helped.
    这是没办法的。
13. Don't worry. You couldn't help it.
    别着急，你自己也没有办法。
14. It's difficult to say what's exactly wrong just now.
    现在还说不好到底是什么问题。

15. It doesn't sound serious.
看起来病情并不严重。
16. It is not serious.
病情不严重。
17. I know how you must feel.
我知道你的感觉。
18. I am sorry to hear that you don't feel well.
听说你感到不舒服，我很难过。
19. I'm sure you'll be completely recovered.
我肯定你会彻底痊愈的。
20. Just a little patience.
请耐心坚持一下。
21. Cheer up. I think things will come all right.
振作起来，我想一切都会好的。
22. Let's hope for the better.
乐观些/想开些。
23. I'm sure you'll be fine.
我确信你会好的。
24. I hope it won't last long.
但愿不会病得太久。
25. I am sure you'll be all right in no time.
我相信你很快就会康复。
26. I believe you'll soon get over it.
我相信你很快就能健康起来。
27. I hope you'll be well soon.
希望你早日恢复健康。
28. I'm glad to see you are doing so well.
我很高兴看到你恢复得这样好。
29. We'll have you fixed up in no time.
我们很快就能给你治好的。
30. I hope you'll be feeling better soon.
我希望你很快就会好转。
31. It won't take long to recover.
不会太久就恢复了。
32. If you need any more information, come and see me.
如果你需要了解更多的情况，请来找我。
33. I think you'll recover soon.
我想你将很快恢复健康。
34. Don't worry.
不必担心。

35. The most important thing is to adjust yourself and have self-confidence.
    最重要的事情是调整心态，树立信心。
36. It's not serious.
    病情不严重。
37. Your condition has been controlled in general.
    你的病情基本稳定。
38. Don't worry. It'll be all right soon.
    请别担心，过一会儿就没事。
39. Please trust our medical staff.
    请相信我们医护人员。
40. Don't be afraid. I think you can stand it.
    不要害怕，我想您能承受得住。

## B. Situational Conversation(情景会话)

### (1)

Nurse: Hello, Mr. Zhang. I notice you are depressed this time, aren't you?
护士: 张先生，你好。我注意到你这次入院心情很不好，是吗？
Patient: Well, I feel life is meaningless. I don't believe chemo-treatment. It's hopeless.
病人: 哎，活着没意思。我不相信化疗能起作用。
Nurse: You feel life is so hard because you are going to take the "hopeless" chemo-treatment.
护士: 你认为活着很艰难是因为你将要接受你认为的"毫无希望"的化疗。
Patient: That's it. And I think I'm a big trouble. I don't want to lead a painful life. How it would be better to get euthanasia!
病人: 是的，我是个"大包袱"。我不想这样痛苦地活着，我想安乐死。
Nurse: Mr. Zhang, I can understand your feeling. But do you know there are many patients suffering from the disease as you or even worse than yours. It's a wonder that they survive for years.
护士: 我能理解你的心情，张先生。可是，还有很多像你一样的癌症病人，甚至病情比你更严重，他们都奇迹般地活下来了。
Patient: Really?
病人: 真的吗？
Nurse: Of course. There is a patient who has been striving against cancer for years. He is living in No.201 bed. He came here for periodical chemo-treatment. At the very beginning, doctors thought he could be alive only for a half year. However, it has been eight years since he suffered from cancer. Moreover, his condition is not bad. He is taking treatment, meanwhile, sticking to working. People named he "anti-cancer star".
护士: 当然。我们医院的 201 病床就住着这么一位患者，他和癌症抗争了许多年。他这次入院来接受定期的化疗。最初，医生都认为他只能活半年，然而，今年已经是第八个年头了。并且，他的身体状况还不错。他一边坚持治疗，一边坚持上班，被人称为“抗癌明星”。

Patient: Oh, he is so luck. Where did he get such an excellent doctor?

病人：哦，他真幸运，他在哪找的“妙手神医”？

Nurse: There is not only one luck patient like him. Actually, as for a patient, the best doctor is himself. The most important thing you should do is adjust yourself, set life confidence and be a good cooperator. Everything will be better soon.

护士：像他这样幸运的病人不只一个，对于病人来说，最好的医生是自己。你要做的最重要的事情是调整心态、树立信心，好好配合治疗。这样，你很快就能康复。

Patient: Thank you for bringing me the courage. I will be a good cooperator.

病人：谢谢你给我勇气。我会好好配合治疗的。

Nurse: You're welcome. I'll introduce that "anti-cancer star" to you. Would you like to chat with him?

护士：不用谢。要我介绍那位“抗癌明星”给你吗？你们可以好好聊聊。

Patient: My pleasure. I'm glad to make a new good friend.

病人：好的，好高兴能认识一位新朋友。

**(2)**

Nurse: Good morning, Mr. Wang. Please sit in the chair. I'll make the bed for you. How did you sleep last night?

护士：早安，王先生。请您坐在椅子上，让我来为您整理床铺。昨晚您睡得好吗？

Patient: Well, it's so bad. My sleeping time is less than five hours.

病人：哎，糟透了，我的睡眠时间还不足5小时。

Nurse: Are you not accustomed to a new place or anything bothering you?

护士：您是不是对新环境不适应？还是有什么烦心的事？

Patient: I'm old and always get sick. How could I keep quiet?

病人：我年老多病，怎么能静下心来。

Nurse: It's common for older people to get sick. Don't be too depressed. Moreover, the disease can be cured. Nowadays, the average age of people is getting longer. If you lead a delightful life, it's natural to live as old as eighty or ninety years old.

护士：通常老年人容易生病，别难过了。再说，您的病很快就会治愈。现在人的寿命越来越长，像您这样，只要心情舒畅，活到八九十岁没有一点问题。

Patient: Right! With the condition of living getting better, everyone hopes to have a healthy and long life. But it's hard for me to get asleep while lying in bed.

病人：真的！生活条件好起来了，每个人都希望健康地活着。可是我躺在床上很难入睡。

Nurse: You'd better relax yourself and avoid exciting TV shows and novels before going to bed. In addition, you can listen to light music or drink a cup of hot milk.

护士：你放松点，睡前不要看刺激性的电视或小说。另外，可以在睡前听听轻音乐或喝杯热牛奶。

Patient: Really? I'll take your advice. Thank you.
病人： 是吗？我会这样做的，谢谢你。
Nurse: You're welcome.
护士： 没关系。

## （3）

Nurse: Mr. Smith，what is the matter with you? You look so bad!
护士： 史密斯先生，你怎么了？你看上去不太好。
Patient: Hello，nurse，I have been sick for two weeks. I'm afraid I will fall behind work.
病人： 你好，护士。我已经病了两个星期了，我担心我落下的工作。
Nurse: Don't worry，Mr. Smith. The most important thing for you is to receive treatment. I bet you'll catch up with others in two weeks after your discharge.
护士： 别担心。现在你最重要的事情是接受治疗，我相信你出院两周就能赶上别人的。
Patient: Thank you for your encouragement. I might need to work extra hard then. Nurse，why are antibiotics of no help in treatment of the common cold.
病人： 谢谢你的鼓励。我想我该加倍努力工作才行。护士，为什么抗生素对感冒不起作用？
Nurse: Because the common cold is caused by any of the more than two hunded kinds of viruses. There is yet no special medicine that can kill them.
护士： 这是因为引起感冒的病毒可以是200多种病毒中的任何一种。目前还没有对付它们的特效药。
Patient: Does the common cold do harm to people?
病人： 感冒对人体危害大吗？
Nurse: Yes. Though most colds run their course in three to ten days，some patients are susceptible to complications，such as sinusitis，ear inflammations and pneumonia.
护士： 是的。虽然大多数感冒可以在3～10天内痊愈，可是有些病人却容易并发鼻窦炎、耳炎、肺炎等疾病。
Patient: Are there any cures for the cold?
病人： 对感冒是怎样治疗的？
Nurse: Colds are usually treated with rest and fluids，in addition to antihistamines，and cough medicines when necessary.
护士： 感冒通常的治疗方法是休息加上补液，此外还会用些抗组胺药，必要时用点治咳嗽的药。
Patient: What is influenza then?
病人： 那流感又是什么？
Nurse: Influenza is an infection disease of the respiratory tract caused by the influenza virus. It infects human beings worldwide.
护士： 流感是由流感病毒引起的呼吸道传染病，它的传染范围很大。
Patient: Its symptoms are much more serious than those of common colds，aren't they?
病人： 它的症状比普通感冒要严重得多，是吗？

Nurse: Generally speaking, yes. The disease is characterized by fever, cough, and considerable muscle aching and is sometimes complicated by secondary bacterial pneumonia.

护士: 一般来说，是的，流感的特点是发炎、咳嗽、肌肉疼痛，有时伴有继发性肺炎。

Patient: What's the best way to treat it then?

病人: 那最好的治疗方法是什么？

Nurse: Bed rest and plenty of fluids constitute the best treatment.

护士: 卧床休息和大量补充体液是最好的治疗方法。

Patient: Thank you for your advice.

病人: 谢谢你的建议。

Nurse: Oh, yes. You'll get a chest X-ray examination this afternoon.

护士: 哦，对了，你今天下午要去拍胸片。

Patient: I'll get ready for it.

病人: 我已经准备好了。

Nurse: Don't forget to bring your old films and I'll wheel you to the radiology department.

护士: 别忘了带上你的旧片子，我会用轮椅推你到放射科。

## (4)

Nurse: Ms. Du, can you tell me why you seem so unhappy?

护士: 杜太太，看你的样子很不开心，能告诉我为什么吗？

Patient: I feel bad all over. I don't think my disease can be cured. It's better for me to be dead.

病人: 我浑身不舒服，很难受。我看这个病好不了。不如死了算了。

Nurse: Who told you that your disease couldn't be cured, a doctor or a nurse?

护士: 谁说你的病看不好了？是医生，还是护士告诉你的？

Patient: No. It's my own thought. I have gone to several hospitals, but it didn't help.

病人: 不是。我去过好多医院都没看好，是我自己这样想的。

Nurse: I think you will recover from your disease because the doctors haven't told you that you couldn't be cured. The results of your physical examinations are normal, which indicate that your uncomfortable feelings are caused by your depression. Many patients, who suffer from the same disease as you, have recovered and been discharged from our hospital. You must have faith in yourself. The doctors and nurses will help you to recover from your illness.

护士: 既然医生没告诉你病看不好了，就表明你的病是有希望治好的。你的各项检查报告显示你的不适感并非由器质性疾病引起，而是抑郁症的一种典型临床表现。像你这样的抑郁症我们遇到的不少，他们都痊愈出院了。你要对自己有信心，医生、护士会帮助你战胜病魔的。

Patient: But, I'm too sick to go to work and look after my family. On the contrary, my family has to accompany me in the hospital to take care of me. I feel worthless. I prefer to die.

病人: 可是我身体不好，不能工作，也不能照顾家人，反而拖累他们，要他们一天到晚陪着我，照顾我，我觉得自己真是没用，还不如死了算了。

Nurse: I can feel that you are a person who loves your family very much and takes high responsibility for your family. As you know, no one can escape from being sick during one's lifetime. Your family members look after you when you are sick because they love you very much. You should treasure yourself for them. It's better for you to cooperate with your doctor to recover quickly. You should repay your family's love a health body. If you only want to escape in a pessimistic way, you will not only let them down, you will also bring them too much pain.

护士：我可以感到你是一个很爱家人、很有责任感的人。患病是每一个人都无法避免的。你的家人在你患病后悉心照料，说明他们深爱着你。所以你应该好好珍惜自己的身体，积极配合医生治疗，争取早日把病看好，以健康的身体来回报家人的爱。如果你只是采取消极的方法来逃避，不仅辜负了家人对你的一片心，更给他们带来了痛苦。

Patient: You are right. But what can I do for my recovery?

病人：你说得对。但是我该怎样做才能使自己尽快好起来呢？

Nurse: It's simple. Go out of your room and be sociable with other people. Take part in the various activities in the unit. It will help you to enrich your hospital life, divert your attention from your illness, relax your body, and can also help you to interact with other people. This will prepare you to return to your family and society in the future. Above all, you should take the medicines according to the doctor's order. Please let me know if you have any discomfort after you take the medicines. I will help you. It's okay for you to ask any other nurses in our unit for help at any time you need it. They will be pleased to help you.

护士：很简单。只要你从现在开始让自己走出病室，融合到群体中去，尽量参加病区组织的各项活动。这不仅可以丰富你的住院生活，分散你的注意力，忘掉病痛，放松身心，还可以促进你与他人的沟通交往，使你今后能更好地回归家庭与社会。当然，除了这些，最重要的是你要按医嘱服药。服药后如有任何不适可以告诉我，我会给你提供帮助。平时如有什么问题也可以询问任何一位护士，她们会很乐意为你服务的。

Patient: I see I will cooperate with you and try not to think too much any more.

病人：明白了。我会积极配合治疗的，也不会想得太多了。

# Part Two

## Nursing Cases

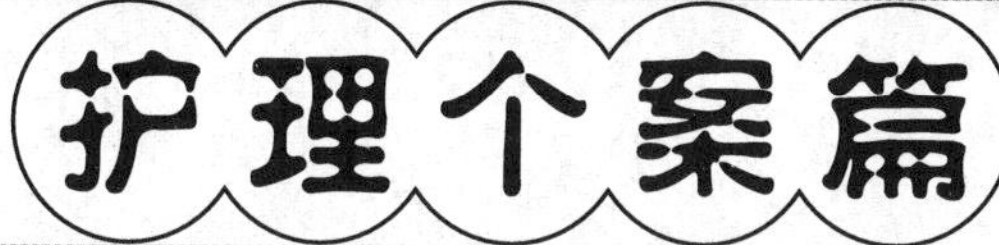

# 1. Receiving a New Patient

# 接收新病人

## （1）

Nurse： Is this Mr. Li? Welcome to our ward. Please take this bed. Everything is ready. Let me help you get into bed.

护士： 你是李先生吗？欢迎你来我们病房。请睡这个床。一切都准备好了。让我帮助你上床吧！

Patient： Thank you very much. I'd like to sit a while before lying down. Where have you put my clothes?

病人： 十分感谢。我想先坐一会儿再躺下。你把我的衣服放在哪里了？

Nurse： They have been given to your relatives at the Admission Office. They have been told to bring them back for you to wear when you leave the hospital.

护士： 住院处已交给你的家属了。已告诉他们在你出院时带回来给你。

Patient： I've forgotten to bring my cup.

病人： 我忘记带杯子了。

Nurse： Don't worry. Here is a little teapot for you. The ward attendant will bring you hot water twice a day. I hope that will be enough for you.

护士： 别着急。这里有小茶壶备你用。病房工人每天给你送两次热水。我想够了吧。

Nurse： Now take a rest. I'll come back later to tell you something about our hospital and its regulations.

护士： 现在该休息了。等一会儿我再来，告诉你一些我们医院的情况和有关制度。

Patient： Good. Thanks a lot.

病人： 好。多谢你。

（The nurse returning）

（护士返回）

Nurse： This is No. 3 ward of the Internal Medicine Department. Your bed is No. 302. Dr Zhang is the chief of this ward but Dr Li is responsible for your treatment. He is kind and considerate. So you are in good hands.

护士： 这是内科三病房，你是 302 床。病房主任姓张，但李医生负责你的治疗。他人很好，并且很负责。你会得到很好的照顾。

Patient： When are my relatives allowed visiting me?

病人：我的家属几时可以来探视？

Nurse：From three to four in the afternoon.

护士：每天下午3～4点钟。

Patient：An hour is too short. Why do you limit the visits only to one hour?

病人：为什么探视时间仅限制为一小时？我感到太短了。

Nurse：It is necessary to give patients a quiet environment for their treatment and rest. Besides, longer visits will be too tiring for them. Your meals are: breakfast at seven, lunch at twelve, and super at six in the evening. The doctors make their morning rounds at nine. Another round is made in the evening.

护士：这是因为必须让病人有安静的治疗和休养环境。时间太长会使病人感到疲劳。这里吃饭的时间是早饭7点，午饭12点，晚饭在傍晚6点。医生在上午9点查房。另外一次查房在傍晚。

Patient：Where is the washroom?

病人：盥洗室在哪里？

Nurse：We will show you after a little while. On the way, we will also show you our nurse's station and the treatment room.

护士：等一会儿我们带你去看。顺便还要让你认认护士办公室和治疗室。

Patient：Thank you. Oh, I have also forgotten to bring my bowls and chopsticks. What can I do?

病人：谢谢。啊，我还忘记带碗筷了。怎么办？

Nurse：Never mind. The hospital furnishes everything for your meals. These have to be sterilized every time they are used. The doctor has ordered a soft diet for you. We will put you on the regular diet when your condition has improved.

护士：不要紧。医院为你们准备好了餐具。每次用后都消毒。医嘱给你软食。在你病情改善后给你正常饮食。

Patient：That's fine. I hope I will not get any injections. I've never had them before.

病人：好。我不希望打什么针。我过去从未打过针。

Nurse：Don't be afraid. It feels just like a mosquito bite. Anyway, you may not even need injections. The doctor may prescribe other treatment for you.

护士：别怕。打针就像蚊子叮一下。而且，你可能不打针。医生也许给你用其他方法治疗。

Nurse：My name is Wang Ying. I am the head nurse of this ward. Press this button any time you need me. But someone will always come if I am not there.

护士：我叫王英。我是本病房的护士长。如果要找我，可按一下电钮。如果我不在，其他人也会来的。

Patient：Thank you for all the information. You have made me feel much easier.

病人：谢谢你的介绍。你使我感到很安心。

Nurse：When I have time I will come back to find out more about your condition and what we can do to make you comfortable. See you later.

护士：等我有时间时再来进一步了解你的情况，我们会让你感到更舒服些。再见。

Patient: Good-bye. Thank you.

病人： 谢谢。再见。

**（2）**

Nurse: Good morning. Welcome to our ward. Can I help you?

护士： 早晨好。欢迎来到我们病房。我能帮你什么忙吗？

Patient: Yes，please. I'm Mrs. Watson and this is my son Richhy who drove me here. I've come for my operation.

病人： 是的，麻烦你啦。我叫华森，这是我儿子瑞科，他开车送我来这里做手术的。

Nurse: Ah，yes...erm. I'll take your appointment letter.

护士： 哎，是的，嗯，把你的住院预约证明给我吧。

Patient: Thank you. It's a lovely place. Is it new?

病人： 谢谢你。很不错的地方，是新的吗？

Nurse: Yes，we're very proud of it. It was inaugurated by her Royal Highness last December. Would you like to take a seat and help me with a few details?

护士： 是的，我们对它感到非常自豪。开幕仪式是由英女皇去年十二月主持进行的。请你坐下，帮助我把几个细节问题搞清楚可以吗？

Patient: Yes，of course. What do you want to know?

病人： 是的，当然啦。你想知道什么？

**（3）**

Nurse: Good evening，Mr. Lee. Let me go through the pre-admission information with you. Who accompanied you to the hospital?

护士： 晚上好，李先生，请让我为你做入院前告知。谁陪你来医院的？

Patient: My daughter Mary is here with me.

病人： 我的女儿玛丽在这陪我。

Nurse: Why have you come to the hospital，Mr Lee?

护士： 李先生，你哪里不舒服来医院？

Marry: My father fainted after having dinner.

玛丽： 我父亲晚饭后晕倒了。

Nurse: What time did he faint?

护士： 他什么时间晕倒的？

Marry: About 6：30pm.

玛丽： 大概晚上 6：30。

Nurse: It's 9：30pm now. That's about three hours ago. Did you take him to see a doctor before coming here?

护士： 现在是晚上 9：30，那是 3 个小时前。来这前你带他去看医生了吗？

Marry: Yes. We brought him to the GP next to our block. The doctor said that it was better to take him to the hospital for a check.

玛丽： 是的，我们带他去看了我们街区附近的全科医生。医生建议他到医院做个体检。

Nurse： Did the doctor give you a letter?
护士： 医生有没有给你一封信？
Marry： Yes. Here it is.
玛丽： 有，给你。
Nurse： OK. Thank you. I will give it to our doctor when he sees your father. Does your father have any drug allergy?
护士： 好，谢谢，我会在我们的医生为你父亲检查后给他。你父亲对什么药过敏吗？
Marry： Dad，do you have some gastric problems?
玛丽： 爸，你的胃有问题吗？
Patient： Yes，I am allergic to pain killers like aspirin.
病人： 是的，我对止痛药很敏感，例如阿司匹林。
Nurse： Any other known allergy?
护士： 还知道别的过敏吗？
Patient： No.
病人： 没有。
Nurse： What about food allergy?
护士： 有食物过敏吗？
Marry： What do you mean by that?
玛丽： 那是什么意思？
Nurse： That means certain food that can cause adverse reactions，like vomiting，itching，diarrhoea.
护士： 是指某种食物能够引起有害反应，例如呕吐、发痒、腹泻等。
Patient： Not really. But I need to watch my diet because of my diabetes.
病人： 不确定，但我需要注意饮食，因为我有糖尿病。
Nurse： Right. As this is a hospital，we like to advise that cash and valuables are kept properly. If necessary，they can be kept in our hospital safe.
护士： 对。由于这是医院，我们建议你保管好你的钱和贵重物品。如果需要，可以放在医院保险箱里。
Marry： I think we can bring back the valuables with us. Not necessary for the safe.
玛丽： 我想我们可以带回随身贵重物品，不需要保险箱。
Nurse： I need to ask about your past medical history，Mr. Lee. Ever been admitted to a hospital or undergone any surgery.
护士： 我需要问一下你的用药史，李先生，你曾经住过院或做过手术吗？
Patient： Yes，for appendicitis.
病人： 是的，因为阑尾炎。
Nurse： When was the operation?
护士： 什么时间做的手术？
Patient： More than ten years ago.
病人： 10多年以前。
Nurse： Where was the operation?

护士：你在哪做的手术？

Patient：A hospital.

病人：A 医院。

Nurse：OK. What about recent medical problems?

护士：好，你最近的医疗问题是什么？

Patient：I have DM.

病人：我有糖尿病。

Nurse：Yes，your daughter mentioned that earlier. When were you diagnosed as diabetic?

护士：对，你女儿刚刚提过，你什么时候被诊断为糖尿病？

Patient：Last year.

病人：去年。

Nurse：Are you on medication for diabetes currently?

护士：你目前服用治疗糖尿病的药物吗？

Patient：Yes.

病人：是的。

Nurse：Do you have any medicine with you now?

护士：你现在身边带有你的药吗？

Marry：Yes. This is my father's packet of medicine.

玛丽：是的，这是我父亲的药包。

Nurse：Let me hold on to this also. Besides diabetes，do you have any other medical problem，Mr. Lee?

护士：让我也记下这些药。李先生，除了糖尿病，你的身体有没有别的问题？

Patient：No，except for my gastric problem. But I am not taking any medication for that now.

病人：没有，除了我的胃病。但是我现在没有因为这个服用过任何药物。

Nurse：Are there any other information or special requests that you may want to add?

护士：有没有其他信息或特殊要求你想补充的？

Patient：No.

病人：没有。

Nurse：Thank you，Mr. Lee，for the information. Doctor Wang will see you soon.

护士：谢谢李先生提供的信息，王医生一会儿将过来看你。

## （4）

Nurse：Hello，Mr. Lee. Welcome to Ward 10. Before the doctor sees you，let me make a quick assessment. I need to get your weight and height. You are limping. Are you able to stand up for a while?

护士：你好，李先生。欢迎来到 10 号病房，让我为你做一个快速评估。你需要测一下体重和身高。你有点跛行，能站一会儿吗？

Patient：Yes. Should not be a problem.

病人：可以，应该没问题。

Nurse：All right. Height 1.55m，weight 56kg. Very good，Mr. Lee. You may sit on the bed.

Let me check your pulse and breathing. So, what happened to you?

护士：好，身高 1.55 米，体重 56 公斤。很好，李先生，你可以坐在床上。让我为你测一下脉搏和呼吸，那么，你感觉怎么不舒服？

Patient: I felt uncomfortable after dinner and fainted in the toilet. I fell and that's how I injured my right knee.

病人：我晚饭后感觉不舒服晕倒在厕所。我觉得因此伤了右膝。

Nurse: Oh yes, you were limping just now. Don't worry, we will give you a thorough check-up here. How old are you, Mr. Lee?

护士：是的，刚才你走路蹒跚。不用担心，在这儿我们将为你进行全面检查。李先生，你多大年纪？

Patient: I am seventy one this year.

病人：我 71 岁。

Nurse: Really? You look younger than your age. How do you make it?

护士：真的吗？你看起来很年轻，怎么保持的？

Patient: Nothing special. Just plain common sense. Eat well and sleep well. Also, an apple a day keeps the doctor away.

病人：没有什么特别的，只是普通简单的道理。吃得好睡得好。也就是一天一个苹果让医生走开。

Nurse: Ah, good, so you take fruits. How many hours do you sleep a day?

护士：哈，好，你经常吃水果。你每天睡几个小时？

Patient: I usually sleep early. By 9: 30p.m., I will be in bed. And I feel very fresh when I wake up at 6: 00a.m. in the morning. I don't need afternoon naps.

病人：我总是睡得很早，一般晚上 9：30 上床，当我早上 6 点醒来时，感觉精神饱满。我不需要午后小睡。

Nurse: Have you ever fainted before?

护士：你以前曾晕倒过吗？

Patient: This is the first time. I am always healthy.

病人：这是第一次，我一直很健康。

Nurse: You can keep your eyeglasses in the drawer beside your bed. Do you have dentures?

护士：你可以把眼镜放在床边抽屉里，你有义齿吗？

Patient: No, these are my natural teeth. But some have dropped out over the years.

病人：不，这些是我自己的牙。但是有些已经掉了好几年了。

Nurse: Very well, Mr. Lee. Our ward doctor will see you soon.

护士：很好，李先生，我们病区的医生一会儿将来看你。

# 2. Emergency

# 急诊

Nurse: What seems to be the problem?

护士：您哪里不舒服？

Patient: Nurse, I have a sharp pain in my upper abdomen.

病人：护士，我上腹部忽然疼痛。

Nurse: When did it begin?

护士：什么时候开始的？

Patient: About three hours ago.

病人：约3小时前。

Nurse: Have you ever had any pains like this before?

护士：您以前这样痛过吗？

Patient: No, never.

病人：不，从来没有过。

Nurse: Show me the pain location.

护士：指给我哪痛。

Patient: Here.

病人：这儿。

Nurse: What kind of pain it is? Intermittent or persistent?

护士：是怎样的痛？是间歇的还是持续的？

Patient: It's a kind of sharp. It was off and on, but now it hurts all the time.

病人：是剧痛。本来是一阵一阵的，可是现在持续痛。

Nurse: Do you feel nausea?

护士：你觉得恶心吗？

Patient: I feel vomiting.

病人：我想吐。

Nurse: let's take a white blood count and a blood analysis test, a kind of test for acute pancreatitis.

护士：让我们做个白细胞计数和淀粉酶试验，这是一种专为查急性胰腺炎的试验。

Patient: OK, thank you.

病人：好吧，谢谢。

# 3. Pharmacy

# 药房

Patient: Good morning, nurse.
病人：早上好，护士。
Nurse: Good morning, madam. What can I do for you?
护士：早上好，女士。请问有什么需要我帮忙的吗？
Patient: Can you fill the prescription for me ?
病人：请按药方帮我抓药好吗？
Nurse: Of course. Please give me the prescription.
护士：当然可以。请把您的药方给我。
Patient: Here you are.
病人：给你。
Nurse: Just a moment, please. Your prescription will be ready in a few minutes.
护士：请稍等片刻。好了，您要的药全在这儿了。
Patient: Thank you very much.
病人：谢谢。
Nurse: Don't mention it. By the way, you got the prescription from Dr. Johnson, didn't you?
护士：别客气。顺便问一下，您这个药方是约翰逊医生给您开的吗？
Patient: Yes, indeed.
病人：是的。
Nurse: Did he tell you how to take the medicine?
护士：那么他有没有告诉您怎么服用这些药物？
Patient: No. He didn't say anything about it.
病人：没有，他什么都没说。
Nurse: All right. Let me tell you what you have to do. Take two of these tablets three times a day after meals.
护士：好的。我给您解释吧。这些药片每日3次，每次2片，饭后服用。
Patient: How about this cough syrup?
病人：那么这个止咳糖浆怎么服呢？
Nurse: First shake the bottle. Take two spoonful of the cough syrup three times a day.
护士：先把瓶子摇晃几下。每日3次，每次2勺。

Patient: Thank you very much.

病人：非常感谢。

Nurse: You're welcome. I hope you will recover in no time.

护士：不客气。祝您早日康复。

# 4. How to Use Different Medicines

# 药品服用方法

Patient: How do I take the tablets?

病人：我怎么服用这种药片。

Nurse: Take two tablets each time，four times a day.

护士：每次 2 片，每天 4 次。

Patient: How do I take the sucking lozenges?

病人：我如何服用这种含片？

Nurse: Please put one under your tongue，don't swallow it.

护士：放在舌下一粒，别咽下去。

Patient: How do I take the liquid medicine?

病人：我怎么服用这种液体药物呢？

Nurse: Just drink it.

护士：吸吮就行了。

Patient: How do I take the pills?

病人：这种药丸怎么吃？

Nurse: Please dissolve one pill in water and then drink the water.

护士：服用前放到水中融化。

Patient: How do I take the syrup?

病人：我怎么服用这种糖浆？

Nurse: One teaspoon each time，three times a day.

护士：一次一勺，每天 3 次。

Patient: How do I take the drug?

病人：这种药怎么服？

Nurse: Drink one line（half a line）each time，three times a day. Shake it well before taking it.

护士：每次一格（半格），每天 3 次。服用前充分摇动。

Patient: How do I take these pain-killer?

病人：这种止痛药怎么用？

Nurse: Take one tablet of this pain-killer if you are in pain，but no more than once every four hours.

护士：感觉疼痛的时候吃一片，每 4 小时不能超过一次。

Patient: How do I use this suppository?

病人： 这种栓剂怎么用？

Nurse: Insert one into your anus (vagina) every night.

护士： 每晚塞入肛门(阴道)一个。

Patient: How do I use this adhesive?

病人： 这种药膏怎么用？

Nurse: This is a special adhesive for easing the pain. Apply it to the painful area and change it every two days.

护士： 这是一种缓解疼痛的药膏。将它敷在患处，每两天换一次。

Patient: How do I use this lotion?

病人： 我如何使用这种药水？

Nurse: Apply this lotion to the itching spot with this cotton swab.

护士： 用棉棍将药水涂在痒的地方。

Patient: How do I use this powder?

病人： 这种药粉如何使用？

Nurse: Please dissolve the powder in hot water. Soak your hand (foot) in it for twenty minutes twice a day.

护士： 将药粉溶解在热水中，将您的手(脚)泡在水里 20 分钟，每天两次。

Patient: How do I use the eye-drop and ointment?

病人： 我如何使用这种眼药水和药膏？

Nurse: Put the eye-drop into your right eye four to six times a day, one to two drops each time. Squeeze a bit of ointment on your eyelid every night.

护士： 将眼药水滴入眼中，每天 4～6 次，每次 1～2 滴。每晚在眼皮上挤一点药膏。

Patient: How do I apply the nose drop?

病人： 这种滴鼻剂怎么用？

Nurse: Bend your head as far back as possible and then drop some in the nostril.

护士： 尽可能地仰头，滴入鼻孔中少许。

Patient: How do I apply the ear drop?

病人： 我如何使用这种滴耳剂？

Nurse: Tilt your head to the side; put one to two drops into your ear. Press the tragus for a few seconds.

护士： 把头偏向一侧，向耳中滴 1～2 滴。按压一会儿耳屏。

# 5. Bronchial Asthma

# 支气管哮喘

Nurse: Hello, Miss Li, do you feel better now?

护士：你好，小李，现在感觉好点了吗？

Patient: Much better, thanks. But, I don't understand what caused the acute episodic asthma this afternoon because I was fine this morning.

病人：谢谢你，好多了。但我就搞不懂上午还好好的，怎么下午哮喘就发作了。

Nurse: There are many factors that can trigger asthma attack. Allergy is one of the primary factors.

护士：哮喘的发作有多种诱因，其中过敏是哮喘发作的主要诱因之一。

Patient: Was mine caused by allergy?

病人：那我的哮喘发作是属于过敏引起的吗？

Nurse: Yes. According to your history, you are possibly allergic to some kinds of paint.

护士：是的。从你的发病情况来看，你很可能对油漆过敏。

Patient: Why do I have a problem while many other people don't when they are exposed to paints?

病人：那为什么别人接触油漆没关系，我就不行呢？

Nurse: That is because you have a different physical make-up. In other words, you have an allergic tendency toward paint. After contacting with paint, the allergen in the paint can trigger the body cells to produce special substances which can cause the constriction of the bronchial muscle and results in symptoms such as dyspnea and chest distress. So, you must remember not to touch paint in the future.

护士：那是因为你的体质具有特异性，也就是说具有对油漆的过敏性。在接触过油漆后，油漆内的过敏原使你体内会产生一些特殊的细胞物质，这些物质导致支气管平滑肌收缩，从而引起呼吸困难、胸闷等症状。所以你今后一定要记住不能再接触油漆类物质了。

Patient: Does this mean that if I do not touch paint, I will no longer get asthma?

病人：那是否意味着我今后只要不接触油漆就可能避免哮喘发作呢？

Nurse: Generally speaking, besides paint, there are many other substances such as pollen, dust mites, fungi spores and animal fur, etc that can trigger asthma. Some people may have hypersensitive reaction after eating fish or shrimps or eggs.

护士：一般来讲，除了油漆以外，还有一些容易引起过敏的物质，如花粉，尘螨，真菌孢子和动物的毛、屑等。有些人在摄入鱼、虾、蛋后也会引起过敏。

Patient: So I should not eat fish, shrimp and eggs in the future, right?

病人：那我以后是否不能再食用鱼、虾、蛋类食物呢？

Nurse: No. Not all people are hypersensitive to these foods. You must have eaten fish or shrimps or eggs before and did not have any allergic reactions. Therefore, you should watch if you are allergic to pollens, dust mites, fungi spores, and animal fur. Try to avoid the substance to which you have shown allergic reactions.

护士：也不是的，并非所有的人对这类食物都过敏。正如你以前肯定食用过鱼、虾、蛋类食物，但并没有引起发病。在你今后的生活和工作中，应注意观察自己是否对花粉、尘螨、真菌孢子、动物的毛或屑等过敏。尽量避免接触已知的致敏物质。

Patient: I see. Thank you for your advice.

病人：知道了，谢谢你给我讲这些知识。

# 6. Cough Up Sputum Instructions

# 排痰指导

Nurse： Hello，Mr. Zhang，how are you feeling today?

护士： 你好，张先生，今天感觉怎样？

Patient： I feel there is sputum in my throat but I cannot cough it up.

病人： 我觉得喉咙口有痰，但就是咳不出。

Nurse： How much water do you normally drink when you are at home?

护士： 你平时在家每天喝多少水？

Patient： I don't like to drink water，and only drink it when I feel very thirsty.

病人： 我不喜欢喝水，只有感到口渴时才喝。

Nurse： Oh! That isn't good for sputum expectoration. There are many self-care strategies to promote sputum expectoration. Drinking water is one of these strategies. You should make sure to drink 1200 to 1500ml of water every day.

护士： 哦，看来这样对你的排痰是很不利的，一般来讲，促进排痰有很多自我护理的方法，多喝水就是其中一种。你每天最好保证喝1200～1500ml的水。

Patient： Why do I need to drink so much water?

病人： 为什么要喝这么多水？

Nurse： Because sufficient water can dilute the sputum and make it easy to spit out. Drinking water can also increase the discharge of urine that contains metabolic wastes. Furthermore，it can also prevent the flu.

护士： 因为只有补充充足水分，才可以稀释痰液，以助排痰。同时通过多饮水可增加排尿量，帮助排出体液内废物。此外，多喝水还有利于预防流感。

Patient： Oh! It sounds like drinking more water is good for me. But how can I drink so much water?

病人： 原来喝水有这么多的好处，那我该怎么做才能完成这么多的饮水量？

Nurse： It is not so difficult once you get in the habit of drinking water（i.e. drinking some water even when you don't feel thirsty）. You can drink regularly，for example，right after you get up in the morning，two hours after your meals，before you go to sleep，and after urinating at night. Drink more when you are in an air-conditioned room where the air is usually drier.

护士： 你只要养成主动喝水的习惯（即不要等口渴以后再喝水），完成这点饮水量并不会太困难的。如你可以有规律地把喝水的时间安排在早晨起床后、三餐以后的2

小时、睡前、夜间起床小便后。如果你待在空调房间的话，还应适量增加饮水量。因为空调房间的空气比较干燥。

Patient: Are there any other means to promote expectoration?

病人：那除了多饮水之外，还有别的方法帮助排痰吗？

Nurse: Of course. Let me teach you how sputum can be spit out by coughing correctly.

护士：有呀，现在我就可以教给你一种正确的咳嗽排痰的方法。

（The nurse demonstrated to the patient.）

（护士示范了正确的咳嗽排痰方法。）

Nurse: OK. Now try it yourself.

护士：好了，现在请你来做一遍吧。

（The patient tried it under the guidance of the nurse）.

（病人在护士的指导下完成了正确的咳嗽排痰方法。）

Nurse: Well done. Keep doing this from now on. Now，have some rest，I am going to visit other patients and will be back to help you with nebulization therapy and to pat your back.

护士：你做得不错，以后就可以这样做了。现在我先去看其他病人了，过会儿再来给你做雾化吸入和捶背，你先休息吧。

Patient: Good，thank you.

病人：好的，谢谢你。

# 7. Oxygen Safety Instruction

# 安全用氧

Nurse: (bringing all the things needed to the bedside for oxygen therapy) Hi, Mr. Zhao, I'll give you some oxygen since you are feeling distressed. This will make you feel more comfortable.

护士：（带着准备齐全的吸氧用物来到床边）赵先生，你好，你现在感觉胸闷，我给你吸点氧气，这种治疗会让你舒服一些。

Patient: OK.

病人：好的。

Nurse: (skillfully setting up the oxygen inhalation therapy system) Mr. Zhao, I have connected the oxygen system for you. How are you feeling now?

护士：（非常熟练地完成了吸氧治疗操作）赵先生，氧气给你接上了，你感觉如何？

Patient: (looking at the flow meter of the oxygen tank) I feel short of breath. Why do you give me so little oxygen?

病人：（看了一眼流量表）我现在气都接不上来，你怎么就给我开一点点氧气。

Nurse: Oh, Mr. Zhao, you do not understand. According to you present condition, you must be given the oxygen in a low flow level. I have adjusted the flow rate for you. You shouldn't change it by yourself. Please rest. I'll see you after a while.

护士：哦，赵先生，你误会了。根据你的病情，你需要低流量吸氧，我已经给你调节好流量了，你可不能自行调节哦。你先休息，过会儿我再来看你。

(One hour later, when the nurse came back, she found that Mr. Zhao had a red face, was talking a lot, and the oxygen flow had been adjusted to 8 liters per minute.)

（一小时后，护士来到床边，发现赵先生面色潮红，多语，氧气流量已被调至8升/分。）

Nurse: Mr. Zhao, what's the matter with you? Are you OK? (The nurse adjusted the oxygen flow to the previous rate.)

护士：哦，赵先生，你怎么啦？（护士随手把氧气流量调至原来的刻度。）

Patient: Why am I feeling worse than before?

病人：我怎么感觉比刚才更糟糕了？

Nurse: You shouldn't have increase the oxygen flow by yourself. Because your breathing is stimulated by the reflex of hypoxia, if you inhale excessive oxygen in a short period of time, hypoxia might be improved transiently, but retention of carbon dioxide will get worse. What we are doing now is called controlled oxygen therapy which can prevent respiratory suppression，correct hypoxia and carbon dioxide retention. Do you understand my explanation?

护士：你的氧气可不能调高呀。因为你目前的呼吸主要通过缺氧来反射来刺激的。如短时间内吸入过多氧气，虽然缺氧得到短暂改善，但二氧化碳潴留会更加重。我现在给你施行的就是控制性氧疗，这样既可避免呼吸抑制，又可纠正你的缺氧和二氧化碳潴留。我这样解释，你理解吗？

Patient: Oh，I see. I'll not adjust the oxygen by myself again.

病人：哦，原来是这样，我懂了。我再也不会自行调节流量了。

# 8. Tuberculosis

# 肺结核

Nurse: Mr. Wang，how are you? You will be discharged tomorrow，and these are your medicines after you leave the hospital.

护士： 王先生，你好，你明天可以出院了，这是你出院带的药。

Patient: Why do I need so many medicines?

病人： 怎么这么多药？

Nurse: Well，these are the medicines for only one month. You should take these continuously for six to nine months. The specific length that you need to take these will be determined by your monthly out-patient check up.

护士： 是的，这里仅仅是你一个月的用药量。你回去后仍需坚持服药 6～9 个月。具体时间则需根据你每月门诊随访情况而定。

Patient: Aren't I healed? Why should I take medicines for so long? Can the length be shortened?

病人： 我现在不是已经好了吗？怎么还要服这么长时间的药物？能否缩短一些时间？

Nurse: Mr. Wang，I understand your concern. When we treat pulmonary tuberculosis，we must follow the therapeutic principles of early start，combination，sufficient quantity，regularity and full course treatment. That's to say，we must strictly follow the drugs，methods and courses required by the chemotherapy program. Patients cannot stop taking medicines by themselves off and on，and they shouldn't change the therapeutic program. The therapeutic program needs to be full course. This is the only way patients can be cured clinically and biologically.

护士： 王先生，我非常理解你。但在治疗结核病时，我们必须遵循早期、联合、适量、规律和全程的治疗原则。也就是说，必须严格按照化疗方案规定的药物、方法、时间用药，不可无故随意停药或随意间断用药，也不可更改治疗方案，要坚持治满疗程。只有这样，才能同时达到临床治愈和生物学治愈。

Patient: But I don't understand what“being cured clinically and biologically”implies?

病人： 我不明白什么叫临床治愈和生物学治愈？

Nurse: Tuberculous pleuritis can be cured by means of absorption，fibrosis，and calcification，etc. If after treatment，the clinical symptoms of tuberculosis completely disappear，the local lesion becomes stable，and no tubercle bacilli are emitted，but there are some surviving bacilli. In this case，the surviving bacilli may be active，breed，and spread again. This is what is called being "cured clinically". Contrary to this, a "biological cure" means the local lesion is completely eliminated, absorbed or taken away by surgical operation. No tubercle bacilli exist in the lesions.

护士： 结核性胸膜炎的主要愈合方式有吸收、纤维化、钙化等。如经过治疗使病灶稳定，并停止排菌，结核毒性症状完全消失，但病灶内仍可能有结核菌存活，并有再次活跃、繁殖而播散的可能，这种情况即为临床治愈。而生物学治愈是指病灶彻底清除，包括完全吸收或手术切除，并确定病灶内已无结核菌存活。

Patient： There's so much knowledge related to tuberculous pleuritis. Now I realize the importance of taking medicines for the full period prescribed. But I'm afraid I may forget to take the medicines.

病人： 哦，原来结核性胸膜炎的愈合也有这么多学问。我现在终于明白了坚持用药的重要性，但真正实施时我还是担心自己会忘记。

Nurse： Don't worry about it. I have already made you a schedule for taking the medicines. Isoniazid and Rifampin should be taken on an empty stomach, so you should put the medicines on the nightstand and take them immediately when you get up in the morning. Pyrazinamide should be taken after meals, so you should put the medicine on the dining table.

护士： 你不用担心。我已经给你制订了一个服药计划表。你看，异烟肼和利福平需要空腹口服，你就把药物放在床头柜上，你早上一起床就服。而吡嗪酰胺需在餐后口服，药物可放在餐桌上，每次在用餐后即服药。

Patient： Very good, you are so considerate. I won't forget to take the medicines. Thank you very much.

病人： 太好了，你考虑得真周到。这样我肯定不会忘记服药了，谢谢你。

# 9. Hemoptysis

# 咯血

Nurse: (His bed nurse, Miss Zhou, comes to his beside with smile) How do you do? I am your bed nurse. My last name is Zhou and Doctor Zhang is your doctor. Please call me any time if you need help.

护士：（床位护士小周面带微笑来到床边）你们好，我是床位护士，我姓周，你们就叫我小周吧。以后有什么事可以找我，我会尽我所能去做。你的床位医师姓张。

Patient: OK, thank you. (Suddenly coughing, spitting out five-mouthful scarlet-colored blood, the patient and his family members become very nervous.)

病人：好的，谢谢你的介绍，麻烦你了。（说着病人又一阵咳嗽，并咯出 5 口鲜红色的血液，患者及家属均表现出十分紧张的神色。）

Nurse: (after taking care of the patient) Do you feel better now? You should lie in bed quietly, and try to relax and don't be too nervous. Emotional stress may increase the tension of the vagus nerve, resulting in a spasm of the laryngeal muscle which narrows the respiratory tracts. The blood clot in the airway will be difficult to be removed by coughing. This might result in suffocation and produce more serious consequences.

护士：（在安置好病人后）现在舒服点了吧，你先安静躺着，注意一定要让自己身心放松，不要紧张。因为情绪紧张后会使迷走神经的张力增加而导致喉肌痉挛，致使呼吸道变窄，气道内的血块不易咯出而影响呼吸，甚至会导致窒息，从而产生更严重的后果。

Patient: (with a suspicious appearance) Oh.

病人：（表现出疑惑的神情）哦。

Nurse: You are now in the acute stage of the disease because the amount of blood you spit out is not so little. You should lie in bed and don't talk and move too much. I'll tell you something you should pay attention to. If you have any questions, you can ask me, OK?

护士：因为你现在还处在疾病的急性期，并且咯血量较大，所以你需要绝对卧床休息，尽量减少说话，少活动。还有些注意事项你先听我讲，如有疑问可轻轻地问我。好吗？

(Patient nodded slightly.)

(病人微微点头,表示默许。)

Nurse: First, patient with hemoptysis must cough gently and shouldn't cough as you did a few moments ago. Because coughing with too much force will lead to increased pressure of the thoracic cavity and aggravate bleeding. There are other factors that can increase the pressure of the thoracic cavity, such as holding your breath, defecating with force, etc. So you should try to avoid those behaviors. Attention should be paid especially to defecating. Because lying in bed weakens the movement of one's intestines and most people are not accustomed to defecating in bed, therefore people in bed are prone to have constipation. However, constipation can be avoided by eating food rich in fiber, drinking lots of water, avoiding spicy foods, and performing stomach massages every day.

护士: 首先咯血病人的咳嗽一定要轻轻地,不能像你刚才那样。因为用力咳嗽会导致胸腔内压力增高而加重出血。其他可导致压力增高的因素还有用力屏气、用力大便等。所以你要尽量避免,尤其是排便问题更应引起重视,因为一方面卧床休息会导致肠蠕动减弱,另一方面,可能你还不能习惯于床上排便,所以很容易产生便秘。在通常情况下,可通过进食富含纤维素的食物,多饮水,避免进辛辣等刺激性食物,注意每天腹部按摩来保持大便通畅。

Patient's wife: My husband likes eating very hot food, will this affect his disease?

病人妻子: 我们老赵平时喜欢吃偏烫食物,这对他的疾病有影响吗?

Nurse: This is a topic that I want to discuss with you. At the present time, lukewarm, cool, light liquid or semi-liquid food is suitable for your husband. Hot food is not good for the prevention of bleeding.

护士: 这就是接下来我要跟你们说的话题。目前赵先生最好进食温、凉、清淡的流质或半流质食物。因为食物的温度偏高不利于止血。

Patient's wife: Thank you for telling us so many things.

病人妻子: 谢谢你跟我们讲这么多。

# 10. Spontaneous Pneumothorax

# 自发性气胸

Nurse: Hello, Wang Lei. I'm nurse Zhang. You can regard me as your old sister if you wish, because I'm a litter bit older than you.

护士：你好，王磊，我是你的床位护士，我姓张。我的年龄比你稍大，假如你愿意，你可以把我当成姐姐。

Patient: I wish you were my sister and could stay beside me. I'm afraid to move or even breathe with this tube in my chest. Could you tell me something about my problem?

病人：现在，我真愿意有你这样的姐姐守在我边上。身上插了这么一根管子，我动都不敢动，也不敢呼吸了，你能给我讲讲吗？

Nurse: Well, the human lung is composed of many pulmonary alveoli which exchange gas with outside air, thus supplying oxygen for human body. Because of some congenital and postnatal reasons, some pulmonary alveoli in your lung merged together and formed a big bubble and its wall became very thin. It broke suddenly when you exercised vigorously or breathed rapidly. This allowed the gas to fill into the thorax and accumulated until it affected the normal function of your lung and resulted in your breathing difficulties.

护士：好的，人体的肺组织是由很多很多肺泡组成的。正是这些肺泡与外界之间进行着气体交换，人体才能得到源源不断的氧气供应。你的肺中，有一小部分肺泡由于先天和后天的因素，融合在一起，形成一个大泡泡，壁也变得很薄。在剧烈运动或频繁的吸气换气的情况下，突然破裂，气体就直接进入胸腔，越积越多，最后限制了正常肺组织的功能，你就出现呼吸困难的症状了。

Patient: Oh, I know. Then what is this tube for?

病人：喔，原来我的肺中还有这么一个大泡。那插这根管子有什么用呢？

Nurse: The drainage tube is inserted to your thoracic cavity and it help to expel the gas from inside. Then, your lung may be expanded normally after the gas is removed. Do you hear the sound in the drainage bottle?

护士：这根胸腔引流管直接通到你的胸腔里，把积在其中的气体排出来。气体排出后，你的肺部就又可以舒张了。你听到下面引流瓶内的水泡声了吗？

Patient: Yeah, but I can't move with the tube there.

病人：是的。可是，管子插在那儿我就不能动了！

Nurse: You can make some body movements on the bed, but you should not get out of bed these days. In addition, the tube should not be bended or folded. Otherwise it will not drain smoothly. Moreover, you should not turn your body too much to prevent the tube from dropping out. If you need to go out to take some tests, such as a chest X-ray, you must call me. I will clamp the tube down temporarily. If the tube drops out, it will worsen your condition because the thoracic cavity will open again.

护士：并不是完全不能动，这几天你可能不能下床，但可以在床上进行一些肢体活动。不过要特别注意这根管子，不要弯曲折叠，以免引流不畅。翻身幅度不能太大，以免管子脱落。假如要出去做检查，如 X 线检查等，一定叫我，我可以暂时把管子夹闭，否则，管子脱落，使密闭的胸腔又开放了，那会加重病情的。

Patient: When will the tube be taken out?

病人：什么时候这根管子能够拔掉呢？

Nurse: It can be taken out when the gas inside has been drained out, the X-ray shows your lung functions are normal, and you do not feel chest pain any more.

护士：等到你胸腔内的积气排出，并且 X 线片证实肺部膨胀良好，你的胸闷症状也完全改善后，这根管子就可以拔掉了。

Patient: Could I exercise like playing ball and running after I leave the hospital?

病人：出院后我还可以打球、跑步运动吗？

Nurse: I'm sorry there must be some limit to vigorous exercises. Also, you should avoid lifting weight, acute coughing and holding your breath. You also need to keep a regular bowel movement.

护士：很遗憾，可能对一些剧烈运动会有些限制了。同时你还要避免抬举重物、剧烈咳嗽、屏气，也要保持大便通畅。

Patient: After hearing your explanation, I don't feel nervous any more.

病人：听了你的讲述后，我的心里踏实多了。

# 11. Mechanical Ventilation

# 机械通气

Nurse： Mr. Wang，you have been under the oxygen therapy for two hours now，how do you feel?

护士： 王先生，你已经吸了两个小时的氧气了，感觉如何？

Patient： （waving his hands impatiently）Not so good. I still feel distressed. I am having a hard time breathing. It just feels so exhausting.

病人： （较烦燥地甩甩手）不行，我还是觉得很闷，透不过气来。我总觉得呼吸时特别累。

Nurse： I understand. Try to rest for a moment. I'll call the doctor now.

护士： 我知道了。你先休息一会儿，我马上去向医生汇报。

（The nurse came back to the patient again.）

（护士再次来到病人床边。）

Nurse： Mr. Wang，the doctor has come by to check on you. Following his order I am going to put you on a non-invasive breathing machine. It will help you breathe，so you can feel more comfortable.

护士： 王先生，医生刚才来看过你了。我现在遵医嘱准备给你使用无创呼吸机，让呼吸机来帮助你呼吸，这样你可能会感觉舒服点。

Patient： （waving his hand nervously）No，no. I don't want to use the machine. I'll be better in a moment.

病人： （很紧张地摇摇手）不要，不要，我不要上呼吸机。我待会儿就会好起来的。

Nurse： （smiling）Mr. Wang，don't be so nervous. This isn't the same kind of respirator we used in the past. It is a mini-respirator，and with few unfavorable effects. We will put a face mask on you and all you need to do is to breathe normally.

护士： （微微一笑）王先生，你别紧张。这种呼吸机不是我们以前所用的那种呼吸机。这是一种小型的呼吸机，对你影响不大。使用时，我们会给你佩戴一个面罩，你所要做的就是跟平常一样呼吸就行了。

Patient： （puzzled）Really?

病人： （很疑惑地）是吗？

Nurse： Yes，you see，here is the respirator.

护士： 是的，你看，我已经把呼吸机带来了。

Patient： （turned his head to look at the machine）Oh.

病人： （转头看了一下）哦。

Nurse: Mr. Wang, let me adjust the parameters of the respirator and the tube connections first, then I will help you to put on the mask, is that all right?

护士：王先生，我现在把呼吸机的参数调好，把管道连接好以后给你把面罩戴上，好吗？

Patient: (reluctantly) OK. Let's give it a try.

病人：（无奈地）那就试试吧。

Nurse: (finished the operation dexterously) Mr. Wang, are the straps of the mask on properly?

护士：（动作熟练地完成了操作）王先生，固定带的松紧合适吗？

(The patient nodded his head.)

（病人点点头。）

(The nurse helped clean the patient's bed.)

（护士帮助病人整理床单。）

(The patient pointed to the face mask with a stressful expression.)

（病人表情很痛苦，用手指着面罩。）

Nurse: (took off the face mask) What's the matter?

护士：（协助把面罩取下）怎么啦？

Patient: It is not working, I feel even more distressed. I rather go back to the oxygen therapy.

病人：不行，不行，我觉得更闷了。我还是像刚才那样吸氧气吧。

Nurse: Mr. Wang, many patients have experienced the same feelings when they first put on the mask. If you endure for a few minutes, you will get used to it. Let's try it again, OK?

护士：王先生，刚开始上这种呼吸机时，好多病人会出现与你一样的情况。你只要坚持几分钟就会适应的。我们再来试一下，好吗？

Patient: (sighed) OK.

病人：（叹气）好吧。

Nurse: (helped the patient to put on the mask again, and patted his shoulder) Mr. Wang, breathe normally, don't hold your breath. Right, that's it. Not bad. I will stay here to observe you.

护士：（再次帮病人把面罩固定好，拍拍病人的肩膀）王先生，就跟平时一样呼吸，不要刻意屏气。对，就像现在这样，不错，我在这儿看着呢。

(The patient nodded.)

（病人点点头。）

Nurse: (observed for about five minutes) Mr. Wang, how are you feeling now? Do you feel better?

护士：（站在床边观察了 5 分钟）王先生，现在感觉如何，是否比刚才好多了？

(The patient nodded.)

（病人点点头。）

# 12. Peptic Ulcer

# 消化性溃疡

## (1)

Nurse：Mr. Li，I know as a taxi driver，you must be very busy every day.

护士：李先生，我知道作为一名出租车司机，你平时一定很忙碌。

Patient：Yes，during working hours，I often can not eat regularly. Sometimes I get stomach aches.

病人：是的，在工作时间，我经常不能准时进餐，有时还会感到胃痛。

Nurse：That's one of the symptoms of a gastric ulcer. Besides taking antiacid drug，you must following the diet therapy.

护士：这是胃溃疡的临床表现之一。你除了服用抗酸药外，更要注意饮食治疗。

Patient：Could you tell me what is the diet therapy?

病人：你能告诉我什么是饮食治疗吗？

Nurse：Diet therapy is one of the most important parts of treating a gastric ulcer. You should have a well-balanced diet，eat slowly，chew thoroughly，and have small snacks such as soda biscuits between meals. You should also avoid irritating foods such as caffeine，nicotine，and alcohol.

护士：饮食治疗是胃溃疡治疗最重要的部分之一。你应该每日进食均衡膳食，细嚼慢咽，两餐之间吃些小点心，像苏打饼干。同时，你也应该避免进食刺激性食物，如咖啡因、尼古丁和酒精。

Patient：Yes，I know，but I'm very busy every day. Sometimes I forget these rules. What should I do?

病人：是的，我知道。但是我每日工作很忙，时常会忽视这些。现在我怎么做才好呢？

Nurse：I believe a healthy lifestyle will quicken your recovery. You should maintain a good mood，get enough rest，have a light diet，and avoid taking inappropriate medicine such as aspirin，which will irritate the gastric mucosa. Meanwhile，you must give up smoking and drinking，because they stimulate gastric acid secretion.

护士：良好的生活方式会加快你的康复。你应该保持良好的心情，充足的休息，清淡饮食，避免不合理用药，如阿司匹林，会刺激你的胃粘膜。同时，你必须戒烟戒酒，因为它们会刺激胃酸分泌。

Patient：Yeah，I know. But I am afraid that giving up smoking and drinking is too difficulty for me because they have become part of my life.

病人：是啊，我理解。但是戒烟、戒酒对我来说恐怕太难了，抽烟喝酒已成为我生活的一部分。

Nurse：Yes，I understand，it is not easy. But I also believe you can do it if you have strong determination.

护士：是的，我理解，这并不容易。但是我也相信只要你有坚强的意志你就会做得很好。

Patient：Thank you for your encouragement. I will try my best.

病人：谢谢你的鼓励，我会尽力而为。

Nurse：Great. Please don't hesitate to ask me if you have any questions. Let's plan your recovery plan together.

护士：很好。如果你有任何问题都可以问我，请不要犹豫。让我们共同制订你的康复计划。

Patient：What is a recovery plan?

病人：什么是康复计划呢？

Nurse：This is a good question. There are six things you should remember:

1. Maintain a healthy lifestyle as I mentioned earlier.
2. Follow the doctor's orders.
3. Take the medication regularly.
4. See the doctor in the clinic every month.
5. Stick to the treatment plan even after your symptoms have disappeared.
6. See your doctor as soon as possible if you have black stool or severe stomach pain that can't be relieved.

护士：你问得好，我告诉你以下6点你就知道了。

1. 保持上面提及的良好生活方式。
2. 严格遵从医嘱。
3. 规则服药。
4. 每月定期门诊随访。
5. 遵守治疗方案，哪怕你的症状已经消失。
6. 如果你出现黑便或胃痛难以缓解时，就要尽快找医生。

Patient：Thank you very much. I've learned a lot about gastric ulcer. It is very useful and I will follow your advice.

病人：非常感谢。我学到很多有关胃溃疡的知识。这些非常有用，我会按照你的建议去做。

Nurse：You are welcome. I hope you recover soon.

护士：不用谢。祝你早日康复。

**（2）**

Nurse：Where is your pain?

护士：你觉得哪里痛？

Patient：In my stomach.

病人： 胃痛。

Nurse： Show me exactly where it is.

护士： 请告诉我准确的位置。

Patient： Here.

病人： 这里痛。

Nurse： Do you feel pain after meals?

护士： 是饭后痛吗？

Patient： Yes. It happens after every meal.

病人： 对。每顿饭后都会痛。

Nurse： How soon does the pain come on after each meal?

护士： 饭后多久痛？

Patient： About half an hour.

病人： 大约半小时。

Nurse： Do you feel painful when you are hungry?

护士： 饥饿时痛吗？

Patient： Yes.

病人： 是的。

Nurse： Do you feel better after eating something?

护士： 吃点东西以后是否感到好些？

Patient： Yes，a little.

病人： 是，稍微好些。

Nurse： What kind of pain do you feel?

护士： 你感到是怎样的痛？

Patient： It is like a burning sensation.

病人： 像烧灼样感觉。

Nurse： When do you feel pain the most?

护士： 你感到什么时候最痛？

Patient： In the middle of the night.

病人： 在半夜里。

Nurse： Have you vomited?

护士： 有呕吐吗？

Patient： Yes，several times.

病人： 是的。我吐了几次。

Nurse： What did you vomit，food or blood?

护士： 你吐的是什么？食物还是血？

Patient： It was food with a little blood.

病人： 是食物，带一点血。

Nurse： Was the blood red or black?

护士： 吐的血是红色还是黑色？

Patient： Just like coffee.

病人：很像咖啡。

Nurse：According to your symptoms, it looks like you have peptic ulcer. We shall have to take an X-ray picture of stomach and intestine. If the X-Ray picture shows you have peptic ulcer, you'll have to come to the hospital to undergo treatment. In the meantime, the doctor will prescribe some medicine to make you comfortable.

护士：按你的病情像是消化性溃疡。我们将给你做胃肠X线检查。如果胃肠X线检查有消化性溃疡，你应该来医院接受治疗。医生将给你些药，让你舒服些。

**(3)**

Nurse：Hello, Ms. Li. Are you feeling better after five days of treatment ?

护士：李女士，经过5天的治疗您现在感觉好一些了吗？

Patient：A little better. But I feel the results of the treatment are coming too slow. Have you been giving me the right medicine?

病人：好是好一点了，但我觉得治疗效果太慢，是不是你们给我的药不对啊？

Nurse：Ms. Li, the medicine we've given you are for gastric acid control and to protect the gastric mucous membrane. They are appropriate for your illness.

护士：李女士，现在我们给您使用的都是针对您疾病的抑酸药、保护胃黏膜的药物。

Patient：Why am I recovering so slowly?

病人：那为什么恢复这么慢？

Nurse：Ms. Li, you are suffering from a peptic ulcer, which is caused by the digestion of the gastric mucous membrane by your own gastric acid. It's a chronic disease. Healing the ulcer and completely relieving the pain can only be achieved after lengthy treatment. You have only been treated for five days. It is not enough time to completely recover yet.

护士：李女士，您所患的疾病是由于胃肠黏膜被消化液自身消化而造成的溃疡，是一种慢性病，需要坚持长期治疗后溃疡面积才能慢慢修复愈合，疼痛才能完全缓解。现在才刚治疗5天，不可能这么快病就好了。

Patient：But I have stayed in the hospital for five days and there are so many things in my company waiting for me to handle. Please prescribe some better medicine for me so that I can be discharged sooner.

病人：可是我已经住院5天了，公司有一大堆事情等着我处理。你们再给我用些好药，让我尽快治好出院。

Nurse：The medicines we are using are the best. Relax. Anxiety is not good for recovery. It stimulates the secretion of gastric acid and makes your ill-ness even worse.

护士：我们现在给您用的药已经是最好的了。您不要着急，情绪焦虑对疾病治疗恢复不利，反而会刺激胃酸分泌增加，加重病情。

Patient：According to what you have said, it's difficult to cure my illness?

病人：照你这么说，我的病很难治好了？

Nurse：No, don't be so pessimistic. Currently there is a patient in our ward who has the same disease as you. He has almost recovered completely and is preparing for discharge. I will introduce him to you later，and you can talk to him about the treatment. Is that all right?

护士：不是的，你不要对治疗这么没信心。我们病房现在正好住了一位和您患有同样疾病的先生，他经治疗后已基本痊愈，准备择日出院。等会儿我介绍您和他认识，你们可以交流一下治疗情况，好吗？

Patient：OK. Has he really recovered?

病人：好吧。他真的好了吗？

Nurse：Really. Now the most important thing for you to do is to relax and try to be cheerful. I have a comic book. I'll let you read it and hope it will help you relax. I'll come back to see you after a while. If you feel uncomfor table，please tell me or press the call button. OK?

护士：是真的。你现在最主要的是放松心情，保持愉快良好的情绪。我这有一本《笑话大全》给你看，希望对你有所帮助。我一会儿再来看你，有什么不舒服告诉我或者直接按铃招呼我，好吗？

Patient：OK.

病人：好的。

# 13. Gastroscopy Examination

# 胃镜检查

Nurse： Mr. Ding，your bleeding has been stopped after the treatment in the last several days. Now we are going to give you an endoscopy examination. Is that OK?

护士： 丁先生，你经过这几天治疗后出血已止。我们准备给你做一次内镜（胃镜）检查，好吗？

Patient： I'm feeling quite good now. It is no need to have a gastroscopy examination.

病人： 我觉得我已经好了，不用做胃镜了。

Nurse： Mr. Ding，the gastroscopy examination can confirm the reason and exact location of the hemorrhage，so that we can prescribe the right treatment for you.

护士： 丁先生，胃镜检查可以明确你出血的原因及出血的部位，以便对症下药。

Patient： Is it necessary? I've heard that the examination is very uncomfortable.

病人： 必须要做吗？听说做胃镜很难受的。

Nurse： Well，it is better to have it done. It may be a little uncomfortable，but before the examination，the doctor will give you anesthesia in your throat to relieve your discomfort. When the gastroscopic tube is inserted to your throat area，you should follow the examiner's instruction to swallow it as you would swallow noodles. Good cooperation with each other can shorten the time and reduce the discomfort of the examination.

护士： 最好还是做。检查时是有一点难受，但是检查人员在检查前会给你的咽喉部麻醉一下，以减少你的不适。胃镜插到咽喉部后，你可以根据检查人员的口令像平时吞面条一样往下吞咽，检查者会同步插入胃镜，相互配合可减少插管时间从而减轻不适感。

Patient： I'm afraid I may not cooperate with the doctor very well because of being uncomfortable. I'm also concerned about hemorrhaging after they insert the tube into my stomach. Which doctor will perform the procedure for me?

病人： 我很担心自己因难受而不能配合好，还担心胃镜插入后会引起出血。不知道明天哪位医生给我做？

Nurse： I see. Please don't worry. The catheter of the gastroscopy is very thin and the doctor who will perform the examination is very skillful. He will to minimize the discomfort and it will not cause any hemorrhaging. We have more than thirty patients receiving this procedure every day，and almost none of the patients have bleeding problems. Also，the doctor who will perform the examination for you tomorrow is the chief surgeon He is the most experienced doctor at our hospital. So don't worry.

护士：噢，你的担心可以理解，不过你放心，现在的胃镜管很细。给你做检查的医生技术又很熟练，不会让你很难受的，更不会引起出血。每天都有30多位病人来做检查，几乎没有一位病人有出血现象，而且明天主任将亲自给你做。他是我们医院最有经验的医生，别担心。

Patient: Well, what should I do to prepare for the examination? Can I take food after the examination?

病人：那好吧，那么检查前需要做哪些准备工作，检查后是否可以进食？

Nurse: Food and water are not allowed six hours before the examination. You should take a dry towel with you to wipe saliva. You can eat food two hours after the examination. Taking food too early may lead to choking and asphyxia because of the throat anesthesia which can affect swallowing.

护士：做检查前需要禁食禁水6小时，并准备一块干毛巾以擦拭唾液用。术后2小时方可进食，过早进食可因咽部麻醉未消失，吞咽功能未恢复而造成呛咳窒息等情况。

Patient: But how much do I have to pay for it?

病人：做胃镜检查要多少钱？

Nurse: Two hundred and fifty yuan.

护士：250元。

Patient: It's too expensive. You know, Miss Qiu, my family is not doing well financially. Could you consult with the doctor to replace the examination with a cheaper one?

病人：太贵了，邱小姐你也知道我家庭的经济条件不好，能不能和医生商量一下换一种便宜点儿的检查项目？

Nurse: OK. Please wait for a moment. I'll ask the doctor now.

护士：好的，你先等一会儿，我去问问医生，好吗？

(After a while)

(过了一会儿)

Nurse: Mr. Ding, I've asked the doctor. The doctor insisted that you should have a gastroscopy examination.

护士：丁先生，我已经问过医生了，医生认为还是做胃镜比较好。

Patient: You only want to make money, not consider the situation of your patients.

病人：你们就知道赚钱，不考虑病人的具体情况。

Nurse: Don't be so angry, Mr. Ding. It is because of your family financial situation, we select the gastroscopy examination which will reveal the pathological changes clearly and directly. Therefore, other unnecessary examinations can be avoided, and thus to minimize your economic burden.

护士：丁先生，你不要生气。我们也正因为考虑到您的家庭情况才选择能直接清晰看到病变部位的胃镜检查，避免做不必要的其他检查，加重你的经济负担。

Patient: Well, OK.

病人：那好吧。

Nurse: Now, you can have a rest, Mr. Ding. I will accompany you later for the examination.

护士：丁先生，你现在先休息一会儿。等会儿我陪你一起去做胃镜检查。

# 14. Acute Pancreatitis

# 急性胰腺炎

Nurse： Mr. Wu，do you still have abdomen pain?

护士： 吴先生，腹部还疼吗？

Patient： (sighing lightly) I don't have pain any more. But the doctor said I couldn't eat anything，even a drink of water，I'm afraid I will be crashed.

病人： (轻轻叹口气)疼倒是不疼了。只是医生说了暂时还不能吃任何东西，哪怕一口水也不可以喝，我怕身体会垮掉。

Nurse： Yes. Nobody，even as strong as you，can sustain more than several days without eating food and drinking any water. But don't worry，we will provide you with intravenous nutrition liquid. The doctor told you not to eat and drink anything is to allow your pancreas to recover. If you ingest anything，even a little water，you pancreas will swell up，and may even rupture. You know，this kind of pain is very severe，which you have already experienced.

护士： 是的。任何人，即使是像你这么魁梧的人，若是连水都不能喝的话，也是支撑不了几天的。但我们会给你提供静脉营养液，所以你不用担心。医生嘱咐你"禁食"是为了让你的胰腺得到恢复。你吃任何东西，哪怕是一口水，都会使胰腺肿胀，甚至穿孔。你知道，这种疼痛是相当剧烈的，你也经历过。

Patient： Yes，it's hard to bear.

病人： 是的，难以忍受。

Nurse： When the pancreatitis is getting better，you can have food again. First，you can drink some water，five to ten ml each time，five to six times a day. If you are omfortable，you can have some rice soup instead of water，twenty to thirty ml. each time，five to six times a day. You can have vegetable soup，fish soup，and fresh juice as an additional meal. Next you can eat semi-liquids (such as porridge and lotus root starch)，and soft diets (such as wonton and noodles).

护士： 等到胰腺炎症逐渐消退后，你就可以进食了。先从喝水开始，每次5～10ml，一天5～6次。没有不舒服的话，可改喝米汤，一次20～30ml，一天5～6次，中间可加餐：如菜汤、鱼汤、新鲜果汁。然后逐渐过渡到半流质(如稀饭、藕粉)、软食(如馄饨、面条等)。

Patient： Thanks. I see. What should I pay attention to in my diet in the future?

病人： 谢谢，我知道了。那么我以后吃东西需要注意些什么呢？

Nurse： You should abide by one principle: have small quantities but frequent meals. Do not overeat and avoid high proteins and high fat diets. What cause you to become sick this time was your bad eating habits. Also, you must stop smoking and drinking.

护士： 你只需注意遵从一个原则：少食多餐，切忌暴饮暴食和高蛋白高脂肪大餐。你这次发病就是不注意饮食引起的。还有你一定要戒除抽烟、喝酒的不良习惯。

Patient： OK. I'll take your advice by giving up smoking and drinking, and having a reasonable diet. Thanks a lot, nurse.

病人： 好的，我一定听取你的建议，戒除烟酒，合理饮食。谢谢你，护士小姐。

# 15. Diarrhea

# 腹泻

## （1）

Nurse： Mrs. Wang，why do you eat so little food? Is it because you don't like the taste or you just don't have any appetite?

护士： 王太太，您怎么就吃这么一点儿东西？是不合口味，还是没胃口？

Patient： Neither.

病人： 都不是。

Nurse： Would you like to tell me the real reason?

护士： 那么您能告诉我为什么不肯多吃一点呢？

Patient： Oh...，I'm afraid I'll cause too much trouble for you. You see，I can't take care of myself yet.

病人： 嗯……我怕给你们添麻烦，因为到现在我的一切都还不能自理。

Nurse： So this is why you don't want to eat more! Oh，don't worry about that，it's not necessary. I'm your nurse and I'm supposed to take care of you. It is my job to do everything for you，including helping you to clean up after defecating. If you don't eat or drink，you will not have enough nutrition and will not recover quickly. You will not have energy to take care of yourself which will make it more uncomfortable for yourself and family members. Do you remember your perianal eczema was rather severe when you were first admitted to the hospital，and that we had to clean the area and apply medicine for you several times a day，and we never had any complaint?

护士： 您少吃少喝的原因是这样啊。噢！不必担心这些，那是不必要的。我是您的责任护士，为您做一切护理包括帮助您清洁排便都是我的工作。您若不按时吃喝，没有足够的营养，病就不会很快好起来，也就没有力气自理大小便。那样不仅给自己，也给家人带来很多不便。您记得刚入院时您的情况吗？您的肛门湿疹很严重，我们一天好几次给您擦洗、敷药，从来没有嫌麻烦。

Patient： (nodded) Yes.

病人： (点点头) 是的。

Nurse： So you must eat as much food as possible. Don't worry about causing any trouble for me. I'll come to you right away when you call me.

护士： 所以您一定要尽量多吃些有营养的食物。不要担心给我带来麻烦，只要您需要，我会立即来到您身边的。

Patient: OK. But how should I control my stool and urine?

病人：好吧！那我该如何控制大小便呢？

Nurse: You ought to take your meals on schedule and eat as much as you can. Drink adequate amount of water and relax. You will begin to have stool and urine like a normal person.

护士：您只要定时进餐，并尽量多吃一些，适当控制喝水，精神放松些，就会和正常人一样定期排便的。

Nurse: I see. I'll try to relax myself and not to worry about these things.

病人：明白了，我会尽量放松的，不会再顾虑那些了。

**(2)**

Nurse: When did your diarrhea start?

护士：你什么时候开始腹泻？

Patient: It started last night.

病人：昨天夜里开始。

Nurse: Do you remember how many times you went to the toilet?

护士：你记得去了多少次厕所吗？

Patient: I can't remember exactly. It must have been over ten times.

病人：记不准。要超过10次。

Nurse: What kind of stool did you notice，watery or mucous?

护士：你注意大便的样子了吗？是水样还是黏液样？

Patient: At first it was watery，but now I notice some mucus.

病人：开始是水样，现在有黏液。

Nurse: Do you feel abdominal pain when you go to the toilet?

护士：你上厕所时有腹痛感吗？

Patient: Yes.

病人：有。

Nurse: Have you vomited?

护士：吐没吐？

Patient: No，but I feel nauseated.

病人：没有，但我感到恶心。

Nurse: We will take a sample of your stool for examination. What did you eat last night for supper?

护士：我们要取点你的大便标本做检查。昨天晚饭你吃了些什么？

Patient: I had rice，some vegetables，a little meat and a glass of orange juice.

病人：我吃了些米饭、蔬菜、一点儿肉还喝了一杯橘汁。

Nurse: Was the orange juice fresh?

护士：橘汁新鲜吗？

Patient: It tasted fresh.

病人：味道新鲜。

Nurse： Your condition doesn't seem serious，but we must give you intravenous infusion to prevent dehydration. We will also give you some antibiotics. You should drink plenty of water and follow a liquid diet. If your diarrhea stops tomorrow，you can take some semi-liquid food. I think you will recover in no time.

护士： 看来你的病不重，但为了防止你脱水，我们必须给你静脉补液。我们还要给你用点抗生素。你要多喝水，进流质饮食。如果你明天不泻了，可进半流质饮食。我想你将很快恢复健康。

# 16. Diabetes

# 糖尿病

## （1）

Nurse： I notice you have several boils on your body.

护士： 我看到你身上有几个疖子。

Patient： Yes，I have had these boils for some time. They would often subside a little，but they have never healed completely.

病人： 是的。这几个疖子已经长了一些时候了。有时会好一点，但从来没有完全消退过。

Nurse： Is there anything else that bothers you besides the boils?

护士： 除掉疖子外，你还有什么不舒服？

Patient： I feel tired，and I itch all over.

病人： 我感到疲乏和全身发痒。

Nurse： Have you lost weight recently?

护士： 最近体重减轻了吗？

Patient： I think I have.

病人： 我想是减轻了。

Nurse： How is your appetite?

护士： 你的食欲怎样？

Patient： I have a very good appetite，and I feel hungry all the time.

病人： 我胃口很好，总感到饥饿。

Nurse： Do you drink lots of water and go to the toilet often?

护士： 你是否喝水很多？常去厕所？

Patient： Yes，I drink lots of water，but I still feel thirsty. And，I have to go to the toilet often.

病人： 我喝水很多，但仍感到口渴。我去厕所十分频繁。

Nurse： How long have you had these symptoms?

护士： 你有这些症状多久了？

Patient： More than six months.

病人： 半年多了。

Nurse： We would like to take your urine and blood samples to check their sugar contents.

护士： 我们要取你的尿样和血样，检查其中糖的含量。

Patient: Dr. Li told me I had diabetes.

病人: 李医生说我患有糖尿病。

Nurse: Yes, I know. Are there any diabetics in your family?

护士: 这个我知道，你家里有人患有糖尿病吗？

Patient: Yes. My mother has it.

病人: 我母亲有糖尿病。

Nurse: Dr. Li has ordered that you should follow a diabetic diet and insulin therapy. Here are instruction for diet and the therapy, which by the way, you'll have to administer yourself at home. We'll help you if you find any difficulties. Here are some antibiotics for your boils. I am sure you will feel better soon.

护士: 李医生讲你应该用糖尿病饮食及胰岛素治疗。这是给你的糖尿病食谱和治疗的方法，这样你可在家里为自己注射药物。你如有困难，我们将予以协助。这里是给你治疗疖子用的抗生素。我想你一定会很快好起来的。

## (2)

Nurse: Mr. Ni, it's nice to see you have come around. Your wife and daughter were scared to death. How do you feel?

护士: 倪先生，你可醒了，把你的夫人和女儿吓坏了，感觉怎么样？

Patient: I'm exhausted and don't feel like moving all.

病人: 就是没有力气，不想动。

Nurse: Don't worry and make sure you have a good rest. Your blood glucose has decreased to 18.6 mmol/L today. And let me take your body temperature. Oh, very good, 38.0℃. You should drink one glass of water, about 100 ml per hour. You will need less fluid infusion if you can drink more water. It can decrease the workload on your heart.

护士: 没关系的，你好好休息。你今天的血糖已降到 18.6 mmol/L。我来帮你测个体温。现在是 38.0℃，很好，你现在要多喝水，每小时要喝掉这么一杯，大约是 100ml，你能喝水就可以少输液，这样可以减轻心脏负担。

Patient: OK. I will try.

病人: 好的，我尽量喝。

Nurse: Have a rest I will see you later.

护士: 你先休息吧，过会儿我来看你。

Patient: Thank you.

病人: 谢谢。

(Two days later, Mr. Ni recovered almost completely, with temperature of 37.5℃and fasting blood glucose of 10.6 mmol/L.)

(又过了两天，倪先生已基本恢复，体温 37.5℃，空腹血糖 10.6 mmol/L。)

Nurse: Mr. Ni, you look very well today. Now let me measure your 2-hour-after-meal blood glucose. Well, it is 15.4 mmol/L.

护士: 倪先生，你今天气色真好，我现在给你测定餐后两小时血糖，是 15.4 mmol/L。

Patient: Why is the blood glucose level always much higher after meals?

病人：为什么餐后血糖比空腹要高那么多？

Nurse: It's one of the characteristics of Type II Diabetes. Because of the malfunction of your islet, there isn't enough insulin to decrease your blood glucose which leads to higher post-meal blood glucose.

护士：这是II型糖尿病的特点。由于你的胰岛功能差，食物吸收以后，没有足够的胰岛素把血糖降下来，因此餐后的血糖会比空腹高很多。

Patient: I see. Is there any way to decrease it?

病人：原来是这样，那有什么办法降下来吗？

Nurse: Yes. It will surely drop back to normal range if you keep taking the medicine. It is not good if you don't follow the treatment or take medicines.

护士：你只要坚持正规用药，血糖是可以降下来的。像你原来那样不吃药、不治疗是不行的。

Patient: But I feel pretty well these days, nothing uncomfortable.

病人：可是我的感觉真得很好，没有任何不舒服。

Nurse: This is another characteristic of Type Ⅱ Diabetes. Patients usually feel nothing wrong in the early stage. Some people don't know it before complications occur. The post-meal hyperglycemia will do great harm to a patient's heart, blood vessels and nerves. For example, your urine test shows your kidney has some damage. You should have your ocular fundus checked tomorrow.

护士：这又是Ⅱ型糖尿病的特点。在早期可以没有任何不适，等到出现并发症时才发现有糖尿病。餐后高血糖的危害是非常大的，会对人的心脏、血管、神经产生损害，比如你的尿液检查表明肾脏已有损害，明天再去做个眼底检查。

Patient: OK.

病人：好的。

(The patient returned the room after having his ocular fundus checked the following day.)

（第二天，倪先生做了眼底检查后回到病房。）

Nurse: Mr. Ni, here is the result of your ocular fundus examination. You ocular fundus problem is serious. You should have an operation when your blood glucose drops to normal.

护士：倪先生，你的眼底检查结果出来了。你的眼底病变比较严重了。需要手术治疗，等你的血糖降下来就可以手术了。

Patient: That serious? I have had a very bad eyesight for more than a year. I thought it was an aging related problem.

病人：有这么严重？不过我的眼睛看不清已经有一年多了。我以为是老花眼也没在意。

Nurse: The ocular fundus damage results from your long period of poor blood glucose control. Operation is necessary. It will improve your eyesight a lot. But first you must keep your blood glucose in a normal range.

护士：你的眼睛是由于长期血糖控制不佳引起的眼底病变，必须手术治疗，治疗后的效果是比较好的，但是手术前你的血糖要控制好。

Patient: I didn't suppose it was so severe. I was told "Fa-Lun-Gong" could cure my disease.

Considering diabetes is a chronic disease. I thought I could get rid of the medicines, improve my health and avoid trouble if I kept practicing it. Now I recognize because I have delayed my treatment, it has let to more damage to my health.

病人：后果真的很严重，我原来一点也不懂。听别人说练功后可以治疗疾病，我想糖尿病是慢性病，练了功可以不吃药，省了很多麻烦，又可以强身，一举两得。现在看来是耽误了自己的治疗，引来不必要的身体伤害。

Nurse: Yes. Diabetes is a life-disease, which can not be cured completely at the present time. But complications can be prevented by means of medications. If you can stick to the treatment and keep your blood glucose under control from now on, you should be able to live normal just like others.

护士：是的，糖尿病是一种终生性疾病，目前尚无办法根治，只有靠药物长期控制预防并发症。从现在起你只要坚持治疗，控制住血糖，还能像正常人一样生活。

Patient: It seems the old saying"one is never too old to learn"is correct. I will keep this in mind. I will believe in science and the doctors, and stick to medical treatment the rest of my life.

病人：看来人是需要活到老学到老，我会记住这次教训，相信科学，相信医生，坚持终生治疗。

## (3)

Nurse: Mr. Li, I have heard that you are fond of desserts and alcohol, right?

护士：李先生，我听说您很爱甜食和饮酒，是吗？

Patient: Yes, I can't go to sleep without a drink. I know that diabetes patients should not drink, but I can't resist the temptation of wine.

病人：是的，不喝酒我就睡不着觉。我知道患糖尿病不能喝酒，可是我就是挡不住酒的诱惑。

Nurse: Right now your blood glucose is high and you also have cataracts. If you don't give up drinking and don't stop eating desserts, complications will become worse. Why don't we find a way together to curb your desire for wine and dessert?

护士：您现在的血糖处于高水平，又并发了白内障，如果再不禁酒，不控制饮食，并发症会更多更重。我们能否想个办法共同努力控制饮酒和甜食呢？

Patient: That's fine. What I need is your instructions and help.

病人：好的，我正需要你的指导和帮助。

Nurse: Then let us do some interesting things like listening to music, playing chess and reading novels to divert your attention from alcohol and desserts. We can plan an appropriate diet menu for you. We can also request that the nutritionist prepare food with good color, aroma, and flavor for you to stimulate your appetite. I'm sure you are capable of controlling wine and desserts intake.

护士：那好，让我们来找一些有兴趣的事做，像听音乐、下棋、看小说等等，分散您对酒和甜食的注意力。然后我们为您制订合理的食谱，让营养师把食物加工得色香味俱全，刺激您对食物的欲望，相信您会有能力控制饮酒和甜食的。

Patient： Sure, I'll do my best to cooperate with you. Another question is that I have cataracts in both of my eyes. My left eye is almost totally blind and the eyesight of my right eye is very poor. This makes it very inconvenient for me to get around. Can they be treated?

病人： 行，我一定努力合作。还有一个问题想请教一下，我的双眼都患了白内障，左眼几乎全看不清了，右眼的视力也很差，使我行动非常不便，不知能否治好？

Nurse： They can be treated. We can ask the eye doctor to see you after your blood glucose level become normal. A simple operation (laser beam or ultrasonic therapy) will enable you to see again.

护士： 可以治的，只要血糖控制正常了，我们可以请眼科医师来给您会诊，一般只需做一个简单手术（激光或超声雾化）就能帮您重见光明的。

Patient： That's great. I'll cooperate with you to have my blood glucose controlled and then schedule for the eye operation as soon as possible.

病人： 太好了，我一定好好配合你们尽快控制血糖，争取早日安排眼科手术。

Nurse： Fine. Let's work hard together.

护士： 好，让我们共同努力。

# 17. Hyperthyroidism

# 甲亢

Nurse： Would you like to sit with me in the garden?

护士： 我们去花园坐一会儿，好吗？

（The patient nodded and went with the nurse to a stone bench in the garden.）

（病人点点头，随护士来到花园石椅边。）

Nurse： Sit down，please（they sat down on the bench face to face）. Could you tell me the one thing you want the most these days?

护士： 请坐吧（护士、病人面对面坐下）。你能告诉我这段时间您最想做的一件事情吗？

Patient： To have the disease cured and go home as soon as possible because my son is going to take the college entrance examinations next month.

病人： 当然是尽快治好病，早点出院，因为儿子下个月就要参加高考了。

Nurse： Oh. I see you have a great deal of anxiety and hope everyone cooperates with you，right? But is it possible? The financial personnel must follow the routine procedure and your roommates just want to listen to the radio to alleviate their boredom. Try to see from their point of view so you won't be so angry.

护士： 噢，所以你心里很急，希望所有人都能与你合作，这可能吗？财务科必须履行常规手续，而你的同室病友希望用收音机摆脱寂寞。交换位置，替他们想想，你就不生气了。

Patient： But I can't stand it. The more I think about it，the angrier I become. It seems everyone is hostile to me.

病人： 可是我忍不住，越想越生气，觉得所有人都跟我过不去似的。

Nurse： I understand what you are going through. But I must tell you anger and a hot temper won't do any good to your health. My advice is when you are at the verge of getting angry，you should remember the most importance thing for you is a quick recovery，so you can go home to look after your son when he is taking the college entrance examinations. It's no use getting angry with others or over trifles. This way of thinking may help to calm you down.

护士： 我完全理解你此刻的心情。但我必须告诉你，发脾气、生气对你的疾病尽早康复很不利。我的忠告是，当你要发火生气时就想"没关系，比起儿子要高考，需要我回家照顾这件事来讲，这些事不值得我发火"，这样你就能平静下来了。

Patient： You think this will work? I will try. Come to think of it. I should not have lost my temper and quarreled over such trivial matters.

病人： 管用吗？我试试看吧。其实想想这几天发生的事都是不值得生气的。

# 18. Gout

# 痛风

Nurse： Hello，Mr. Qiao. I'm your primary nurse. You can call me Xiao Zou. I reviewed your medical history，and noticed that you have had high blood uric acid for some time. Why didn't you come to see the doctor sooner?

护士： 乔先生你好，我是你的责任护士，我姓邹，你可以叫我小邹。我看了你的病史，发现你的尿酸升高已经有一段时间了，为什么没有来看医生？

Patient： Although my blood uric acid level was high，I didn't feel anything wrong with me. Anyway，I did pay attention to my diets. So far，I only eat bean products，vegetables and mushrooms. I have not touched any animal internal organs or seafood for some time.

病人： 我以为尿酸有点升高，又没有什么不舒服是没关系的。而且我也注意了饮食，动物内脏、海鲜都不敢吃，我只吃豆制品、蔬菜、菌类、蘑菇等。

Nurse： Yes，as you said，it's important for patients with high blood uric acid to pay attention to their daily diet. But you've known only part of the information. As you indicated，seafood and animal internal organs contain high purine，and you don't eat them. But，this is not enough. For example，mushroom and soybean also contain lots of purine，and these foods should not be recommended for you to eat. In addition，spinach，hyacinth beans and peas，are also high in purine. They are also not the proper food for you.

护士： 是的，尿酸升高的病人是要注意饮食。但是你只了解了一部分。动物内脏和海鲜的嘌呤太高不能吃，但是，你还了解得不够，像一些菌类、黄豆也含很高的嘌呤，所以豆制品也不能多吃。除了这些，蔬菜中菠菜、扁豆、豌豆也含很高的嘌呤，也不能多吃。

Patient： I can't eat any of these! What can I eat?

病人： 这些都不能吃，那我能吃些什么呀？

Nurse： Well，its true that the diet for patients with gout is greatly restricted. The seafood，meat and strong tea contain high purine which you should avoid. Are you shouldn't have too much alcohol related drinks，especially the beer. The alkaline foods such as eggs，milk，potato，most vegetables and oranges are recommended. They increased the PH value of your urine which can prevent the uric acid from forming crystals and can also facilitate the excretion of it.

护士：确实，痛风病人的饮食受到很大的限制。一般的鱼虾、肉类、浓茶都含比较高的嘌呤，酒也不能多喝，特别是啤酒。你可以吃一些碱性食物，如鸡蛋、牛奶、马铃薯、大部分的蔬菜、柑橘类水果等。这些碱性食物能使尿液的 pH 值上升，从而可以促进尿酸的排泄，防止尿酸盐结晶。

Patient: If I can't eat so many things, will I be malnourished?

病人：什么都不能吃我不是要营养不良吗？

Nurse: I didn't mean you couldn't eat anything, rather you should control the amount and selection of your food. Considering your body weight is 76.5kg and your height is 170cm, you are over-weight. Your high uric acid level and excessive weight mean that you should control your food intake. As I calculated, you may have 70g of protein and 400g of rice each day. With this amount of food intake, it will meet your physiological needs and you will not become malnourished.

护士：不是让你什么都不吃，而是有控制、有选择地吃。你体形偏胖，你的身高是 170cm，体重达了 76.5 公斤，已经超重，再加上尿酸升高，更需要控制热量，减少饮食量。我已经帮你算过了，你每天的蛋白质摄入量为 70 克，米饭大约可以吃到 8 两，就能满足你每天的生理需要量，而不会出现营养不良。

Patient: Listening to your advice, I've learned a lot and I will pay attention from now on..But my foot really hurts now. Can you take care of this problem as soon as possible?

病人：听你这么一说，我了解了很多，以后一定会注意的。但是我现在的脚比较痛，有什么办法能尽快缓解？

Nurse: Here is the medicine, Colchicine, for your acute gout arthritis. Take one pill per hour. You must stop taking it if diarrhea occurs.

护士：这是秋水仙碱，是治疗痛风性关节炎急性发作的特效药。你每过一小时服一片，出现腹泻立即停药。

Patient: Could I take two pills each time? It might help me get better sooner.

病人：我能不能吃两片，可以好得快一点。

Nurse: No. You should never do that. This drug has some toxic effects. It is only used at the acute stage of gout. You should stop taking it the moment you feel better.

护士：千万不可以的，该药的毒性比较大，只能在痛风的急性发作期才能用，而且一旦症状缓解就要立即停药。

Patient: I see. I will follow your advice.

病人：我明白了，我会按你说的去做的。

(Four hours later, Mr. Qiao was able to walk around without much pain at his joint. The nurse returned to the ward.)

（4 小时后，患者关节疼痛症状缓解，行走自如。床位护士再次来到了病房。）

Patient: This drug really works! I don't feel much pain now. You see, the swelling on my foot has gone also. Could I buy some more of this drug for future use?

病人：这个药真灵，我现在也不太疼了。看，脚也不肿了，我以后能不能自己买了吃。

Nurse: I'm afraid not. As I said, this drug has big side-effects and is only permitted to be taken at the acute stage of gout attack. At chronic stage, two kinds of drugs can be used. One is to facilitate the excretion of the uric acid, such as Probenecid, and sodium bicarbonate. When taking these drugs, make sure to drink water no less than 2000ml per day. The other is Allopurinol. This drug will limit the synthesis of uric acid.

护士： 不可以，刚才我已经说过了，这个药毒性大，不能经常吃，只有在急性发作期才能用。平时你可以吃一些促进尿酸排泄的药，如丙磺舒、碳酸氢钠。用药期间注意多饮水，每天至少2000ml。还可以服一些抑制尿酸合成的药，如别嘌醇。

Patient： OK. I understand. I will watch my diets, and take these drugs after discharge, than I will not need to come back to the hospital again because of the pain.

病人： 好，我知道了，回去以后我会坚持控制饮食，同时服用一些治疗的药物。那样，我以后就不会再疼得需要住院治疗了。

Nurse： Yes. I'm sure you can do it.

护士： 是的，相信你一定能够做到的。

# 19. Acute Hepatitis

# 急性肝炎

## （1）

Patient: I will be discharged from the hospital tomorrow. I know that patients suffering from hepatitis need a lot of rest. But I don't know how long I should rest before I can work normally?

病人：我明天要出院了。我知道得了肝炎要多休息，不知道要休息多长时间才能正常上班？

Nurse: Congratulations，you certainly need to pay attention to rest after leaving the hospital. You should pay attention to both physical and mental rest. You should increase the time for rest and decrease the consumption of physical strength to relieve the burden of your liver.

护士：恭喜你可以出院了。出院以后你的确要注意休息，包括精神休息和身体休息。要增加休息时间，减轻体力消耗，减轻肝脏负担。

Patient: What is a mental rest?

病人：什么是精神休息呢？

Nurse: Mental rest means that mentally you should relax and maintain a peaceful mind. Set aside your office work，study，housework，and social activities temporarily.

护士：精神休息就是说你的精神要放松，心情要平和。工作、学习、家务、人际方面的事情要暂时放开。

Patient: Without work，study，social activities，life would become very boring.

病人：不工作、不学习、不交际，岂不是很闷。

Nurse: Life wouldn't be very boring. You could listen to music，keep a diary or do light weight gardening. But you must not do things that will preoccupy yourself excessively，such as chatting on line，playing card games，playing game machines，etc.

护士：不会啊，你可以听听音乐、写写日记、养养花草。但是精神过分集中的事情不要做，比如上网聊天、打牌、玩游戏机等。

Patient: OK. What should I pay attention to the physical rest?

病人：好的。那么身体方面的休息要注意些什么呢？

Nurse: You are suffering from acute hepatitis. Ninety five percent of patients with this disease can be cured according to the statistics. However, excessive fatigue and inadequate sleep will influence the recovery. So at least for the first month after you leave the hospital, you must rest at home. You must not go to work. Your life must be regular. After one month you can do some moderate work such as washing dishes, dusting and tiding the room. If your job workload is not very heavy, you may try to work. At the beginning you could work for half a day and gradually restore full-time job according to your recovery condition. If your workload is heavy, then you should consult with your supervisor to temporarily shift you to an easier job. You must avoid excessive fatigue in the first six months after you leave the hospital.

护士：你患的是急性肝炎。据统计，95% 的急性肝炎能治愈，但是过度劳累、睡眠不足都会影响恢复。所以你出院后至少一个月内要在家休息，不能上班，生活要有规律。一个月后可以做一些力所能及的事情，如洗碗、擦灰、整理房间等。如果你上班的工作量不是很大，你可以试着去工作，从半天开始，根据身体状况逐渐恢复至全天工作。如果上班工作量较大，你最好去跟领导商量，暂时更换一个较轻松的岗位。在出院后的半年内，一定要避免过度劳累。

Patient: OK. I will consult with my boss. He is quite nice.

病人：好的，我去跟领导说说，他是很有人情味的。

Nurse: Another important thing is you must have midday nap which should last about 30 minutes to one and half an hour. This is the best method to relieve fatigue and restore physical strength. Furthermore, it is better to turn to your right side, and maintain a 45 degree angle while you sleep.

护士：还有一点很重要，就是在你恢复期内，要尽量安排午睡，这是解除疲劳、恢复体力的极佳方法。午睡时间以 0.5～1.5 小时为好。另外，睡觉以右侧卧位为宜，使身体与床面成 45 度角。

Patient: Why?

病人：为什么呢？

Nurse: Because this lying position puts the liver under the celiac artery and allows the blood to flow down to the liver. It is more beneficial for the transport of nutritious substance from artery to the liver.

护士：因为这种卧位使肝脏位于腹腔动脉的下方。动脉血液走下行路线流向肝脏，这对动脉血为肝脏输送营养物质十分有利。

**(2)**

Nurse: Mr. Zhang, how do you feel today? How is your appetite?

护士：老张，你今天感觉怎么样？胃口好吗？

Patient: Well, my appetite today is better than the last couple of days. My wife stewed a turtle for me for lunch and I ate the whole thing. She is going to prepare some tasty food for me this evening as well.

病人：今天感觉不错，胃口比前两天好多了。中午家里给我炖了一只小甲鱼，我一口气就把它吃光了。晚上我太太准备再给我做些好吃的来。

Nurse: Is that right! Your wife is so nice.

护士: 是吗？你太太真贤惠。

Patient: Yes, my disease has made her suffer very much. She has to work and takes care of me. How long do I have to stay in the hospital? If it's too long, my wife will become sick due to the hard work.

病人: 是的，我这次生病可苦了她了，除了上班还要跑医院。我这病还需住院多长时间？长此以往我太太要累垮的。

Nurse: Take it easy, Mr. Zhang, so far you have only been here for one week. Your doctor is treating you with the best program. An important thing I need to repeat is that your disease is still in the progress stage. Your food should be very light and too much fat is no good. Supplement of nutrition is good, but at the present time you'd better not eat food containing high protein such as turtles, ells, eggs etc. After you have recovered and the index of your liver function is normal you may then be supplemented with protein.

护士: 老张，你别心急。你住院还不到一个星期，医生正在用最好的方案给你治疗。不过有一点我要跟你重申一下，目前你的疾病处于发展阶段，饮食要清淡不宜太油腻，增加营养固然是好的，但目前不要进食太多高蛋白食物，像甲鱼、鳗鱼、鸡蛋等暂时不要吃，等你的病慢慢恢复了，肝功能指标正常了，再适当补充蛋白质好吗？

Patient: Oh, I forgot what you had told me before. I will not eat those food for now.

病人: 噢！我忘了你跟我说过的了，那我暂时先不吃了。

Nurse: This is very important. You must keep it in mind. You haven't had bowel movement for two days, so you should eat some fruits and vegetables rich in fiber such as celery, and cane shoot etc. You should also drink proper amount of water. In addition, you may massage your abdomen area around the belly button in a clockwise direction three times a day, five to ten minutes each time, this can promote bowel movement. I will also ask your doctor to prescribe some medicine for your bowel movement.

护士: 这一点非常重要，你务必要牢记。这两天你没有解大便，可以吃一些粗纤维的蔬菜和水果，譬如芹菜、茭白等。适当多喝点水。还有，每天可在脐周顺时针方向按摩3次，每次5～10分钟，这样可以促进排便。我会请医生开一些促进排便的药物给你。

Patient: Thank you, Miss Wu. I will ask my wife to cook some vegetable dishes tonight.

病人: 谢谢你，小吴护士，今天晚上我让太太烧些蔬菜来。

# 20. Cardiac Murmurs

# 心脏杂音

Nurse: Hello，Mr. Li，you seem a little bit concerned about this test. Can you tell me what you are worried about?

护士：李先生，您看上去对做这项检查有点担忧，能告诉我您担心什么吗？

Patient: Yes. I was told that I had cardiac murmurs during the pre-employment physical examination. How could I have heart disease? If it is true，the hiring company will definitely turn me down and I would be finished.

病人：是的，我体检时发现心脏有杂音，我怎么会有心脏病的？如果查出来心脏有问题，招聘单位一定会不要我。那我一切都完了。

Nurse: Oh，I see. I understand your feeling completely. The test today has a lot to do with your heath and your job search，right?

护士：噢，原来是这样。你此刻的心情我非常理解，因为这项检查关系到你的身体健康和就业前景，是吗？

Patient: Yes. I feel as if I am waiting for a trial verdict.（Rubbing his hands while talking to the nurse.）

病人：你说得很对。我感到简直像在等待一场审判。（边说边用力搓着双手。）

Nurse: Don't worry too much. Cardiac murmurs do not necessarily mean that you have a heart disease. It might be just a temporary physiological condition. Did you have a physical examination before entering college? What were the results then?

护士：您不必太担心，不是所有的心脏杂音都表示有器质性心脏病的，也可能是暂时的生理性的。您经历过高考体检，当时情况是怎样的？

Patient: Oh，yes，the doctor told me then that I had a cardiac murmur. But he believed it was a physiological condition. This time I am afraid I will not be so lucky. Otherwise，why was I asked to take the Doppler echocardiograph?

病人：当时那个医生好像也说过我心脏有杂音，是生理性的。不过这次也许不那么好运气了，否则，为什么要我做多普勒超声呢？

Nurse: The purpose of having you take the Doppler echocardiograph is to obtain a more accurate diagnosis. There are two possible results from the test：either to confirm or to rule out heart disease. Therefore，it is possible for either one of the results.

护士：做多普勒超声是为了明确诊断，它会有两种结果：一是确诊心脏有问题；二是确定心脏没有问题。对您来讲两种可能都是有的。

Patient：Oh，I see. They asked me to take a test does not mean that I have a disease. It can help to rule out some possible problems. For me，there is a 50% chance. It does not mean everything is over. I feel much better now. Thank you so much.

病人：护士小姐，我明白你的意思了。做检查并非肯定有疾病，也是为了排除问题，有病和没病的可能各占 50%。所以我不见得真的一切都完了。经你这么一说，我心里感觉好多了。非常谢谢你。

Nurse：You are welcome.

护士：不客气。

# 21. Chronic Heart Failure

# 慢性心力衰竭

Nurse： Mr. Zhang，you looked unhappy these couple days. What's on your mind?

护士： 张先生，我看你这两天总是闷闷不乐，有什么心事吗？

Patient： I am old and because my heart is not good，I had to be hospitalized several times a year. What's the point of living?

病人： 唉！我年纪大了，心脏又不好，一年要住好多次医院，活着还有什么意思？

Nurse： Do not worry too much. You were able to fight it through in the past，right? Can you recall what caused you to be hospitalized the past few times?

护士： 不要太担心！前几次不都过来了吗？现在你能回忆一下前几次住院是因为什么原因吗？

Patient： The first time was because I stopped the medicines on my own. Twice like this time，were because I had a cold，and once was due to fatigue.

病人： 第一次住院是因为我自己停药才发病的。有两次和这次一样都是因为感冒，还有一次是太疲劳。

Nurse： Actually cold and fatigue are the most common inducing factors for heart failure. Other than that，high salt intake and excitement can also induce heart failure. Because of that，you must have enough rest，avoid being too tired，and stay warm to prevent catching cold. Your diet should have low salt and easy to digest，also eat less in quantity but more frequently. Reduce intake of sodium-rich foods such as pickled foods，carbonized beverages and canned goods. You should eat more fruits and vegetables to keep your bowel movement.

护士： 其实像你所说的疲劳、感冒是心衰最常见的诱发因素。除此之外，吃得太咸、情绪激动等也会诱发心衰。因此，你必须注意休息，避免过度劳累，要注意保暖，预防感冒。饮食宜清淡低盐，易消化，而且要少量多餐，避免过饱。少吃含钠丰富的食物，如盐腌食物、碳酸饮料、罐头食品等，多吃蔬菜与水果，保持大便通畅。

Patient： I often like to eat salty fish，pickled vegetables. I see now these types of food are not good to my heart. I also like cooler temperature and often catch cold. If I follow your instructions，I will not be admitted to the hospital so often，right?

病人： 我平时很喜欢吃咸鱼、咸菜，看来这些对我的心脏是有害的，而且我很贪凉，所以经常感冒。如果我能照你说的去做，我就不会经常住院了，是吗？

Nurse: Yes, if you can stay persistent, you'll be able to reduce the frequency of hospitalization.

护士：是的，如果你能坚持的话，就可以减少住院的次数。

# 22. Quit Smoking

# 戒烟

Nurse： Hello，Mr. Pang，you're such a hard worker. You're sill working even in the hospital.

护士： 庞先生，您真勤奋，住院了还忘不了办公。

Patient： I can't help it. Since I've been sick，the company hasn't been able to function normally. As you see，there are so many documents that haven't been read for the past three days.

病人： 没办法，我这一倒，公司的运作都成了问题，你看三天的文件都等着我批。

Nurse： So your health is very important. Because of the myocardial infarction，you must get sufficient rest otherwise your prognosis will be affected.

护士： 所以，你的健康是很重要的。不过，得了心肌梗死，关键是休息，不然对你的预后影响很大。

Patient： Yes，I know that. But I so busy. I have no time to rest and have to smoke two packs of cigarettes to work through the night. I don't know what I should do now I'm suffering from this disease.

病人： 我也知道，可我生意忙，应酬多，往往是两包烟就熬上一个通宵。得了这病以后不知怎么办！

Nurse： I understand. But this kind of lifestyle is not good for your health. Smoking can increase the rate of sudden death in coronary heart disease（CHD）by fifty percent. Fat and high calorie foods，which you usually eat，also increase the risk of early CHD.

护士： 我理解，但是你以前的生活方式都是不利于健康的。吸烟将促使冠心病猝死的危险性增高50%，而长期高脂、高热量饮食也是导致冠心病早发的危险因素。

Patient： （Surprised）Really? Before，I only thought smoking could be harmful to the lung. I didn't know it was so harmful to the heart.

病人： （很惊讶）真的？我只知道吸烟会损害肺，没想到对心脏损害也这么大。

Nurse： In addition to affecting the heart，lung and stomach，smoking can also endanger the people around you.

护士： 吸烟的危害可涉及心、肺、胃。同时，你吸烟还会造成周围人被动吸烟，危及他人。

Patient： Wow! I'm not only hurting myself but also hurting everyone else around me. I must give up smoking.

病人： 哇！那我可不是害人又害己了，我一定要把烟戒了。

# 23. Percutaneous Transluminal Coronary Angioplasty

# 经皮冠状动脉腔内成形术

Nurse: Mr. Wang, is your chest pain getting better?

护士：王先生，你胸痛好些了吗？

Patient: (sighed) I feel much better now since they gave me the transfusion. But the doctor told me that I would need surgery immediately. There are certain risks of having heart operations. Therefore, I am worried if I'll ever be able to go back home if the operation fails.

病人：（叹了口气）输了这瓶液后，胸痛已经好多了。但是，刚才医生告诉我，要马上给我做手术，毕竟这是在心脏动手术，风险一定很大。我担心万一手术失败，我是否能回到自己家里？

Nurse: Yes, I understand your concern very much. This procedure has some risk. But, I should tell you that this procedure has much less risk when compared with the surgery because the incision is relatively very small. In this procedure, the physician will insert a tube into the femoral artery after local anesthesia. You will feel very little pain, almost like having an ordinary injection. Also during the procedure you will be fully conscious. I am sure you can handle it.

护士：是的，我非常能理解你现在的担忧。这个手术是有一定的风险，但是，我要告诉你，其实这是一种创伤很小的手术治疗方法，比外科手术风险小多了。手术时只需在你的大腿根部打上麻醉药，然后穿刺插管，就像平时打针一样稍微有些疼痛。我相信你一定能行，而且你在整个手术过程中始终是清醒的。

Patient: I am not afraid of the pain. But since my coronary artery is occluded completely, how can it be reopened? I will die if the blood vessel ruptures.

病人：这些疼痛我倒是不怕，只是我的血管已经堵塞，怎么有可能再打通呢？万一不小心把血管捅破了，我不就没命了吗？

Nurse: Do not worry. We perform this kind of operation almost every week without any incident. The doctor who will perform the procedure for you is a very experienced physician. The patient next to your bed, Mr. Zhang, underwent the same operation last week. He has recovered nicely and is out of bed, moving around.

护士：你放心，我们几乎每个星期都有这种手术，还未发现过类似的情况。况且，给你做手术的医生是一位非常有经验的医生。你瞧隔壁床的张先生，上个星期也做了与你同样的手术，现在已下床活动了。

Patient: Really? This makes me feel much better now.

病人: 哦，听你这么一说，我放心多了。

Nurse: Good. Now let me tell you a little about the procedure so that you'll be able to cooperate better with the medical personnel during and after the procedure. OK?

护士: 为了让你手术中、术后与医生更好地配合，我来给你简单讲一下手术过程及术后的注意事项，好吗？

Patient: That's great. I want to know it.

病人: 太好啦，我的确很想知道这些内容。

Nurse: (Miss Li takes out an illustration for the patient.) Look at this picture, Mr. Wang. One of your coronary arteries is occluded. This has caused myocardial infarction due to lack of blood and oxygen to the myocardium for an extended period. So first, the physician will puncture the femoral artery and insert a catheter into the opening of the coronary artery. He will then take a coronary angiography to determine where the stenosis is and its severity. Finally he will deliver a balloon catheter to dilate and reopen the occluded artery to allow the blood flow. A stent will be planted if necessary. Do you understand my explanation?

护士: (拿出手中的宣教图片)你看这幅图，王先生。你的一根冠状动脉已被堵塞，导致一部分心肌长时间因缺血缺氧而坏死。手术时，医生首先在大腿根部的股动脉处穿刺，将导管送至冠状动脉口，注入造影剂，以明确病变的部位和程度。再根据造影结果，送入球囊导管，加压扩张球囊后，使堵塞的冠状动脉重新开通，恢复血流，必要时还将植入金属支架，使冠状动脉持续扩张。我这样讲解，能让你理解吗？

Patient: Yes, I see. Therefore I will have no more chest pain after the operation because the re-supply of blood to the myocardium. Is this right?

病人: 明白了。手术后我的心肌重新恢复了血液供应，我就不会有胸痛了，是吗？

Nurse: Yes, usually there will be no more chest pain. However, because of the puncture femoral artery, you must stay in bed for twenty-four hours, and keep your leg from moving for twelve hours to avoid bleeding. You may move around in bed after twenty-four hours if nothing is wrong.

护士: 是的，一般情况下不会再发生胸痛。由于术中穿刺大动脉，为了避免伤口出血，术后你还需要平卧位休息 24 小时，动手术的那条腿要限动 12 小时。如果无异常，24 小时后你就可以适当在床上活动了。

Patient: Really? Twenty-four hours? What should I do if I want to urinate?

病人: 是吗？24 小时不动，如果要小便，怎么办呢？

Nurse: You must learn to urinate and feed in bed.

护士: 所以，现在开始，你就要在床上训练躺着排尿和进食。

Patient: OK. I will.

病人: 好的，我会练的。

# 24. Angiography

# 血管造影

Nurse: Mr. Li，do you still feel pain?

护士：李先生，你还是很痛吗？

Patient: Yes，it is still very painful.

病人：是的，还是很痛。

Nurse: If you hurt too much，you may want to moan loudly which may make you feel better.

护士：如果你痛得厉害，可以大声地哼几声，这样感觉会好一些。

Patient: Why do I still hurt so much after the operation?

病人：我刚才已经做了手术，可我怎么还是这么痛？

Nurse: Take it easy，Mr. Li. What the doctor did you today was angiography to check the condition and the location of the venous thrombosis. This is to prepare for the operation later. The doctor also put a filter in your blood vessel to prevent the thrombus from moving to other organs. He did not take out the thrombus. Because the problem is still there that is why you still feel pain. Let me put a pillow under your leg to reduce your pain.

护士：李先生，不要着急，慢慢来。今天医生只是为你做了一个血管造影检查血管栓塞的部位和情况，为手术做准备。同时还在血管内放了一个滤器防止栓子脱落栓塞其他器官组织，并没有取出栓子。由于根本问题还没有解决，所以还会痛。现在我给你腿下垫一个枕头，这样疼痛会减轻些。

Patient: Miss Wang，why did you put a pillow under my leg? I don't feel comfortable putting my leg on it.

病人：王护士，为什么要垫个枕头，我觉得腿搁在上面不舒服。

Nurse: I put the pillow there to raise your leg to promote the blood in your leg to circulate back to your heart. This will reduce the swelling of your leg and make you feel better.

护士：垫了枕头后腿就抬高了，能促进腿上的血回流到心脏。这样腿肿就会减轻点，腿痛也会随之好一些。

Nurse: Mr. Li，please try not to move the leg for at least eight hours to prevent hemorrhage from the punctured site. You may turn your body after eight hours，but do not get out the bed. You need to remain in bed rest for two weeks. If you get out of the bed and move around，it may cause the thrombus to dislocate or the filter in your blood vessel may also move which is not good for your health. So you should do what I told you.

If you feel your chest tighten up, short of breath, or nervousness, you should call me right away.

护士： 李先生，穿刺的腿 8 小时内不要动，以免穿刺部位出血。8 小时后才可以翻身，但还不能下床，要卧床休息两周。下床后血管里的滤器有可能要移位，也可能栓子脱落，对身体是很不利的。所以你要按照我说的去做。如果你感到胸闷、气急、心慌等不适，要马上呼叫我。

Patient: I see. But my back will be aching if I lie in bed and not move for eight hours.

病人： 我知道了。但是我这样 8 小时躺在床上不动会腰酸背痛很难受的。

Nurse: Don't worry. I will teach you how to raise your buttocks. You can use your hands to hold the back headboard or the sides of the bed, bow your waist, and then raise your buttocks. Do the exercise every one to two hours. I will massage your coccyx area to help release your muscle tiredness, and to prevent the formation of bedsores. Now let us try it.

护士： 不要紧，我教你一个自我抬臀的方法。你把双手往后抓住床靠背或抓住两边的床沿，腿屈起来一撑一收腰，臀部就抬起来了。你要 1～2 个小时抬一下。另外，我会定时来为你按摩尾骶部。这样一方面可以解除你的肌肉疲劳，另一方面也可以防止褥疮。现在来试一试。

# 25. Trans-esophageal Echocardiography

# 经食管超声心动图检查

Nurse： Hello，Miss Fang，you look a little pale. Please sit down for a little while，OK? Are you a little nervous?

护士： 方小姐，看起来你脸色不太好，你先坐一会儿，好吗？是不是有点紧张？

Patient： Yes. I am very nervous. Is the trans-esophageal echocardiography a very uncomfortable procedure? Does it take very long? Will I be able to handle it?

病人： 是的，我非常紧张。做经食管超声心电图检查是不是很难受？时间会不会很长？我能受得了吗？

Nurse： We'll give you anesthesia prior to the test. So you won't feel too uncomfortable. When the tube is inserted into the esophagus，you will feel some discomfort. As it reaches the throat，it may make you feel nausea. At this point，when that happens，try to swallow which will allow the doctor to insert the tube smoothly. Once the tube is inserted，there won't be more irritation and you won't feel too much discomfort. The whole procedure takes about ten minutes. I trust you can do it. During the procedure，it will help if you can take deep breaths to relax and reduce tension.

护士： 检查前我们会给你用一些麻醉药，这会让你感觉不是非常难受。当管子插入食管，到达咽喉部时，你会感到有点不舒服，可能会引起恶心反射。这时，你只要配合做吞咽动作，医生插管就会很顺利。管子插入以后就不会再有什么刺激了，你也就不会太难受了。整个过程大约需要 10 分钟左右，我相信你一定可以坚持下来的。在检查过程中，你可以做深呼吸，用以放松身体、减少紧张。

Patient： Really? How?

病人： 有用吗？怎么做？

Nurse： A lot of people find it helpful. During the test，lie on your side，let your legs bent naturally，take deep and slow abdominal respiration. This will help you reduce the feeling of nausea. Here，will you follow my demonstration and give it a try?

护士： 很多人这么做了都有用。检查时，你侧卧，双下肢自然弯曲，用腹部深而慢地呼吸，这样呼吸会帮助你减少恶心感。来，现在请你跟着我的提示做一遍试试，好吗？

Patient： All right!（After several deep breaths）I no longer feel as flustered. Well，can my mom stay with me during the procedure?

病人： 好。（几次深呼吸以后）我好像不像刚才那样心慌得厉害了。嗯……等会儿检查时，我可以让我母亲陪在我身边吗？

Nurse: If you really need her, she certainly can. However, I'll be by your side for the entire procedure to help you relax and cooperate with the doctor. We'll do it together. Is this all right?

护士：如果你真的需要母亲陪在身边，当然可以。不过，整个过程中，我会一直陪在你身边，及时提醒你放松身体，配合医生检查。让我们一起来完成，好吗？

Patient: This makes me feel much better. Then just let my mom wait outside. She won't be nervous this way.

病人：这样我就放心了。那就叫我母亲在外面等着吧，免得她也紧张。

Nurse: You are such a good daughter.

护士：你真是个好女儿。

Patient: Thank you!

病人：谢谢你。

# 26. Transfusion

# 输液

Nurse: (adjusting the rate of the IV drips) Good morning, Mr. Xu. Do you feel any discomfort because the drip rate is too fast?

护士：(边调节补液滴速边说)徐先生，滴速太快了，你有什么不舒服吗？

Patient: No, I am fine.

病人：我现在感觉挺好的，没什么不舒服。

Nurse: Mr. Xu, you see, the rate of intravenous drips is 80 drops/min now. I think you just want to finish the transfusion sooner. Am I right?

护士：徐先生，你看，你现在的滴速是 80 滴 / 分，我想你是想快一点儿把补液滴完，是吗？

Patient: Yes, there is no problem with my heart function. So I increased the rate. I would like to finish the transfusion sooner so I can take a walk and do some exercises.

病人：是的，我的心脏没什么问题，所以我把补液调快了。况且快点滴完后，还可以散散步，多活动活动。

Nurse: I admire your energetic attitude. It's true that proper exercises are very beneficial to older people. But the functions of organs will decrease with aging. Rapid transfusion will lead to the accumulation of fluid in the heart, increase the burden to the heart, and cause many uncomfortable symptoms, such as dyspnoea, rapid heart rate and even heart failure.

护士：我很赞赏你这种活跃的心态。是的，适当的活动对老年人来说非常有益，但是，随着年龄的增长，身体内各脏器的功能也会随之减弱。快速的输液会使大量液体在短时间内积聚在心脏，加重心脏负担，从而引起许多的不适症状，如胸闷，心跳加快，甚至会引起心功能衰竭。

Patient: I think what you said is very reasonable. But I didn't feel any discomfort at all.

病人：你的话，我觉得很有道理。但是，我没有感到不舒服呀。

Nurse: Maybe you can't feel that. But it doesn't mean the burden on the heart is not increased. Just think what will happen to a machine when it overworks? The original purpose of the transfusion is to give your brain cells more nutrition. Do you think it is worthwhile to risk potential heart failure to finish the transfusion a little faster?

护士：可能你自己感觉不到，但这并不意味着你的心脏没有加重负担。试想一下，如果有一部机器一直让它超负荷运转，机器会怎样？本来输液是为了治疗疾病营养脑细胞，但是如果因为输液过快引起心衰，那该多不划算呀？

Patient: (smiling) All right, young lady, I will follow your instructions and not increase the drip rate anymore.

病人：(笑了)好吧，小家伙，就听你的话，我不再调快滴速了。

Nurse: Great. Thank you for your cooperation. I will begin your transfusion as soon as possible so you can have more time to do other activities.

护士：太好了，谢谢你的合作。我会尽量早一点为你输液，以便你有更多的活动时间，好吗？

Patient: Good! Thank you.

病人：好的，谢谢！

# 27. Nursing Support

# 护理援助

Nurse： Mrs. Shi，are you thirsty? Would you like to drink some water?

护士： 石夫人，你口渴吗？喝水吗？

（The patient turned and smiled at the nurse. The nurse gave a glass of water to her，and helped her with the straw. Mrs. Shi drank the water.）

（病人回过头，笑笑。护士把水杯端上，吸管送到病人口边，病人喝着水。）

Nurse： Why aren't you having lunch? Has your son brought your lunch yet?

护士： 你怎么还不吃饭？儿子还没送过来吗？

Patient： No. He works the early shift today and will not finish work until 3 pm. I told him yesterday that I would just buy something for lunch myself. I will go and get something from the dining room in a few minutes.

病人： 今天我儿子上早班，要下午 3 点才下班。昨天跟他说好了，我自己随便买点吃的，等一会儿我去食堂买就行了。

Nurse： Well，I can buy lunch for you after I finish my work.

护士： 哦，我一会儿就下班了，我来帮你买饭好了。

Patient： No，No，I don't want to trouble you too much. I'll do it myself.

病人： 不要不要，太麻烦了，我自己去吧。

Nurse： It's OK. You can't see too well and I'll be worried if you go out alone. What if you fall down on the way? I'll going to give my off duty report now. Just wait for me.（At 11：40，the nurse brought the lunch to Shi Yingying.）

护士： 没关系的，你看东西不清楚，单独出去我也不太放心，若路上摔跤了，那可怎么办。我去交班，你等我噢！（11：40，护士端着饭菜来到石英英床前。）

Nurse： Mrs. Shi，you need food rich in vitamins. I brought you fried tomato with eggs，fresh vegetables and steamed fish. Would you like them?（The patient sat up and looked at the nurse gratefully.）

护士： 石夫人，你需要多吃点富含维生素的食物。我买了番茄炒蛋、空心菜、清蒸鱼，希望你喜欢吃？（病人坐起身，感激地望着护士。）

Patient： They are all my favorites. Thank you very much.

病人： 喜欢，喜欢，真是太感谢你了。

Nurse： Don't mention it. Next time don't hesitate to tell me when you need help. By the way，I think it's better for you to reserve your meals from the hospital cafeteria，so you don't have to depend on your son to bring in your food. If the cafeteria meals are not to your tastes, let me know. I'll contact the cafeteria to make a menu specifically for you. Now, enjoy your lunch.

护士：不用谢，下次碰到这种情况你尽管对我说好了。其实，你还是订医院的饭菜吧，这样就不用你儿子每餐都要记着来送饭。如果你觉得饭菜不合胃口，就对我说。让我来和营养室联系，为你另外配餐。好了，你慢慢吃吧。

# 28. Hypertension

# 高血压

## （1）

Nurse: How are you feeling?

护士：你感到怎样？

Patient: Not very well. I have a headache. Severe dizziness，ringing noise in my ears，sleeplessness and poor memory. And，when I walk too fast，I get short of breath.

病人：我觉得不太舒服。我头疼、头晕得厉害，耳鸣，失眠和记忆力差，而且走路急时就气喘。

Nurse: How long have you suffered from all these?

护士：你有这些不适多久了？

Patient: Maybe eight years as far as I can remember. At first，I didn't pay any attention to them. Then，when my headache got worse，I went to see a doctor. He told me I had hypertension.

病人：我记得大约有 8 年了。开始我没注意，以后当头疼加重时，我就去看病。医生说我有高血压。

Nurse: Let me take your blood pressure.

护士：让我给你量量血压。

（After taking blood pressure）

（量血压以后）

Nurse: It is a little high. Is there any member in your family who also suffers from hypertension?

护士：有点高。你家里还有人患高血压吗？

Patient: Yes. My father has it. My grandfather died of apoplexy ten years ago，probably also due to hypertension.

病人：有的。我父亲也有高血压。我祖父 10 年前死于中风，可能也是高血压引起的。

Nurse: What kind of treatment have you had?

护士：你过去采取过什么治疗？

Patient: I have been given some antihypertensive drugs. They lowered my blood pressure somewhat; but it would go up again whenever I felt tired or worried.

病人：我曾用过降压药。使用后我的血压降低了一点，但是在疲劳或烦恼后，却又高了起来。

Nurse: It is very clear that you must rest more and stop worrying. You should follow a low-salt diet and eat lots of vegetables and fruit，but little meat. Do you smoke?

护士： 这很清楚，你应该好好休息，不要烦恼。必须吃低盐食物，多吃蔬菜和水果，少吃肉。你吸烟吗？

Patient: Yes. But I'm smoking much less now.

病人： 吸的，但现在吸得不多了。

Nurse: How many cigarettes do you smoke every day?

护士： 你现在每天吸多少支香烟？

Patient: About ten.

病人： 大约10支。

Nurse: Do you drink?

护士： 你喝酒吗？

Patient: Yes. I usually drink wine at super.

病人： 噢，我通常在晚饭时喝。

Nurse: My advice to you is to keep off wine and give up smoking.

护士： 我劝你戒酒、戒烟。

Patient: It is difficult for me to give them up. But，I will try my best. Thank you for your advice.

病人： 戒烟酒对我来讲是困难的。但是，我一定尽最大努力去做。谢谢你的忠告。

Nurse: I'm glad to have been of help to you. Good-bye.

护士： 我很高兴能帮助你。再见。

## （2）

Nurse: How can I help you，sir?

护士： 有什么需要帮忙的吗，先生？

Patient: I have a terrible headache.

病人： 我头痛得厉害。

Nurse: When did it begin?

护士： 什么时间开始的？

Patient: About a week ago.

病人： 大约一周前。

Nurse: Does it help you if take aspirin?

护士： 吃阿司匹林管用吗？

Patient: No. They just seem to go away by themselves.

病人： 不管用。疼痛好像是自然缓解的。

Nurse: Have you ever had this kind of headache before?

护士： 您以前有过这样的头痛吗？

Patient: I have headaches off and on last few years，but none as bad as this.

病人： 近几年我经常有断断续续的头痛，但从来没有像这次这么厉害。

Nurse: Have you seen a doctor before? Did he say anything about it?

护士: 您以前看过医生吗？医生说过什么没有？

Patient: Three years ago, I went to the local hospital for a swimming certificate. They told me that I had hypertension.

病人: 3年前我去当地医院做游泳检查，医生说我患有高血压。

Nurse: Have you ever had swollen ankles?

护士: 您的脚踝肿胀过吗？

Patient: Not that I can remember.

病人: 我记不得了。

Nurse: What kind of treatment did have in the past?

护士: 您以前曾做过什么治疗吗？

Patient: I took "hydrochlorothiazide" occasionally.

病人: 我有时候用"氢氯噻嗪"。

Nurse: Let me take your blood pressure.

护士: 我给您量一下血压。

Patient: OK.

病人: 好的。

Nurse: It's one hundred and eighty over one hundred and ten mmHg. That's moderately high. You may need to have a urinalysis, blood urea nitrogen test, and chest x-ray and electrocardiogram examination.

护士: 您的血压是180/110mmHg，中度偏高。您可能需要做尿检、血尿素氮化验，还要做胸部X线检查和心电图检查。

Patient: Is it serious?

病人: 我的病严重吗？

Nurse: You should take the medicine, have a good rest, avoid nervous tension or stress, and give up smoking and alcohol. Come back again next week for the results and another check of your blood pressure.

护士: 你一定要服药了，好好休息，避免精神紧张或思想负担，并要戒烟和戒酒。一周后来复诊，看化验结果和复查血压。

Patient: All right. Thank you.

病人: 好的，谢谢您。

# 29. Migraine

# 偏头痛

Examiner: Are you feeling tired? Please sit down and rest for a moment.

检查者：你感觉累吗？先坐下休息片刻。

Patient: What kind of examination is this?

病人：这是什么检查？

Examiner: It's Transcranial Doppler Ultrasonography. Are you not feeling well?

检查者：是经颅超声多普勒，你有什么不舒服吗？

Patient: I feel dizzy and have a headache.

病人：我感到头晕、头痛。

Examiner: Have you ever had this kind of headache before?

检查者：以前有过这种头痛吗？

Patient: Yes, I do, but not so severe.

病人：是的，但没这么严重。

Examiner: What kind of examination did you have before?

检查者：以前做过什么检查吗？

Patient: CT.

病人：CT。

Examiner: What was the result of your CT examination?

检查者：结果如何？

Patient: Normal.

病人：正常。

Examiner: Please lie down on the bed. I will examine you right away.

检查者：请躺在检查床上，我给你检查一下。

Patient: OK.

病人：好的。

Examiner: What kind of pain do you have? Is it intermittent or persistent?

检查者：疼痛是间歇性还是持续性的？

Patient: Intermittent. The headache is in my left side and you should examine there.

病人：间歇性的。我是左侧头痛，你应该检查这边。

Examiner: Don't worry. The main brain vessels will all be examined. Please get up and sit down for the vertebrobasilar artery examination.

检查者：你放心，环主干的血管都要检查。你现在起来，坐在这儿检查椎基底动脉。

Patient: Do I have a problem?

病人：我有问题吗？

Examiner: The blood supply to your brain is not sufficient.

检查者：是脑供血不足。

Patient: What cause my headache?

病人：那我头痛是怎么回事？

Examiner: The blood supply is relatively insufficient because of cerebral vasospasm. It is the functional change of the blood vessels.

检查者：这是脑血管痉挛所致的相对供血不足，是功能性的改变。

Patient: I see.

病人：我明白了。

Examiner: Here's your report. Show this to your doctor.

检查者：这是你的检查报告，把它给你的医生看。

# 30. Vertebrobasilar Artery Insufficiency

# 椎基底动脉供血不足

Examiner: What kind of discomfort do you have?
检查者：你有什么不舒服？
Patient: I feel dizzy especially when changing body positions.
病人：我头晕，尤其是体位改变时明显。
Examiner: How long have you been like this?
检查者：这种情况有多久了？
Patient: Two or three days.
病人：有两三天了。
Examiner: Lie down on the bed please. I'll examine you.
检查者：请躺在检查床上。我给你检查一下。
Patient: What's my condition?
病人：我的情况怎么样？
Examiner: Your internal carotid artery system is normal. Get up slowly and sit down please. Let me check your vertebrobasilar artery.
检查者：你的颈内动脉系统检查正常。你慢慢起床，坐在这儿。我再检查椎基底动脉。
Patient: Oh, I am feeling dizzy now.
病人：哦，我现在正头晕呢。
Examiner: Take it easy. Let me help you. Do you feel better now?
检查者：别紧张，让我扶你一下。现在感觉好些了吗？
Patient: Yes. Thanks.
病人：好点儿了。谢谢。
Examiner: I will give you a neck rotation test.
检查者：我要给你进行转颈试验。
Patient: What should I do?
病人：你看我该怎么做呢？
Examiner: Relax. Don't be nervous.
检查者：你放松，别紧张。
Patient: What's the result?
病人：检查结果如何？
Examiner: It is insufficiency of blood supply from the vertebral artery.

检查者：是椎动脉供血不足。

Patient：Thank you.

病人：谢谢你。

Examiner：You are welcome. Please see a doctor for treatment. I hope you have a quick recovery.

检查者：不客气。去看医生，接受治疗，祝早日康复。

# 31. Subarachnoid Hemorrhage

# 蛛网膜下腔出血

Examiner: Be careful and do not move. I will check you right away on the stretcher.

检查者：你小心点儿，不要动，就在平车上检查 .。

Patient: Why?

病人：为什么？

Examiner: To avoid another hemorrhage.

检查者：防止再出血。

Patient: Thank you.

病人：谢谢。

Examiner: Keep quiet and don't move your head as long as you can during the examination.

检查者：检查时保持平静，你的头尽量保持不动。

Patient: OK.

病人：好的。

(after the examination.)

（检查完毕。）

Patient: What have you found?

病人：你发现了什么吗？

Examiner: There is vasospasm in your cerebral vessels. Here's your report. You should give it to your physician, now.

检查者：目前有脑血管痉挛。这是你的检查报告，给医生看。

Patient: Thank you very much.

病人：多谢。

# 32. Severe Stenosis in Extracranial Carotid Artery

# 颈动脉颅外段严重狭窄

Examiner: Do you have a headache?

检查者：你头痛吗？

Patient: No, I just feel dizzy.

病人：不痛，就是感到头晕。

Examiner: How long have you been feeling like this?

检查者：这样的情况有多久了？

Patient: It all started the day before yesterday.

病人：从前天开始突然发作的。

Examiner: How long have you suffered from hypertension?

检查者：你高血压有多久了？

Patient: About ten years as far as I know.

病人：我知道有 10 年了。

Examiner: Are there any other members in your family suffering from the same disease?

检查者：你家里还有人有高血压吗？

Patient: Yes, my father has hypertension.

病人：是的，我父亲有高血压。

Examiner: Do you smoke?

检查者：你吸烟吗？

Patient: Yes, I do.

病人：是的。

Examiner: My advice to you is to give up smoking.

检查者：我劝你不要吸烟了。

Patient: OK. What's the result of the examination?

病人：好的，检查结果如何？

Examiner: There is a stenosis at your left extracranial internal carotid artery.

检查者：你的左侧颈内动脉颅外段狭窄。

Patient: Is my condition serious?

病人：我的情况很严重吗？

Examiner: There is an adequate intracranial collateral circulation, the symptom is not very clear. I suggest you take additional examination to confirm the result.

检查者： 因为颅内侧支循环良好，所以你的临床症状不明显，但需要进一步检查。

Patient: What kind of examination do you suggest?

病人： 需要做哪些检查？

Examiner: DSA or MRA. Here's your report, you should give it to your physician now.

检查者： DSA（数字减影血管造影）或 MRA（磁共振血管造影）检查。这是你的检查报告，现在拿去给医生看。

Patient: Thank you very much.

病人： 多谢。

# 33. Transient Cerebral Ischemia

# 短暂性脑缺血

Examiner: How do you feel?

检查者：你感觉怎么样？

Patient: I could not speak and my right hand was weak.

病人：我曾经不能说话，右手无力。

Examiner: When did it happen?

检查者：那是什么时候？

Patient: About twenty hours ago.

病人：20 个小时前。

Examiner: Let me help you to lie down slowly on the examination bed.

检查者：来，我扶你慢慢躺在检查床上。

Patient: OK. What is this examination?

病人：好的。这是什么检查？

Examiner: Transcranial Doppler Ultrasonograph.

检查者：经颅多普勒超声。

Patient: Which cerebral vessels could it detect?

病人：它能检查哪些血管？

Examiner: Main intracranial cerebral arteries.

检查者：颅内大血管。

Examiner: What are you going to do?

检查者：你打算干什么？

Patient: Oh, I just want to take a rest.

病人：哦，我只想休息休息。

Examiner: Here's your report, you should give it to your physician now.

检查者：这是你的检查报告，现在拿去给医生看。

Patient: Thank you very much.

病人：多谢。

# 34. Middle Cerebral Artery Stenosis

# 大脑中段动脉狭窄

Examiner: What kind of discomfort do you have?

检查者：你有什么不舒服？

Patient: Oh，headache，vertigo，poor memorization and the numb of my left hand.

病人：哦，头痛、头晕、记忆力差，左手麻木。

Examiner: How long do you have these symptoms?

检查者：这些症状有多久了？

Patient: More than a month.

病人：已超过一个月了。

Examiner: All right，let me give you an examination.

检查者：好，让我给你检查一下。

Examiner: What diseases have you had before?

检查者：你以往生过什么病？

Patient: I had hypertension and diabetes mellitus at the age of 50.

病人：我 50 岁时查出患高血压和糖尿病。

Examiner: Let me examine your right temporal window carefully.

检查者：让我仔细查一下你的右侧颞窗。

Patient: Do I have any problem?

病人：我有问题吗？

Examiner: There is a stenosis in your right middle cerebral artery.

检查者：你的右侧大脑中段动脉狭窄。

Patient: What should I do?

病人：你认为我该怎么办？

Examiner: You should have a DSA or MRA to confirm the finding.

检查者：你需要进一步做 DSA（数字减影血管造影）或 MRA（磁共振血管造影）检查。

Patient: Why?

病人：为什么？

Examiner: These tests can show the shape change of the intracranial blood vessels.

检查者：它能显示颅内血管的形态学变化。

Patient: Did it cause the numbness in my left hand?

病人： 那我的左手麻就是这个原因？

Examiner: I think so. Here's your report. Please show it to your physician.

检查者： 我认为是这样。这是你的检查报告，拿去给医生看。

# 35. Leukemia

# 白血病

Patient： How could god be so unfair to let me have this disease? I don't want to be treated any more. This disease is incurable anyway.

病人： 老天为什么这么不公平啊！让我生这个病，我不治了，反正这个病也治不好。

Nurse： (spoke softly) I fully understand your feelings. Actually, you are getting much better after the treatment. This is like the darkness before daybreak. The night is almost over and the day will come soon. So you should encourage yourself to cooperate with us on your treatment.

护士： (温和地说)我很理解你的心情。事实上，你的病情经过治疗已经在好转之中。现在你的状况就像黎明前的黑暗，黑夜正在渐渐褪去，黎明的曙光即将来临。所以，你一定要鼓起勇气积极地配合治疗。

Patient： (looked at the nurse dubiously and said with a sigh) But leukemia is an incurable disease!

病人： (将信将疑地看着护士，叹了口气说)白血病是绝症啊！

Nurse： The technology for medical treatment is developing very quickly. There are many treatment techniques for leukemia available now. Please believe that if you can keep high spirits and cooperate with the treatment, you will win this battle. We have had many patients with much worse conditions than yours when they were admitted, and some of them have already recovered and gone back to work. I can give you the telephone number of a patient whom you can call and chat with.

护士： 现在的医疗技术发展很快，对白血病的治疗手段也越来越多。你应该相信，只要你保持良好的情绪，积极地配合治疗，一定会战胜病魔的。我们有很多病人来的时候病情比你重多了，但经过治疗，有的已经治愈正常上班了。我给你一个病人的电话号码，你可以打电话和她聊聊。

# 36. Chemotherapy

# 化疗

## （1）

Patient: Mrs. Xu, I am really concerned. Originally, I thought I would be healed once the tumor was surgically removed. I never thought that I would need chemotherapy which has many adverse effects. I am afraid I will not be able to persist in this treatment.

病人：小许，我很害怕。本来以为肿块切除了，也就好了，没想到还要化疗。化疗有很多副作用，我怕我不能坚持治疗。

Nurse: Surgery is one of the major methods of oncotherapy, while chemotherapy is also a main treatment technology at the present time. It is absolutely necessary to carry out chemotherapy after the surgery to prevent and control the spread or infiltration of the cancer cells. Chemotherapy is a treatment method of using chemicals to control the cancer cells. Compared to surgery, the side effects of chemotherapy should be overcome more easily. It is like climbing a mountain. You will encounter a great deal of difficulties on the way, but if you can bravely confront these difficulties, and persist in climbing, you can surely reach the top and view the beautiful scenery. Chemotherapy works the same way for cancer. Besides, we will help you during the whole process.

护士：手术是肿瘤治疗的主要手段之一，化疗也是目前医治肿瘤的主要辅助治疗。术后为了预防及控制癌细胞的扩散或浸润，进行化疗是非常必要的。化疗也就是应用化学药物治疗的方法。比起手术来说，化疗带来的副作用应该更容易克服。好比爬山，虽然这一路会有很多困难，但只要勇敢面对，坚持一下，一定能到达顶点，看到美丽的风景。化疗也是一样。况且，我们会帮助您的。

Patient: What side effects will chemotherapy have?

病人：那化疗到底有哪些副作用？

Nurse: Chemotherapy has many side effects including gastrointestinal tract reaction such as nausea, vomiting, and constipation; allergic responses; bone marrow depression as drop off white cell and platelet count; damage of liver function; and alopecia. But, not all side effects will occur and not all patients have the same side effects.

护士：化疗有很多副作用，包括胃肠道反应，如恶心、呕吐、便秘；过敏反应；骨髓抑制，如白细胞、血小板下降；肝功能损害；脱发等。但不是所有副作用都会出现，也不是每个人都会有同样的副作用。

Patient: How to prevent these side effects?

病人: 那怎么来预防这些副作用?

Nurse: Before chemotherapy, we will run several examination for you, including blood test, CT, electrocardiogram, etc. to understand your body and your tumor conditions. We will select a most effective treatment plan with the least side effects for you. Your doctor will discuss the detailed plan with you. The doctor will carry out pre-treatment for you before the chemotherapy by using some drugs to prevent vomiting, allergic reactions, and to protect your liver function. In addition, reasonable foods and drinks, good mood and enough sleep are very important too. The majority of the patients receiving chemotherapy have only minimal side effects after pre-treatment. Therefore you don't have to worry.

护士: 化疗前,我们会给您做全面的检查,如验血、拍摄 CT、查心电图等。了解您的全身情况及肿瘤情况,选择效果较好、副作用相对较轻的方案。床位医生会详细跟您谈具体的内容的。医生会进行化疗前的预处理,也就是使用一些预防呕吐、过敏、保护肝功能的药物,最大程度地减轻药物的副作用。另外,合理的饮食、良好的情绪、充足的睡眠也是非常重要的。经过预处理,大部分病人出现的副作用是轻微的。所以,您不用害怕。

## (2)

Nurse: Hello, Mrs. Xia. How are you? It has been over a month since your gastrectomy. Now you will need regular treatment for a period of time. I mean, you will need intravenous chemotherapy for about three to six months. During this period, you will often need intravenous transfusion to complete the chemotherapy. The chemotherapy drugs may hurt your peripheral blood vessels, so it is better for you to have a central vein indwelling catheter.

护士: 您好,夏女士,您胃切除术已一个月了,接下来需要一个阶段的常规治疗,也就是3～6个月的静脉化疗。在这期间,您通常需要通过静脉输液来完成化疗。考虑到化疗药物可能对周边血管造成损害,建议您留置中心静脉导管。

Patient: Catheter? No, I don't want to do it. It is anther operation, isn't it?

病人: 导管?不,我不想做,又要做手术?

Nurse: Oh, no, Ms. Xia. It is just a catheter to be placed from the shallow vein to the deep vein. Don't worry, it is not an operation.

护士: 哦,不是的,夏女士。中心静脉导管是通过浅静脉置入深静脉的导管。您不用担心,不需要做手术的。

Patient: I'm nervous. The needle will stay in my body for a long time, right?

病人: 我有点紧张,那是要把针留在体内好长时间吧?

Nurse: The catheter, made from a special material, is very thin and soft. We will choose a bigger peripheral vein above your brachial area, insert a catheter and push it to the central vein. The tip of the catheter will reach the superior vena cava which is short and thick and has larger volume of blood which will allow the high concentration drugs be quickly sent to all parts of your body. Because the drugs can be effectively diluted in the central vein, the irritation of these drugs to your body vessels will be greatly reduced. Meanwhile, you can also avoid the pain from being punctured every day. Furthermore, you won't even feel the catheter in your vein.

护士：导管是由一种特殊材料制成的，非常纤细柔软。我们会选择肘部较粗的静脉，通过穿刺送入中心静脉导管。导管的前端可至上腔静脉，上腔静脉短而粗，血流量大，高浓度药液进入后可迅速输送至全身，从而有效地稀释了局部的药液浓度，减少了药物对血管的损害，同时，可以避免每天输液均需静脉穿刺的疼痛。导管漂浮在血管内是没有感觉的。

Patient: Oh. But is it painful when puncturing the vein? I am afraid of pain.

病人：噢，那么穿刺的时候痛吗？我特别怕痛。

Nurse: Don't be afraid, it won't hurt much. Have you ever had your blood drawn?

护士：不用害怕，只有一点点疼痛。您抽过血吗？

Patient: Sure.

病人：抽过。

Nurse: Was it painful?

护士：那痛吗？

Patient: Just a little.

病人：还可以。

Nurse: (assessing the patient's blood vessel again) The condition of your blood vessel is very good. We are going to puncture your vein and place a catheter through a needle which is slightly thicker than an ordinary needle. The process takes about three to five minutes. The length of the catheter is strictly regulated and the position of the catheter will be confirmed later by X-ray.

护士：(俯身再次评估血管)您的血管很好。我们给您做一个静脉穿刺，通过穿刺送入导管。只是穿刺比普通的针尖粗一些。置入导管大约需要3～5分钟。导管的长度有严格规定，穿刺完成后，可通过摄片再次确定导管位置。

Patient: It's a lot of trouble to have an indwelling catheter in my vein. How long will it be kept there?

病人：留置导管后很麻烦的，要放多长时间？

Nurse: Currently, the catheter will be kept there for about one year. But the exact length of the time will depend on the need of the treatment and the condition of the catheter. In order to prevent infection, we will change the dressing and the adhesive film, and strictly follow the procedure guidance.

护士：目前使用的导管留置时间是一年，但具体时间还要根据治疗的需要以及导管的使用状况决定。为了预防感染，平时我们会严格按照操作规程进行换药、更换贴膜等导管的维护。

Patient: Thank you. You've told me a lot about this procedure. I have a general understanding about the central vein catheter now. Let me think about it.

病人：谢谢，你讲得非常详细。我对留置中心静脉导管已经有了一个大概的了解，让我考虑一下。

Nurse：OK. Now I'll introduce you to a patient who has had this kind of catheter. You can discuss this procedure with him，OK?

护士：好的，现在我介绍一位已经留置了这种导管的病友给您认识。您还可以与他探讨一些关于这方面的问题。

Patient：OK，thank you. You are so thoughtful.

病人：好的，谢谢，你想得真周到。

# 37. Pituitary Adenoma

# 垂体瘤

Nurse: Good morning. Ms. Wang. If there is anything I can do to help during your stay in our department, please don't hesitate to tell me. I will try my best to help you.

护士：王女士，你好。在你住院期间如果有什么我能帮助你的，请你一定来找我，我会尽力给予你帮助的。

Patient: Thank you. My concern is whether my illness can be cured. I have been going to the gynecologist for a year but nothing helped.

病人：谢谢，我现在就是担心我的病能否治好。看了一年的妇产科，一点儿没用。

Nurse: The key to curing the illness is to find the cause. You have gone through a detour before you come to this point. Now you know that the pituitary adenoma is what caused your problem. We can solve the problem by removing the tumor.

护士：治病关键是找到病因。以前是因为没找到才走了冤枉路，现在好了，知道是因为垂体瘤引起的，只要把瘤切除了，问题就解决了。

Patient: Yes. The cause has been found. But the tumor is in my brain. How scary! It really frightens me to think about it.

病人：哎！病因是找到了，可是脑袋里的问题，多吓人呀！想想心里真的很害怕。

Nurse: That's true. Everyone will experience this psychological process when realizing one is ill, just in different degrees. If you like, I will explain the treatment process of this disease for you.

护士：的确，每个人生了病后都会有这个心理过程，只是程度轻重不一样。如果你愿意，我给你介绍一下这个病的治疗过程，好吗？

Patient: Yes. I would really like to know.

病人：好的，我很希望知道这些。

Nurse: First I want to tell you that this disease is not so complex to treat. In the past few years, our doctors have made great progress on the ability to carry out the surgery. The level of their skill has reached the international standards. You probably did some inquires prior to your admission to our hospital, right?

护士：首先我要告诉你，这个病一点都不复杂。而且这些年我们科的医生们在这个手术上取得了越来越大的进步，已能接近国际水平。相信你在住院前一定也已经打听过了，是吗？

Patient: Yes. I had planed to go to Shanghai for treatment. But after I consulted many experts,

I was told that your department did have a very high standard.

病人： 是的，我曾经想去上海看病。但后来经过多方打听，的确这儿的水平是相当高的。

Nurse： Great! That means you trust us. Once you have confidence，we can help you to conquer the disease much better. Actually，comparing with other neurosurgeries the operation you will receive is fairly simple. And it will not affect your appearance after the operation. The operation will be performed through nasal cavity with very little impairment and you can recover quickly. Unlike other neurosurgery procedure that requires shaving off the hair，you will be able to keep your beautiful long hair.

护士： 太好了，这么说，你已经相信我们了。只有你具有了这样的心态，我们才能和你一起更快、更好地战胜疾病。其实，你的手术相对脑外科的其他手术来说，已经是相当简单了。而且手术后一点都不影响你的外貌，因为这个手术是通过鼻腔进行的，损伤很小，恢复很快，不用像其他开颅脑手术那样剃掉头发，所以你的美丽长发可以继续保留了。

# 38. Preoperative Education (Cholelithiasis)

# 术前指导(胆石症)

Nurse: Ms. Wang, I've heard that the head surgeon, Doctor Li, will operation on you next Monday. I can sense you are worrying about it, right?

护士: 王女士,听说李主任下周一要给你动手术了。我感觉到你有点担忧,是吗?

Patient: Yes. You know I've rarely seen doctors before. But now I will have an operation. How can I not be worried?

病人: 是的,我从小到大都很少看医生。如今要做手术了,怎么不担心?

Nurse: Would you like to tell me what you are worrying about in detail? Maybe I can help you.

护士: 你能具体跟我讲讲你所担心的事吗?或许我能给你帮助。

Patient: (thought for a moment) I want to know if the operation is very painful. I'd also like to know how long I have to stay in the hospital after the operation, because my work won't allow me to take a long absence.

病人: (略思索片刻)我想知道手术是不是很疼?术后大约要在医院待多久?因为我的工作不允许我请长假。

Nurse: To your first concern, you need not worry at all. Anesthesia techniques have developed a lot. The anesthetist will administer some drugs to you before the operation. Then you will fall asleep and feel nothing. When you wake up, the operation will already be finished. As time passes, the effect of the anesthetic will gradually disappear. At that time you may or may not feel a little pain. But I'm sure you can tolerate it. If the pain is too severe, we will give you some medicine. So don't worry.

护士: 对于第一点,你完全可以放心。现在麻醉学科发展很快,在手术开始前,麻醉师会给你用些药,然后你就会沉沉地睡一觉,什么知觉都没有。等你一觉醒来,手术也结束了。随着时间的过去,麻醉药的药效也渐渐消失,此时你或许有一点疼痛的感觉,但我相信你能忍受。若你疼得实在厉害,我们会给你用药,所以你不必担心疼的问题。

(The patient nodded her head.)

(病人点头表示明白。)

Nurse: As for how long it will take you to recover after the operation, you can be discharged in a week if everything goes well. Now let tell you something about what we should do before the operation. First, you must take good care of yourself not to catch cold or have a fever. Second, you should practice in bed using a bedpan from now on in order to be accustomed to it after the operation.

护士：至于术后恢复需多长时间，一般顺利的话，一周后你可以出院。现在让我给你讲讲术前应注意的问题。首先你在术前应好好休息，避免着凉，防止感冒、发烧。其次你得在床上练习使用便盆，免得术后不习惯。

Patient: Why do I have to practice to use a bedpan?

病人：为什么要练习在床上使用便盆？

Nurse: Because after the operation you will be too weak to get up to go to the toilet.

护士：因为手术后你很虚弱，不能下床如厕，只能用便器。

Patient: OK, I see. I will cooperate with you. Thanks.

病人：噢，我明白了，我一定好好配合。非常感谢你。

Nurse: It's my pleasure. I wish you a successful operation.

护士：不客气，祝你手术顺利！

# 39. Postoperative Education (Cholelithiasis)

# 术后指导(胆石症)

Nurse: Good morning, Ms. Wang, do you sleep well last night?

护士: 早上好，王女士，昨晚睡得好吗？

Patient: Not very good. I'm aching all over.

病人: 不是很好，浑身疼痛。

Nurse: I'm sorry to hear that, Lying still on your back for a whole night is difficult for anybody. You can try to turn over slightly. You just need to be careful not to let the drainage tube come off or twist. It can encourage bowel movement and promote you to pass gas. Come on, let me give you a hand to turn your body to the right side and put a soft pillow behind your back. How do you feel about this?

护士: 很遗憾你没睡好。一动不动地平躺一整夜，谁都受不了。你可以试着在床上轻翻身，只要留意不要让引流管滑脱或扭曲就行。在床上翻身可以促进肠蠕动，促使肛门排气。来，现在让我协助你向右翻，在背部给你垫个软枕，你感觉怎么样？

Patient: Fine, I feel better now. Thank you. Nurse Zhang, may I eat something?

病人: 好的，这样感觉好多了。张护士，我能吃些东西吗？

Nurse: Not now. You are not allowed to eat anything, until you pass gas. At that time you can have some liquid food, such as water, rice soup, fish soup, juice, etc. Then depending on your condition we will change your food from semi-liquid diet to soft diet, to regular diet. But I should remind you that you should have small and frequent meals, and avoid greasy food such as viscera, eggs yolks, and fat meat. Otherwise you will have dyspepsia and diarrhea. You can have fish, chicken, lean meat, etc. Fresh vegetables and fruits are good for you.

护士: 现在不能。要等到肛门排气才可以，那时你可以进一些清水、米汤、鱼汤、果汁等流质。以后根据你的情况再逐渐进半流质、软食直至普通食品。但是提醒你的是：少量多餐，不食油腻的食物，如动物内脏、蛋黄、肥肉等。因为这些食物会使你消化不良、腹泻。你可以选鱼、鸡、瘦肉等，另外，新鲜蔬菜、大量水果对你身体有益。

Patient: OK. I've got it. But nurse Zhang, would you mind writing this down on a piece of paper in case I forget?

病人: 噢，我明白了。不过张护士，能麻烦你给我写在纸上吗？我怕忘了。

Nurse: Of course. By the way, you should have a good rest after you are discharged from the hospital.

护士： 当然可以。顺便说一句，出院后你还得注意身体。

Patient: OK. I'll will. Health is the first concern.

病人： 好的，我会记住的，毕竟健康才是第一财富。

# 40. Facial Paralysis

# 面瘫

Nurse: Do you know your husband often tell us how gentle, soft, kind-hearted, understanding, smart, and admirable you are. It is obvious that your beauty is in the heart of your husband more than your appearance. Your health is the most important in his eyes. (Nearby Mr. Wang nodded and smiled full of love.)

护士：你知道吗？你的丈夫经常在我们护士面前称赞你温柔贤惠、善解人意、聪明可人。可见，你的美丽在你爱人心目中已不仅仅在于你的外表了，你的健康才是他眼中最美的风景。(旁边王先生坚定地点点头，会心的眼神中充满爱意。)

Patient: But, when I eat, I have no feeling in my right cheek.

病人：可是，我吃东西时右侧颊部麻木，没有感觉。

Nurse: Oh, it is OK. This is a normal phenomenon. But in order to prevent mouth ulcers and infection, you must rinse your mouth after eating to get rid of the food waste. Can you persist in doing this?

护士：没关系，这是正常现象。但是为了防止你口腔内溃疡或感染，每天饮食后必须漱口，清除口腔内的食物残渣。你能坚持吗？

Patient: (The uneasiness assailed her heart quickly and she asked in a low voice.) I work in a bank. How can I face my colleagues and customers with such an image? They will sneer at me.

病人：(另一种不安袭上心头，随即又轻声问道)我在银行工作，这样的形象怎么能面对我的同事和客户？他们肯定会暗笑我。

Nurse: Don't worry. I have already asked your doctor about this. What cause your facial paralysis and insensibility is an unavoidable effect from the surgery. Fortunately it is a reversible trauma. Nevertheless, nerves are delicate, and they need a long process to recover. After six months you will return to your pervious appearance.

护士：放心吧！我已详细问过你的主刀医生，你面瘫和面部麻木的原因只是手术中不可避免的碰触，是一种可塑性的创伤。不过，神经是娇嫩的，恢复需要一个过程。半年后，你会以一如既往的美丽展现在你同事的面前。

# 41. Injury and Fracture

# 外伤和骨折

## (1)

Nurse: How did it happen?

护士：你怎么受伤的？

Patient: When I was riding my bike to my office, a bus came from behind and struck me.I fell down and felt a severe pain in my left leg.

病人：我骑车上班，一辆汽车从后面撞了上来。我立即跌倒，感到左腿剧痛。

Nurse: When did it happen?

护士：这在什么时候发生的？

Patient: An hour ago.

病人：一小时前。

Nurse: Did you faint?

护士：你昏倒了吗？

Patient: I think I did for a little while.

病人：是的，但时间很短。

Nurse: Could you stand on your legs and walk after the accident?

护士：出事以后你能站起来走路吗？

Patient: No, I couldn't stand up at all.

病人：不行。我一点也站不起来了。

Nurse: Can you bend your knees?

护士：膝盖能弯吗？

Patient: I cannot bend my left knee.

病人：左膝不能弯。

Nurse: Did you receive any treatment before you came to the hospital?

护士：来医院前做过什么治疗吗？

Patient: No. I was brought straight here immediately after the accident.

病人：没有。出事后我被立即送到了这里。

Nurse: Please point out where it hurts the most.

护士：请告诉我哪里最疼？

Patient: Here.In my left lower leg.

病人：　这里。就在左侧小腿。

Nurse：　I see. It looks swollen.Let us send you to the X-ray DEPARTMENT. We'll see if there is a fracture in your leg.

护士：　唔，你的小腿已经肿了。我们送你到放射科去检查一下你的小腿是否有骨折。

（After the X-ray）

（X线检查后）

Nurse：　The X-ray shows that the bone in your leg is broken.But don't worry. Dr. Zhang will make a cast for you.I Think the bone will knit in ten weeks if there is no complication.

护士：　X线检查表明你的小腿有骨折。但不要紧张。张医生会给你上石膏的。我想，如果没有并发症，10周后断骨将接上。

Patient：　Is there anything I should pay attention to when I go home?

病人：　我回家后应注意些什么？

Nurse：　Yes.There are two things you must remember.First，you should move all the joints in your foot from time to time，and check the color of the toes.And second，if you feel any pain or numbness in your toes，please immediately notify me or Dr. Zhang.

护士：　你应该注意两件事。第一，经常活动趾关节，并注意脚趾的颜色。其次，若足趾感到疼或麻木，立即找我或张医生。

Patient：　I'll try to remember.Thank you.

病人：　我一定记住。谢谢你。

Nurse：　You are welcome.

护士：　别客气。

## （2）

Nurse：　How were you injured?

护士：　你是怎么受伤的？

Patient：　I was hit by a stone，banging my forehead quite hard. The first aid wrapped a bandage around it to stop bleeding.

病人：　我被石头砸伤了，前额部碰得很重，那个急救人员用绷带给我缠上止住了血。

Nurse：　Did you lose a lot of blood?

护士：　出了很多血吗？

Patient：　Not too much.

病人：　不太多。

Nurse：　Were you unconscious?

护士：　你晕过去了吗？

Patient：　No.

病人：　没有。

Nurse：　The wound is rather large，so the doctor will stitch it up.

护士：　这伤口相当的大，得找医生把它缝上。

Patient：　Will it hurt ?

病人：　痛吗？

Nurse： Oh，no. It won't be painful. Have you had an anti-tetanus injection lately?

护士： 不，不会痛的。你最近打过抗破伤风注射液吗？

Patient： I think the only one I have had was about five years ago.

病人： 我记得5年前打过一次。

Nurse： Well，I think you'd better have another one.

护士： 我认为你需要重新打一次。

Patient： Whatever you say.

病人： 按你说的做吧。

**（3）**

Nurse： What seems to be the problem?

护士： 你哪里不舒服？

Patient： Well，I was knocked by a stone to the ground，and when I got up，my left arm and elbow were grazed，and now I have a pain in my ribs.

病人： 唉，我被撞倒在地，从地上爬起来时，我发现我的右臂和肘部也擦伤了。现在我感到肋骨有点疼痛。

Nurse： I'll just take a look. Where does it hurt?

护士： 让我检查一下吧。你哪里痛啊？

Patient： It's hard to say. It hurts all over.

病人： 这很难说清楚，好像浑身都痛。

Nurse： Does it hurt when I do this?

护士： 我按这儿，你痛不痛？

Patient： Ouch! The pain is very bad when you press here.

病人： 哎呀！你一按这儿我就痛得要命。

Nurse： You arm and elbow seem to be all right. But，to be on the safe side，you'd better go to the X-ray Department. When the X-rays are ready，bring them back to me to examine.

护士： 你的胳膊和肘部好像没什么问题。但是出于安全考虑，你还是最好去做X线检查。检查之后，把X线片马上拿过来让我看看。

Patient： OK. See you later.

病人： 好的，那么待会儿再见吧！

Nurse： See you then!

护士： 待会儿见！

# 42. Postoperative Rehabilitation (Fractured Cervical Spine)

# 术后康复（颈椎骨折）

Nurse： How are you? Did you sleep well last night?

护士： 你好！昨晚睡得好吗？

Patient： Yes，I feel at ease after the surgery.

病人： 睡得很好！手术以后我就安心了许多。

Nurse： The surgery was a success. From now on，the most important thing we should do is the functional training. I'll teach you every day. Please follow my instructions.

护士： 现在手术成功了，接下来最重要的就是功能锻炼了。每天由我来指导你，请配合！

Patient： Thank you. I'll try my best.

病人： 谢谢！我一定会努力的。

Nurse： OK，let's begin. Raise your arms and grasp the rings，you should do at least 100 times every day. You may divide them into four to five sections.

护士： 那好，我们先来做第一个动作，双上肢上举抓住吊环，每天 100 次，可以分 4～5 个时间段进行。

Patient： OK（making great efforts to raise her arms）. My arms feel so heavy.

病人： 好（努力举起双臂）。我感觉双上肢特别重。

Nurse： You will have this feeling in the first several days，but you will feel easier later.

护士： 这是刚开始锻炼时的感觉，以后你会感觉越来越轻的。

Patient： （couldn't hold on the rings）I couldn't do it. How come it seems my brain can not control my hands?

病人： （双手抓不住吊环）不行了，我怎么觉得大脑支配不了我的双手了？

Nurse： This is the phenomenon of the injured nerve caused by fracture of the cervical spine. The only way you can recover the function of the nerve is by keeping daily training. But it looks like this exercise is too hard for you now，so let's change to another method. I will give you a small water bottle. Try to hold it and pass it between your two hands. Can you do that?

护士： 这就是颈椎受伤后神经受损的表现，只有每天坚持练习，才能恢复功能。这个动作现在对你来说有一定的难度，那我们换一种方法。现在我给你一个小矿泉水瓶，你试着用手把它抓住，然后在双手间传递，这样行吗？

Patient： （practicing to pass the water bottle）Oh，this method is better.

病人： （双手练习握矿泉水瓶）哎，这个办法真好。

Nurse： You should continue the exercise until you are tired.（after 5 minutes of exercise）Do you feel tired now? You can take a rest. I'll do some passive movement for your knees and ankles. The joints that you can't move by yourself，will need this kind of passive movement. You can ask your family numbers or paramedics to help you. This exercise can keep the function of your knees and ankles.

护士： 这样每天坚持练习到疲劳为止。（锻炼 5 分钟后）你有点累了吧，现在让你稍作休息，我帮你做下肢膝关节和踝关节的被动运动。你自己不能动的关节都要做像这样的被动运动，有时间可请护理员或家属协助你运动，这样才能保持膝关节和踝关节的功能。

Patient： OK，I'll do the exercise frequently.

病人： 好的，我会经常练习的。

Nurse： Now let me help you to do the toe extension exercise，try your best to extend the toes.（five seconds later，the patient's right toes have an inconspicuous movement.）Yes，very good，continue to move your toes like this.

护士： 下面我再帮助你锻炼足趾背伸运动，自己努力跷足趾。（5 秒钟后右足趾稍微动了一下。）对，很好，就像这样继续活动足趾。

Patient： Oh，my god，it almost requires all my strength.

病人： 太费力了，我几乎用了全身的劲。

Nurse： But with your effort，the toes actually move. It's a good start. You have the great possibility of recover if you persist. You are the most determined woman I have ever met.

护士： 但通过你的努力，脚趾确实动起来了，这就是良好的开端，只要你坚持下去，恢复的希望就很大。你是我见过的最坚强的女性。

Patient： Thank you very much. You give me the hope of recovery.

病人： 非常感谢，你让我看到了康复的希望。

# 43. Lumbago and Acupuncture

# 腰疼与针刺疗法

Patient: I feel painful in my shoulders and lower back. My shoulders have bothered me for a long time. But the pain in my lower back started only a week ago. Is there anything you can do to relieve my pain?

病人：我觉得腰及肩部有些疼痛。我的肩已疼了很长时间，但腰疼只有一周。你能帮助我止疼吗？

Nurse: Yes. But, let me examine you first.

护士：好，让我先检查一下。

(After examination)

（检查完毕）

Nurse: We will try acupuncture and see what happens. Are you afraid of needles?

护士：我们想给你针刺治疗，看看是否有效。你害怕扎针吗？

Patient: No.

病人：不怕。

Nurse: That's good. When I insert the needle into a certain point, you may have the sensation of soreness, numbness and something like an electric shock. If you feel these sensations, it shows that the treatment is effective. Now, I am going to start. Take it easy and don't move. How do you feel when I rotate the needle?

护士：那很好。当我把针刺入穴位时，你会有酸、麻和触电似的感觉。如果你有这些感觉，说明针刺有效。现在我开始给你针刺。别紧张，别动。我捻针时你有什么感觉？

Patient: I feel sore and some numbness.

病人：我觉得发酸和有点麻木。

Nurse: I am also going to try cupping therapy on you after the needles are removed. You will only feel a little heat but no pain.

护士：拔针以后我再给你拔罐治疗。你会感到有些热，但是一点也不疼。

(After the treatment)

（拔罐治疗以后）

Nurse: How do you feel now?

护士：现在你感觉如何？

Patient： Much better. How long should I undergo this treatment?

病人： 好多了。我要治疗多久？

Nurse： Once a day for a course of ten days. It should be able to relieve you of your pain.

护士： 一个疗程要10天，每天一次。这样可以治愈你的疼痛。

# 44. Holistic Nursing Care (High Level Paraplegia)

# 整体护理(高位截瘫)

Nurse： Mr. Liang，please open your mouth and let me brush your teeth，OK?

护士： 梁先生，请你张开嘴，让我来帮你刷牙、漱口，好吗？

Patient： (sadly) No，there is no need.

病人： (沮丧地)不必了。

Nurse： The situation of your health makes everyone feel sad，but there is still hope. The chief doctor is going to perform the operation on you the day after tomorrow. Your condition will have some influence on the success of the operation. Please tell me what you are thinking and let me share your concern，OK?

护士： 你现在的状况确实使大家都很痛苦，但并不是毫无希望呀！后天主任就要给你动手术进行复位。你的状况对手术会有一定的影响，告诉我你在想什么，让我来为你分担些，好吗？

Patient： Can I stand up again after the operation? Just tell me the truth，please.

病人： 手术会让我重新站起来吗？请告诉我实话。

Nurse： Spinal surgery technique progresses very quickly in our country and the doctor who will perform the operation on you is a noted authority in this field. Your condition will definitely become better after the operation. Your tactile sensibility will be improved. At least you can sit in the wheelchair like Ms. Zhang Haidi. You will still be a health man if you believe you can do it and cooperate with us.

护士： 好的。国内脊柱外科手术发展得很快。给你做手术的医生又是国内最权威的。术后肯定比现在的状况要好，起码知觉要多一些。像张海迪那样坐在轮椅上不一样能成为强者吗？

Patient： OK.(The patient opened his mouth and the nurse did the oral care for him.)

病人： 好吧。(病人张开了嘴，护士为他做口腔护理。)

Nurse： Now you may have your breakfast. Mrs. Liang，you can feed him now.

护士： 漱完口你该吃早餐了，梁太太，你来喂他，好吗？

Patient's wife： OK.(Mrs. Liang，began to feed the patient carefully and the nurse left.)

病人妻子： 好的。(梁太太开始细心地喂病人早餐，护士暂离。)

(That afternoon，Mrs. Liang went to the nurse and told her that her husband's urinary catheter had slipped out and it needed to be reinserted. The nurse asked the doctor in charge to come to

reinsert the catheter for the patient and also to give him some instruction.）
（下午，病人妻子找到床位护士，说病人的导尿管脱落了，需要重插，床位护士找来了床位医生为病人重新插好导尿管并给予指导。）

Nurse: The catheter can temporarily relieve the patient's abdominal distention. But, we should not relay on it forever. We should clamp it for half an hour every two hours, to fill the bladder, and train the urination reflex. Early bladder training will promote his self-urination control. Your burden will become less. Let's try it, OK?

护士：尿管只能暂时缓解病人腹胀，但不能“依赖”它。最好每两小时夹管半小时，让病人的膀胱充盈，培养其排尿的条件放射，这样及早促进病人自己控制排尿，你的负担就减轻了。怎么样？试着练几次，好吗？

Patient's wife: Fine. I'll try. Miss, I would like to talk to you in private if you have time.

病人妻子：好的，我尽力试试。小姐，你有空吗？我想跟你单独谈谈。

Nurse: No problem, please come to my office.（The patient's wife went to the office along with the nurse.）Sit down, please.

护士：好吧，去我办公室吧。（病人妻子随护士进了办公室。）请坐。

Patient's wife: Thank you.（sitting down, facing the nurse and keeping silent for a moment）.

病人妻子：谢谢。（坐下，护士在其对面坐下，沉默片刻）。

Nurse: Mrs. Liang, you are very brave. I'll help you no matter it is psychological or how to take care of your husband.

护士：梁太太，你很坚强。我很愿意帮你，无论是精神上还是在对病人的护理上。

Patient's wife: Thank you（silent, sobbing）. I'm in a dilemma and don't know what to do when I think that I'll have to face a paralyzed husband the rest of my life. I have my work and my dreams. But now...

病人妻子：谢谢（沉默、流泪）！我很矛盾，一想到今后我将一辈子面对一个瘫痪在床的丈夫，简直不知所措，我有自己的理想和事业，而现在……

Nurse: Yes, everyone will be at a loss when facing such a situation like yours. However, we must face the reality. The most important thing you should do now is to support and encourage your husband. We should work together to help him go through all problems successfully before, during, and after the operation. The better the result of the operation, the fewer the problems you will have to face. I'm ready to help you at any time. Please trust me.

护士：是的，任何人遇到如此巨大的灾难都将不知所措。然而我们毕竟还是要面对现实的，现在最关键的就是要支持和鼓励你丈夫，我们必须共同努力帮助他渡过术前、术中及术后的全部“难关”。手术效果越好你今后所面对的难题也就愈少。我会始终在你身边，随时帮助你，支持你，相信我。

Patient's wife: （holding the nurse's hand tightly and saying）I believe you.

病人妻子：（紧紧握住护士的手，连声说）我相信你。

# 45. Multiple Periosteoma

# 多发性骨膜瘤

Nurse: Mr. Wang, have you thought about how sad your wife and son would be if you give up treatment and let the cancer spread?

护士：老王，你想过没有，如果你放弃了治疗，任癌细胞肆意蔓延，你妻子、儿子会如何伤心吗？

Patient: It is because they have to take leaves after my previous operations and accompanied me day and night, I don't want to trouble them again.

病人：正因为我每次术后他们都要请假，日日夜夜守护我，陪伴我，所以我才更不该拖累他们。

Nurse: But have you ever thought about that they did this was because of their love and hope for you. How could they work and live if you give up treatment? They will be worrying about you all the time. If you left them forever, how can they not feel sad and sorrow all their lives? Please think about these!

护士：可是，你想过没有，他们是为爱和希望才这样做的。如果你放弃了治疗，他们又如何能安心地工作和生活呢，他们将时刻惦记你的生命安危。一旦你离开了他们，他们能不悲痛欲绝抱憾终身吗？请想想这些！

Patient: Amputation means that I'll become a crippled person. I cannot accept this fact.

病人：截肢意味着我变成了一个残疾人，我无法接受这个事实。

Nurse: Yes, losing a leg is a bitter experience physically and mentally. But you must face this cruel reality in order to keep you alive and keep the integrity of your family. Besides, you may install an artificial leg after the operation, it will not be too much difference compared with before if you recover well.

护士：是的，失去一条腿，无论从肉体上还是心理上都将很痛苦。但是想想这是为了保全生命，保持家庭的完整，只好忍痛接受这一残酷的事实。何况还可以装假肢，如果恢复得好和原来相比不会有太多变化的。

Patient: Is there any recurrence of the cancer after amputation?

病人：截肢后癌细胞还会复发吗？

Nurse: It can be prevented if you continue to have chemotherapy and radiotherapy.

护士：只要坚持化疗和放疗应该可以预防复发的。

Patient: It seems that I really don't have many choice. After hearing what you have said, it seems there is some hope for me. Thank you.

病人：看来也只好这样了。听你讲了这么多，我似乎又有了希望，谢谢你。

# 46. Care at the Operation Room

# 术中照顾

Nurse: Are you cold?

护士： 你觉得冷吗？

Patient: No.

病人： 不冷。

Nurse: Do you have rhinitis? Do you want to raise the pillow higher?

护士： 你有鼻炎吗？需要加高枕头吗？

Patient: No，Thanks. But I feel the cold air blowing on my face. I have a stuffed-up nose from that.

病人： 谢谢，枕头倒不需要加高，就是这儿有冷气吹到我鼻子里，我一吸到冷气鼻子就塞。

Nurse: Should I adjust the room temperature a little higher?

护士： 那我调高一点室温，好吗？

Patient: Thanks a lot. I am not afraid of heat. A little higher temperature will be fine.

病人： 谢谢。我不怕热，就怕冷。

Nurse: You are welcome. Just let me know whatever you want. Everybody's preferred temperature is different. We will adjust it to your liking.

护士： 不用谢，你有什么要求尽管跟我说。每个人对冷热的感受都不同，在这个房间以你的要求来调整。

Patient: Could you adjust the fan so the breeze will not blow directly at me?

病人： 这个风扇能不能不要对着我吹？

Nurse: No problem.（Adjusted the bed location with the work's help.）Is this better?

护士： 可以。（在工人的协助下调整了床的位置。）这样可以吗？

Patient: Thanks，your attitude is really good. I hope that I didn't bother you too much.

病人： 谢谢，你们的态度真好，不影响什么吧？

Nurse: Don't worry about it. You won't feel the breeze after they spread the aseptic sheet during the surgery. We will move the bed back then.

护士： 不会影响什么的，手术时铺好消毒单你就吹不到风了，那时我们再把床移到正中。

（The patient was very grateful and also felt bad about this request. She thanked the nurse repeatedly.）

（患者很感激，有些过意不去，反复地感谢。）

Nurse: Don't worry about it. This is a multi-functional bed which is very easy to move or change direction. Just tell me if you have any problem.

护士：不用担心，床是多功能的，移动很方便。你有什么问题尽管跟我讲。

# 47. Enema

# 灌肠

Nurse: Mr. Zhao, the doctors will operate on you tomorrow, so I will give you an enema around eight o'clock tonight.

护士：赵先生，明天你就要做手术了，今晚8点左右我要为你做一个术前灌肠。

Patient: Oh, my goodness, no. I have bowel movement very regularly. Besides, the operation is not on my abdomen, why do I need an enema?

病人：不用，不用。我每天大便都很正常，况且又不是腹部手术，为什么要灌肠？

Nurse: Although the operation is not on your abdomen, we will perform the operation on your hip joint under continuous spinal cord extradural anesthesia. After anesthesia the part below where the drug is used will have no feeling any more. The sphincter of the rectum will be relaxed, and you cannot control the lower part of your body. If you have stool incontinence during the surgery, the operating area will become contaminated. An enema can help you to remove all the stools. Moreover, after the operation you will be on complete bed rest for several days. During the early days after the operation, it is not convenient for you to use the toilet.

护士：虽然你不是做腹部手术，但你的髋关节手术需用连续硬膜外麻醉的方法。使用麻醉药后，被麻醉平面以下没有知觉，肛门括约肌松弛。你无法像现在一样控制下半身的运动，万一有大便排出，就会污染手术区。灌肠可使肠内的宿便排出体外。况且，你术后需卧床一段时间，手术后开始几天，解大便有可能不方便。

Patient: Why can't I just use two Glycerin suppository?

病人：那你给我用两个开塞露不就行了？

Nurse: Glycerin suppository can only help you remove the stool that is in the rectal area, But enema is different. It fills the suds in your colon by the catheter. This will clean the intestines more thoroughly.

护士：开塞露只能排空接近直肠处的大便，而灌肠则不同，它通过管子将肥皂液灌入结肠中，可以比较彻底地帮助清洁肠道。

Patient: Oh, that's why. To avoid making a fool of myself, I will not eat anything tonight.

病人：喔，原来是这样！那我今天晚餐就不吃了，以免手术中出洋相。

Nurse: That's not necessary. You can eat something light for supper. Then follow the doctor's order that stop eating and drinking afterwards.

护士：这倒不必，今晚你可以吃些清淡的饮食，然后按规定禁食禁水就行了。

Patient: Is enema painful?

病人：灌肠会不会很疼？

Nurse: It may be a little uncomfortable.(turning to Mr. Liu who had the enema before) Mr. Liu, you had the enema before. What do you think about it?

护士：灌肠可能会有一些不舒服。(转向邻床的刘先生)刘先生，你术前也曾做过灌肠，你觉得怎样？

Mr. Liu: Mr. Zhao, no pain at all. Just feel a little distention when filled with the enema solution. I just followed the nurse's instruction, opened my mouth and took a deep breath. It is quite effective, so don't worry.

刘先生：赵先生，一点都不疼，只是灌肠水灌进去时觉得肚子有些胀。我听护士说要张嘴深呼吸，当我试着这样做后效果不错，不用担心。

Nurse: That's right, it is better to keep the solution in your intestines for five to ten minutes. Deep breathing can decrease the feeling of distention. I am quite sure that you can do it very well by following my instructions to clean out the intestines.

护士：确实如此，灌入肥皂液后最好让它在肠道内保留 5～10 分钟，深呼吸可以减轻腹胀，只要你按照我提示的方法去做，保证能顺利完成肠道清洁工作。

Patient: After your explanation, I don't feel as nervous as before. I will do my best to cooperate with you.

病人：经你们这么一说，我没有那么紧张了，我一定尽量配合。

# 48. Appendicitis

# 阑尾炎

## (1)

Nurse: I understand you have a stomachache.

护士: 我看你是胃痛。

Patient: Yes. It is getting terribly painful.

病人: 是的。痛得十分厉害。

Nurse: How long have you had it?

护士: 你痛多久了？

Patient: It started last night, At the beginning, I didn't pay much attention to as I thought it would go away very soon. But it has become worse and worse, and it is now almost unbearable.

病人: 昨天夜里开始的。起初我没注意，我想它一会儿会好的。但是它越来越不好，现在几乎难以忍受。

Nurse: Where is the pain?

护士: 痛在哪里？

Patient: It is in the lower right side of my abdomen.

病人: 就在右下腹部。

Nurse: Do you feel anything else besides the pain?

护士: 除了痛，还有什么感觉？

Patient: I am a little nauseated. But I felt more comfortable when I lay down and bent my legs.

病人: 有点恶心。但当我躺下将腿屈起来时就觉得舒服一些。

Nurse: I am afraid you are suffering from appendicitis. We will have your blood examined. In the meantime, the doctor will come to examine you. If he finds you have acute appendicitis, you will be admitted and be operated on immediately.

护士: 我看你像是得了阑尾炎。我们要给你查血。同时，医生将要对你进行检查。如果他诊断你是急性阑尾炎，你就得住院并立即做手术。

## (2)

Nurse: Hello. What brought you to the emergency room?

护士: 您好，您到急诊室来看什么？

Patient: I've got an awful pain in my belly. And I feel like I'm going to throw up all the time. I feel awful.

病人：我腹部疼痛剧烈，老是想吐，很难受。

Nurse: How long have you had this pain?

护士：腹痛多长时间了？

Patient: It started last night，up here，but this morning it's here and it really hurts.

病人：昨晚开始的，在这边，但是今早在这边，痛得很厉害。

Nurse: Has it moved again?

护士：现在又转移到别的地方了吗？

Patient: No，it been steady for two hours.

病人：不，现在固定了，有两个小时了。

Nurse: Is it there all the time.

护士：一直痛吗？

Patient: No，it just comes and goes，but now it's really killing me.

病人：不，一阵一阵的。现在，痛死我了。

Nurse: Have you had any diarrhea?

护士：拉肚子吗？

Patient: No，I haven't had a bowel movement for 2 days.

病人：没有，我已经两天没有大便了。

Nurse: Is this regular for you?

护士：常这样吗？

Patient: No，I usually have one every day.

病人：不，我平时每天大便一次。

Nurse: How about all this nausea and vomiting?

护士：恶心和呕吐怎么样了？

Patient: Well，it's gotten better. Last night I was vomiting about every two hours，soon after the pain began.

病人：哦，好多了。昨晚大约每两小时吐一次。一痛就吐。

Nurse: Have you had temperature?

护士：发烧吗？

Patient: Last night I took my temperature. It was 38℃.

病人：昨天晚上我量过体温，38℃。

Nurse: Show me where it hurts most right now.

护士：告诉我现在哪最痛。

Patient: Just here.

病人：就在这儿。

Nurse: Please lie down. Let me examine your abdomen. Do you feel pain when I press here? Does it hurt you when I withdraw my hand suddenly? I think that you have appendicitis. You need an operation.

护士：请躺下，让我检查一下你的腹部。我按的这儿痛吗？当我忽然松手时痛吗？我想你是得了阑尾炎，你需要手术。

Patient: Is it serious?

病人：严重吗？

Nurse: Don't worry. Let's ask the doctor for his advise.

护士：别担心，让我们去请教医生。

(3)

Patient: Nurse, I'm not feeling well today.

病人：护士，我今天感觉不舒服。

Nurse: Where don't you feel well?

护士：您哪儿不好？

Patient: I have a pain in my abdomen.

病人：我肚子痛。

Nurse: How long have you had it?

护士：痛多长时间了？

Patient: It started in the morning. At the beginning I thought that I had a stomachache.

病人：早晨开始的，起初我以为是胃痛。

Nurse: How long have it last?

护士：持续了多长时间？

Patient: About three hours, but this afternoon it moved to the right lower part of the abdomen for five hours.

病人：大约 3 小时，但今天下午转移至右下腹，有 5 个多小时了。

Nurse: Have you had any vomiting.

护士：您呕吐吗？

Patient: I have only nausea.

病人：我只是恶心。

Nurse: Constipation?

护士：便秘吗？

Patient: Yes.

病人：是的。

Nurse: Have you any diarrhea?

护士：您有过腹泻吗？

Patient: No.

病人：没有。

Nurse: Any fever?

护士：发热吗？

Patient: I don't know.

病人：我不知道。

Nurse: Let me take your temperature. All right, you have a slight fever.

护士：我给您量一下体温。好了，有点发热。

Patient： Please lie down on the bed. Loosen your belt，please. Let the doctor examine your abdomen.

护士： 请躺在床上，松开腰带，让医生检查您的腹部。

Patient： Thank you.

病人： 谢谢。

Nurse： Don't be nervous and try to relax.

护士： 不要紧张，尽量放轻松。

Patient： All right.

病人： 好的。

Nurse： The doctor said you need to collect a specimen of blood and urine for examination.

护士： 医生说您需要取血液和尿液标本做化验。

Patient： Yes.

病人： 是的。

Nurse： The result of your blood test tells us that your while blood cell counts is $18\times10^9$/L.

护士： 您的验血结果，白细胞 $18\times10^9$/L。

Patient： I see，thank you.

病人： 我知道了，谢谢。

Nurse： The doctor said that you had acute appendicitis.

护士： 医生说您患的是急性阑尾炎。

Patient： Oh gosh.

病人： 噢，天啊。

Nurse： Don't be afraid，you will recover. The doctor said that you have to have an operation. So，please sign your name on the consent from to say that you agree to the doctor operation on you.

护士： 不用怕，您一定会好的。医生说您必须接受手术治疗。现在请您签手术同意书，表示您同意医生为您做手术。

Patient： I'll co-operate.

病人： 我会合作的。

Nurse： Thanks for your co-operation.

护士： 谢谢您的合作。

# 49. Comforting Care

# 舒适护理

Nurse: Mr. Li，can you tell me where you feel uncomfortable?

护士：李先生，你哪儿不舒服，告诉我好吗？

Patient: My whole body is uncomfortable.

病人：我觉得全身不舒服。

Nurse: It is wound?

护士：是伤口疼痛吗？

Patient: No. I'm using the analgesic pump now，but still do not feel well.

病人：不是，我用了镇痛泵。但是还是觉得浑身难受。

Nurse: Maybe you have lay on your back too long. Let me help you to change your position.（The nurse assisted the patient to lie on his side，and arranged the abdominal cavity drainage tube and the gastrointestinal decompression tube to the proper position.）

护士：可能是在床上平卧的时间长了，让我来帮你换个体位，好吗？（护士协助病人翻成侧卧位，并妥善安置好腹腔引流管及胃肠减压管。）

Patient: I dare not turn my body with so many tubes on me. I really feel like pulling them out，especially the gastric tube through my nose.

病人：这么多管子在身上，我都不敢翻身。我真想拔掉这些管子，尤其是这根从鼻子插进去的胃管。

Nurse: You have made through the operation. These tubes are very important to you，because they can help you recover quickly. Don't be afraid，insist for two more days，let's overcome the barrier together.

护士：这么大的一个手术你都挺过来了，这些管子现在对你很重要，它们会帮你尽快恢复的。不要怕，再坚持两天，我会尽力和你一起渡过这个难关的。

Patient: What's the function of these tubes and when will they be removed?

病人：这些管子到底有什么作用？要多久才能拔掉呢？

Nurse: Usually there will be some blood and fluid accumulated in the abdominal cavity after operation. The two drainage tubes placed in the abdominal wall are used to help drain these fluids. After two or three days，when the drainage fluid decreases，the doctor will put out the tubes for you. The gastric tube is uses to drain the gastric juice and some accumulated blood from your stomach. Portion of your stomach has been removed and the remaining portion was connected to the intestines below. In order to heal the wound better and more quickly, the gastric juice must be drained out in time. If the tubes were taken out too early, the fluid would be accumulated in the stomach, and the wound could be split by the weight of the fluids.

护士： 手术一般都会在腹腔内留下积液、积血。插在腹壁上的两根引流管主要是帮助引流腹腔的积血或积液。两三天后，引流液明显减少，医生就可以帮助你拔掉这两根管子了。至于胃管，是引流胃液和一些手术后的血液用的。你的胃部被切掉一部分，并和下面的肠子做了吻合。为了吻合口能愈合得更快、更好，胃本身分泌的胃液必须及时引流出来，否则会影响吻合口的愈合。过早拔掉管子，胃里液体太多，张力大了会让吻合的伤口裂开。

Patient： But the gastric tube irritates my throat. It is really unbearable.

病人： 可是，胃管刺激我喉部的感觉，真难以忍受。

Nurse： Try to take deep inhalation, then exhalation, like what I am doing (giving a demonstration), it will make you feel better. You will feel more uncomfortable if you keep focusing and pay too much attention to these tubes.

护士： 你尝试着深吸气，再呼气，像我一样（示范深呼吸的动作）这样会好一些。如果你的注意力都在这几根管子上，不舒服的感觉就会更明显了。

Patient： Could I ask my wife to bring the radio for me tomorrow?

病人： 明天，可以让我爱人把收音机带来听吗？

Nurse： Of course, I was just about to suggest you to do so. You can do other things as well. Just do not think of the tubes too often.

护士： 当然可以，我正想建议你这样做呢。你还可以做一些其他的事情，只要不经常想这些管子，就会感觉好多了。

Patient： OK, I'll try to overcome the difficulties since they are so important to me.Thank you very much.

病人： 好的。这些管子既然那么重要，我会尽量克服的。谢谢你。

# 50. Peri-operative Nursing Care (Benign Prostatic Hypertrophy)

# 围手术期护理（良性前列腺增生）

## (1)

Nurse: Hello. Mr. Wang, how are you? Are you exercising?（Mr. Wang answered with a nod.） Let me check your drainage bag to make sure the fixed position is right.（Nurse Wu bent over to look at the patient's drainage bag.）Very good. The urine is also pretty clear. Did you drink any water this morning?

护士：王先生，你好！正在下床活动呢。（王先生点头答应。）让我看看引流带固定的位置对不对。（小吴弯下腰查看尿液引流情况。）很好，尿色也很清。早晨喝水了吗？

Patient: I drank a cup of water this morning. Miss Wu, could you help me to ask the doctor if he can operate on me sooner?

病人：早晨喝了一杯水。小吴你能帮我跟医生打个招呼，能早点给我动手术吗？

Nurse: Don't worry, Mr. Wang, the operation is set for tomorrow. Yesterday, I told you about the operating procedures and how you can cooperate with us. Do you still have anything unclear that I can help you with?

护士：王先生，不要着急，明天你就要动手术了。昨天我已给你介绍了手术的方法及配合手术的有关事项。你还有哪些不明白的地方我再给你说说，好吗？

Patient: I understand them well because I have studied the materials you gave me several times. Let me show you.（Mr. Wang began to restate the information about the operation. Nurse Wu listened and made a few corrections from time to time.）

病人：我都明白了。你给我的这些材料我都反复看了好多遍了。我说给你听听。（王先生开始复述手术相关知识。护士小吴边听边给予补充和纠正。）

Nurse: Mr. Wang, you have a good memory. Now, let us practice relaxing, deep breathing, and effective coughing. Please lie down on the bed first.（Nurse Wu helped him to lie down on the bed and he began to practice.）Close your mouth when you take a deep breath. Use your nose to inhale and relax your hands. Good. Let's try again.

护士：王先生，你真是好记性。那我们练习一下全身放松，深呼吸及有效咳嗽排痰。你先躺在床上。（小吴扶王先生上床，王先生开始练习。）深吸气时嘴巴闭起来，对，用鼻吸气，双手不要握拳，手掌自然伸开。好，再来一次。

Nurse: Mr. Wang, your operation tomorrow will need epidural anesthesia, that is, lower body anesthesia. The anesthetic drug will be injected to your spine and you'll have no feelings in your lower half body after the injection, but you will remain conscious. Now I'll teach you how to cooperate with doctor. Mr. Wang, please lie on your side and bend your legs to your chest, use your arms to hold your knees. (Nurse Wu helped Mr. Wang to hold his knees with his arms.) Try to make your back protruding and lower your head. Good, that's right. I'm going to care for other patients now. But I'll be back later to do some preoperative preparation for you. Mr. Wang, you can sit back and chat with Mr. Zhang on bed 26 who had the similar operation as yours.

护士: 王先生,明天手术是硬膜外麻醉,就是半身麻醉。麻药打在腰脊椎骨内,下半身没有知觉,人是清醒的。我现在教你麻醉时如何配合医生。王先生请你身体侧睡,双腿屈曲,靠近胸口,两手抱住膝盖。(小吴指导王先生用两手抱住膝盖。)背尽量后凸,头低下一点儿。好!就这样。我先去看看其他病人,等一会儿我再来为你做术前准备工作。王先生你现在先休息一下,与26床张先生聊聊,他与你的手术是一样的。

(Nurse Wu asked Mr. Zhang to talk to Mr. Wang about his operating experiences. After completing nursing care on the other patients, Nurse Wu came back and finished Mr. Wang's preoperative preparations.)

(小吴请26床张先生与王先生谈谈手术体会。护士小吴在做完其他病人的护理后为王先生做了常规的术前准备工作。)

## (2)

(In the afternoon, nurse Wu came to the ward to take the patient's temperature.)

(下午护士小吴到病房准备为病人量体温。)

Nurse: Hello, Mr. Wang, did you have a good rest at noon?

护士: 王先生,你好!中午休息得好吗?

Patient: Not bad, I didn't sleep, just rested for a while.

病人: 还好。没睡着,躺了一会儿。

Nurse: Are you still nervous about tomorrow's operation? Is there anything else you are concerned?

护士: 是不是明天要做手术,心里有点紧张,还是有什么顾虑?

Patient: Miss Wu, to tell you the truth, when I was admitted I wanted the operation as early as possible. But now, as the operation is near, I'm really nervous. Knowing Mr. Zhang's operation went very well, I'm not concerned about your medical technology. However, Mr. Zhang told me that the balloon of the catheter pressing on the prostate was tied to the thigh which will make one feel pain and discomfort in the perineum area. I'm so scared of pain. I'm afraid that I may not cooperate with you well when you tell me not to move my leg as the catheter is fixed. If I can't endure the pain and move my legs, it may cause the balloon to move from its position and leads to bleeding. What should I do then? Miss Wu, please help me to ask the anesthetist to install a pain control pump.

病人: 小吴,不瞒你讲,我入院时希望早点手术。真的听到要手术了,心里倒真的有点紧张。我看 26 床张先生手术很顺利。对你们这里的医疗技术我是放心的。不过听张先生讲压迫在前列腺窝内的导尿管气囊牵引在大腿上，会阴部会肿痛，挺难受的。我很怕痛，我怕我不能很好地配合。到时候你们嘱咐我固定导尿管的下肢不能动，我怕忍不住，万一把气囊位置移动了，引起出血怎么办？小吴，麻烦你帮我与麻醉师联系一下，看能不能给我安置镇痛泵。

Nurse： Don't worry. I'll contract the anesthetist to come see you.

护士： 放心，我会与麻醉师联系来看你的。

Patient： Thanks and sorry for troubling you.

病人： 好的，麻烦你了小吴。

Nurse： You are welcome. Mr. Wang，let me take your temperature now.（Nurse Wu took Mr. Wang's temperature.）

护士： 不麻烦。王先生，我现在给你量体温。（小吴给王先生量体温。）

Nurse： Your temperature is normal，36.8℃.Don't catch cold when you take a bath later.

护士： 体温正常，36.8℃。等一会儿洗澡时注意不要着凉。

Patient： OK.

病人： 知道了。

Nurse： Mr. Wang，did you have bowel movement between 14：00 yesterday to 14：00 today?

护士： 王先生，昨天下午两点到今天下午两点解大便了吗？

Patient： Just once.

病人： 解过一次。

Nurse： Was it dry?

护士： 大便干结吗？

Patient： No. It was easy to dispel.

病人： 不，很容易就解出来了。

Nurse： Did you use the bedpan? Did you feel comfortable using it?

护士： 使用便器了吗？能适应吗？

Patient： Yes，I can use it.

病人： 使用了，能适应。

**（3）**

（Nurse Wu briefed middle shift nurse，Miss Zhu，at the bedside.）

（护士小吴与中班小朱到床边交接班。）

Nurse Wu and Nurse Zhu： Hi，Mr. Wang，your wife is here too.

护士小吴、小朱： 王先生，你好！你夫人也来了。

Patient's wife： Since my husband is going to have the operation tomorrow，I cooked several nutritious dishes for his supper this evening including braised fish，brine shrimps，tomato with eggs，potato with green peppers，and stirred green vegetables.

病人妻子： 我丈夫明天要手术了，我做了点清蒸鱼、盐水虾、番茄炒蛋、土豆青椒、炒青菜，让他增加点营养。

Nurse Wu：Mr. Wang，your wife is so nice to you. But you should not eat too much this evening because of tomorrow's operation. Eighty percent full would be enough.

护士小吴：王先生，你夫人对你真体贴。不过，由于你明天需要做手术，今天晚饭不要吃得太饱，八分饱就行了。

Patient：OK，I see.

病人：我会注意的。

Nurse Wu：Let me introduce you the middle shift nurse，Miss Zhu.（The patient greeted her with a nod.）She will conduct an enema for you at 8：00 pm. After that you should not eat anything. After 12：00pm，water is also forbidden. Remember that.

护士小吴：这是中班小朱。（病人点头会意。）晚上 8 点她要为你进行术前灌肠。灌肠以后不可以吃东西了，晚上 12 点以后水也不能喝了。不要忘记了。

Patient：OK.

病人：我知道。

## （4）

（On the morning of the operation day，nurse Wu entered the ward to check the preparation for his operation.）

（手术日早晨，护士小吴到病房查看手术准备情况。）

Nurse：Good morning，Mr. Wang，did you sleep well last night? And have you changed to the operating clothes?

护士：王先生，早安！昨晚睡得好吗？手术衣裤换好了吗？

Patient：Yes. I slept very well last night and I have changed to the operating clothes.

病人：睡得很好。衣裤已换好了。

Nurse：Your temperature and blood pressure are all normal this morning. The operation should be fine. So don't worry.

护士：今晨体温和血压都很正常。手术会顺利的。不要紧张。

Patient：I'm not worried. I trust your medical services.

病人：我不紧张，我相信你们的医疗、服务。

（Nurse Wu checked the patient's hair，nails，and skin conditions and made sure that any jewelry，watch，and dentures were removed. Then the operating room worker arrived to meet the patient. Nurse Wu helped Mr. Wang to lie on the stretcher，comforting him and accompanying him leaving the ward.）

（护士小吴边与病人交谈边查看病人的头发、指甲、皮肤情况，首饰、手表、假牙是否取下。这时手术室来接病人。护士小吴扶病人到病车上并边安慰边送出病房。）

## （5）

（The patient returned from the operating room. Nurse Wu helped him to his bed.）

（病人从手术室返回了病房，床位护士小吴帮助病人转移到了病床上。）

Nurse： Mr. Wang，your operation went very well and the anesthetist had installed a pain control pump for you. Now，you need to keep your right leg unbend.（Supporting the patient's right leg）Right. Try not to move or bend your right leg. You can move it after the catheter is released tomorrow.

护士： 王先生，你的手术非常顺利。麻醉师为你安置了镇痛泵。现在，请你右下肢保持外展伸直位。（扶着病人的右腿）对，右下肢尽可能不要移动、屈曲，明天导尿管牵引放松后才能活动。

Patient： OK.

病人： 知道了。

Nurse： How do you feel now?

护士： 你现在感觉如何？

Patient： I am thirsty.

病人： 感觉有点口渴。

Nurse： I will clean and moisten your mouth right now.（Nurse Wu began to clean his mouth.）Do you feel better?

护士： 我马上为你进行口腔清洗，湿润一下口腔。（护士小吴为病人进行口腔清洗。）感觉好点吗？

Patient： Yes，I feel better now.

病人： 好点了。

Nurse： Have a rest.

护士： 你休息吧。

## （6）

（Nurse Wu arrived at the patient's bedside the day after the operation.）

（手术后第一天，护士小吴来到病人旁边。）

Nurse： Hello，Mr. Wang. Thank you for your cooperation. Today the catheter has been relaxed and you can move your right leg now. You can even turn your body over. But you should move slowly and don't do it too often.（instructing him to turn over his body）. Since you have passed gas，you can eat food now，but drink some warm water first.

护士：你好，王先生。非常感谢你的配合。今天导尿管牵引已放松，右下肢可以活动了，你可以自己翻身，但要注意动作缓慢，幅度要小（指导病人翻身活动）。你肛门已排气，可以进食了，先喝口温开水。

（Nurse Wu designed the patient's activity plan，supervised and instructed him to move correctly，guided him to choose the proper diet，from full-fluid to semi-fluid to regular diet，and taught him ways to avoid constipation. The patient had bowel movement easily three days after the operation.）

（护士小吴为病人制订了活动计划，并督促、指导病人正确进行活动。指导病人从流质、半流质、普食中选择合适的饮食，防止便秘。手术后第三天，病人顺利排出了大便。）

## (7)

Nurse: Hello，Mr. Wang. You recover very quickly after the operation. The doctor will remove the catheter for you today.

护士: 王先生，你好！你术后恢复很快，今天要拔除导尿管了。

Patient: That's great! Does this mean I will be discharged soon?

病人: 太好了。是不是我很快可以出院了？

Nurse: Yes. There will be some temporary urinary incontinent after removing the catheter. You should continue the functional exercises following my instruction. It will be recovered soon. Don't be nervous.

护士: 是的。拔除后可能出现暂时性排尿失控情况。你继续按我教你的功能锻炼方法去做，很快就会好的，不必紧张。

Patient: I see and thanks.

病人: 知道了，谢谢你。

Nurse: However，don't be reckless after your discharge. You should avoid lifting heavy objects，sitting for a long time and riding bikes. You should also keep your bowel movement smooth. Make sure to see the doctor when you notice any urinate difficulties. Here are the discharge instructions and our telephone number. Please keep in touch with us.

护士: 不过，出院后不要大意。避免重负、久坐、骑车，要保持大便通畅，尿线变细及时就诊。这是出院后的注意事项及我科的联系电话，随时保持联系。

# 51. Cystectomy

# 膀胱全切术

## (1)

Nurse： Hi，Mr. Zhang，I am your nurse. You are going to receive the operation soon，so I would like to talk to you about the preparation for the surgery，OK?

护士： 张先生，我是你的床位护士。你马上就要手术了，现在我想与你谈谈，行吗。

(Mr. Zhang stared at Nurse Wang for a few seconds but said nothing.)

(张先生抬头望了一下护士小王，未吭声。)

Nurse： Mr. Zhang，you already have a colostomy on your abdomen. You are going to have a radical cystectomy. The ureter will be connected to the pouch of your colostomy. If you do not mind，I would like to check your colostomy，and clean it for the upcoming operation.

护士： 张先生，你腹部已有一个结肠造口，接下来要做的手术是根治性膀胱全切术，要把输尿管接在结肠造口袋内。如果你愿意，我想检查一下你腹部的造口，好为手术做好清洁准备。

Patient： No.（Mr. Zhang shouted very loudly. The nurse was taken aback and his roommates as well as their relatives were also surprised. Nurse Wang felt embarrassed and rushed out of the ward.）

病人： 不。（张先生大喝一声，吓了护士一跳，也使同病室的几位病人与家属惊呆了。护士小王感到很委屈，跑出了病房。）

## (2)

(Nurse Wang ran into the nurses' station where she met the specialized nursing team leader，Teacher Li，who was writing the report for next shift.)（小王跑进护士办公室。遇到正写交班报告的专业组长李老师。）

Nurse： （sobbed）The patient in bed 3 is really a strange guy. I offered the preoperative instructions to him patiently，but he yelled at me in return. I can't stand this guy.

护士： （充满委屈地哽咽道）3 号床病人真怪，我好好地与他讲关于手术的事，结果他却冲我大喊大叫，真受不了。

Teacher Li： Xiao Wang，have you thought about from the point of the patient? He had double blow of losing anus and bladder with only one year. What does this mean to a young man of 23?

李老师：小王，你有没有设身处地地站在病人的位置替他想想。仅仅一年的时间，他面临了失去肛门又将失去膀胱的双重打击，这对一个23岁的小伙子来说意味着什么？

Nurse：I know he is depressed and unhappy，but I was trying to help him. I was advising him about the operation and I was following the health education protocol of the"Nursing Care Plan".

护士：我知道他很沮丧，也很难过，可是我是在帮他呀。我是完全按《护理计划》中制定的健康教育方案去向他讲解有关手术的情况的。

Teacher Li：Well，you were doing your job which is fine. However，don't you think your timing was a little off? The patient was in a physical，psychological，and sociological confusion state. Mentally he was not ready for the radical cystectomy，yet you are doing preoperation nursing on him. That's why he was mad at you.

李老师：是的，你是在按照计划执行没错。可你想过没有，你选择的时机不对，此时的病人正处在躯体、心理、社会诸多问题的紊乱之中。他还没有做好切除膀胱的心理准备，你已经在为他做术前准备了，叫他如何不迁怒于你呢？

Nurse：Oh，I see. Mr. Zhang is self-contempt now and I should deal with his self-pity of losing an organ，and disturbed self-image first. I picked the wrong time to give him the health instructions.

护士：哦，我明白了。这时的张先生很自卑，躯体器官的丧失和自我形象紊乱是我应首先解决的问题。看来，我是没把握好健康教育的时机。

## （3）

（Teacher Li invited Mr. Zhang to have a face to face talk in the nurse's station. Nurse Wang sat beside them.）

（在护士办公室，李老师约来了病人张先生面谈，一旁坐着小王。）

Nurse：I'm sorry，Mr. Zhang，I was too brusque. Could you tell me what you are worried about the most right now? My teacher and I are willing to help you.

护士：对不起，张先生，刚才我太唐突了，能告诉我，现在你最担心的问题吗？李老师和我都非常希望能帮助你。

Patient：（lowered his head and spoke softly）I am finished，absolutely useless. What's the meaning to still be alive?

病人：（低下头去轻声说）我这辈子算是完了，废人一个，活着还有什么意思？

Teacher Li：Mr. Wang，we all will encounter many difficulties in our life. You have to conquer yourself before you can conquer those difficulties，and the key to conquering yourself is to accept the reality. I am very proud of you，a real man，taking all these hardships without letting your parents feel unhappy. However，the capability of one man is limited. We are willing to help you to conquer this hardship.（Mr. Zhang raised his head gradually and listened carefully...）

李老师：张先生，每个人的一生都会遇到很多困难，要战胜困难首先得战胜自己，而战胜自己的关键是接受现实。我很佩服你，像个男子汉，为了不让父母伤心，一切都自己扛着。但个人的力量是有限的，我们想帮你一起跨过眼前的这道坎。（张先生渐渐抬起头，认真聆听着……）

Nurse: That's right. The medical science is progressing very fast. Surgical techniques as well as care equipments are getting much better. The watertight bag for the colostomy is not only able to prevent back flow but can also improve the physiological function. The appearance of the bag is also approaching perfection. It can make you live like a normal man.（Mr. Zhang's eyes were focused on Nurse Wang full of hope. Nurse Wang smiled as she took out the Colostomy Manual，pen and paper，and began to draw something to show Mr. Zhang.）

护士：是啊，现在医学科学发展很快，手术方法、护理工具也日趋完善，造口贴袋不但能防倒流，而且也能完善生理功能，在外观上也能力求完美，可以让你像正常人一样地生活。（病人张先生紧盯着王护士，双眼闪现了希望。王护士会意地笑了，从口袋里拿出造口手册和纸笔，给张先生画了起来……）

# 52. Peritoneal Dialysis

# 腹膜透析

Nurse： Mrs. Wu，how do you do? Based on your present condition the doctor has decided to give you a peritoneal dialysis. Peritoneal dialysis is a process that can help you get the useful substances from dialysis solution and at the same time remove the waste products from your body. Do you know about this procedure?

护士： 吴女士，你好。医生根据你目前的病情决定为你做腹膜透析术（腹透）。通过腹透使透析液中的有用物质进入你的体内，同时将你体内的代谢废物等随透析液排出体外，从而达到治疗目的。你了解这个手术吗？

Patient： I know a little. The doctor talked to me a while ago. He said he will open a small hole on my abdomen and put in a tube there.

病人： 知道一点，刚才医生跟我谈过，说是要在腹部开一刀，然后放上一根管子。

Nurse： Yes. This procedure is called"peritoneal dialysis tube insertion". The procedure can be done under local anesthesia. The doctor will make a small cut（three to four cm）on your abdomen and insert a silica gel tube of forty-one cm long. A small portion of the tube will remain outside the abdomen and be connected with a small tube will be used to perform the peritoneal dialysis.

护士： 是的，这个手术叫腹透管置管术。这种手术只要在局部麻醉下就可以进行了。在你的腹部做一个约 3～4cm 的切口，将一根长约 41cm 的硅胶管放入腹腔内，腹壁外留出一小段，然后外接一根短管即可透析。

Patient： I am a little afraid.

病人： 唷！我听了心里有点害怕。

Nurse： I know you will have some concerns. Please follow me to the demonstration room. I will show you the whole procedure and peritoneal dialysis on the analogous human body.（Demonstrated to the patient in the demonstration room）

护士： 我知道你会有顾虑的。请你跟我一起到示范室去，我将在模拟人身上为你演示整个手术和腹膜透析的过程，让你有一个全面的了解。（在演示室示范）

Patient： I am beginning to understand it. I am feeling better now. Do I need to stay in the hospital to do the peritoneal dialysis all the time? Do I need to do it every day or once every several days?

病人： 噢，现在我有点明白了，害怕的感觉好一点了。那么做腹透需要一直住在医院里吗？是每天做一次，还是几天做一次呢？

Nurse: Peritoneal dialysis is a renal substitute method. You have to do it every day, about three to four times a day. Every time a bag of dialysis solution (2000ml) will be introduced into and remain in the abdomen for three to four hours. In the hospital we will train you and your family members with related knowledge. After you have learned it, you can do it at home. And by then you will be able to do some light housework as well. The tube inside your abdomen will be remained all the time and the small tube should be changed every two to three months. If you want to accept further treatment, such as kidney transplantation, the peritoneal dialysis tube will be pulled out.

护士：腹透作为肾脏替代疗法，每天都需要做。一般一天做透析 3～4 次，每次一袋透析液（2000ml）在腹腔内保留 3～4 小时。在医院内我们会对你和你的家人进行相关知识的培训。等你们完全掌握该操作以后，可以出院在家自行透析，还可以从事力所能及的家务。在腹腔内的透析管一直留在腹腔内，外接的短管一般 2～3 个月更换一次，如果你准备做进一步的治疗，如肾移植，到时可将腹透管拔除。

Patient: Now I am only allowed to eat some vegetables. What kind of diet should I have after the peritoneal dialysis? Can I take a bath?

病人：我现在只能吃一些蔬菜，那么做腹透以后饮食上面要注意些什么？还有，我能不能洗澡？

Nurse: Because you will lose a small amount of protein from the dialysis procedure, you need to eat food with high quality of protein such as milk, eggs and meat. You also need to take vitamins. Water is not limited. So you do not need to eat like before. But be sure the food is clean and avoid infection of abdomen. You can take a shower, but no bath. And when taking a shower, you need to take care of the tube by using some 3M tapes or the nursing bag to protect the opening.

护士：每次透析过程中你都要丢失一部分蛋白质，因此要注意补充优质高蛋白饮食，如牛奶、鸡蛋、瘦肉等，还要补充维生素。水分一般不必限制，因此饮食不再像以前一样受到限制，但要注意卫生，避免腹腔感染。如果洗澡的话，要将腹腔管保护好，可用 3M 肤贴或造口护理袋，一般可淋浴，禁止盆浴。

# 53. Gastric Cancer

# 胃癌

Nurse: Madam Chen, today is our party's as well as your birthday. It is also the day you will challenge the death for the third without showing fear on your face. Our nursing department has brought you a bouquet of flowers to wish you a happy birthday and a successful operation. It is almost the time to wheel you to the operating room. Hope you will not be worried or get nervous.

护士：陈夫人，今天是党的生日，也是你的出生日，又是你不畏困难、不怕死神，第三次与病魔做斗争的日子。我们护理部给你送来一束鲜花，祝你生日快乐，手术顺利。马上到时间了，我们送你到手术室，希望你不要担心，不要紧张。

Patient: Thank you for your concern and emotional support. I am neither worried nor nervous. I will calmly face the third operation. I have great confidence in your professionalism and skills. It is nurses and doctors who supported and helped me successfully went through three of my life and death difficult time.

病人：谢谢你们的关心及对我精神上的支持，我不担心，也不紧张。我会坦然对待这第三次手术的。我对医护人员的敬业精神及技术水平非常信任。这辈子三次的生死抉择，都是护士与医生们的帮助支持使我顺利渡过难关。

Nurse: What a great lady you are! You are still so strong and open mind, and optimistic at your age. You have taught us a good lesson and set an excellent example for our students. In case there might be some pessimistic patients in the future, we will tell them about you, and I'm sure they will be greatly inspired and encouraged to fight their illness.

护士：你真不简单！这年龄你还那么坚强、乐观、开朗。你的言行直接教育了我们，也是我们学习的好榜样。今后遇到有悲观苦恼的病人时，我们一定会把你的经历介绍给他们。我想他们一定会深受启发，增强战胜疾病的信心的。

Student Nurse: Madam Chen, we sincerely admire your courage and adamant. Here is a birthday present for you (gave her a little picture frame). We will bring you back to the ward (recovering room) after the operation. And we will do whatever we can for you in the postoperative care.

实习护士：陈奶奶，我们佩服你的勇气和坚强。这是给你的生日礼物（递上一个小镜框)。等你手术结束,我们会来接你回病室(监护室)。手术后的一切护理工作我们都承包了。

Patient: What a nice group children you are. Thank you all so much for your self-made picture frame. "Wish you a happy birthday, a speedy recovery and a forever smile!" Your blessing will be with me all my life. It has already placed deeply in my heart.

病人: 好孩子,你们太费心了,谢谢你们自制的小镜框。"生日快乐、早日健康、笑口常开"这一祝福将永远陪伴我,它已深深刻在我的脑海中。

# 54. Rectal Cancer

# 直肠癌

Nurse： Mrs. Zhang，the doctor has decided to perform the"Mile's"operation after considering your husband's whole body conditions. Do you know the process of the operation?

护士： 张女士，医生考虑你丈夫的全身状况，决定采用麦氏手术，你了解这个手术吗？

Patient's Wife： Only a little. That is to make an artificial anus in his abdomen，right?

病人妻： 知道一些，就是在肚皮上再造一个肛门，是吗？

Nurse： Yes，the cancer invaded rectum will be excised along with his anus，and will construct an anus like opening on his abdomen wall. This operation is pretty safe.

护士： 是的，将有肿瘤侵犯的直肠部分连同原来的肛门一同切除，在腹壁上再造一个肛门。这种手术挺安全的。

Patient's Wife： Then，the stools will come out of his abdomen all the time and the smell will be terrible. This will affect him，his family members and everyone else around him. I'm afraid he can't accept that.

病人妻： 那样，粪便每时每刻都会从肚皮上流出，气味一定很重，对他个人、家人、周围人都会有影响，我担心他会受不了的。

Nurse： Your understanding and support is the most important thing. Please tell me，if we have the methods to eliminate the odor，would you agree to let him accept the operation and do your best to help him go through the most difficult care period after the operation?

护士： 现在，最需要的是你的理解和支持。首先，你告诉我，如果有办法消除气味等其他影响，你会同意让他接受这样的手术，并全力以赴地帮他度过术后最困难的照顾时期吗？

Patient's Wife： I think I will. What I'm most concerned about is his life. I hope he can live long and well. We love each other very much.

病人妻： 我想我会的。因为我最担心的是他的生命。我希望他能好好地活着，我们很相爱。

Nurse： It looks like that your husband's worry is not necessary. However，we must face the reality. As a nurse in charge，I must teach you how to help your husband to take care of his"artificial anus"and allow him to live the same as before. To have a quality life is the best thing your husband would want.

护士：好的，看来你丈夫是多虑了。但我们还应正视现实，作为床位护士，我必须教会你如何帮助你丈夫护理好"人造肛门"，让他基本活得和以前一样。良好的生存质量才是你丈夫最需要的。

Patient's Wife：Thank you. I will help my husband to take good care of the artificial anus after operation according to what you have told me. Thank you very much.

病人妻：谢谢你，护士小姐，手术后我一定会按你教的方法帮助他护理人造肛门的。谢谢你。

# 55. Counseling (Breast Surgery)

# 担忧疏导(乳房术)

## (1)

Patient: Is the surgery very painful?

病人：手术会很疼吗？

Nurse: No, not during the surgery. But there will be a little pain during the local anesthesia which is less painful than the skin allergy test.

护士：手术时不会疼，但打麻药时有一点点疼，比做药敏试验好一点。

Patient: How long will the effects of the anesthesia last? Will I feel pain after the anesthesia wears out?

病人：麻药的作用能维持多长时间？麻药过后会疼吗？

Nurse: Generally, the anesthetic will last for two hours. If you feel pain during the operation, the anesthetist can give you more anesthetic anytime. And if you feel pain after surgery, your doctor can prescribe pain medication for you. The time interval between the two pain medications is six hours.

护士：一般麻药作用完全消失需两小时。手术中如果你感到疼痛，麻醉师可随时适当添加麻药。术后如果疼痛得厉害的话，可根据医嘱服用止疼片。第二次服用止疼片应与前一次间隔 6 小时。

Patient: Will this surgery affect my breastfeeding in the future?

病人：这手术会影响我将来喂奶吗？

Nurse: Don't worry. In general, it should not.

护士：放心好了，一般不会有什么影响的。

Patient: Is my fibroid tumor benign or malignant?

病人：我的纤维瘤是良性的还是恶性的？

Nurse: The mastofibroma is usually a benign tumor. A routine pathological examination will be done on the removed tumor, and report will be available in three business days. You can pick up the report from the outpatient surgery clinic at that time. Do not hesitate to contact the doctor immediately if there is any problem.

护士：乳房纤维瘤一般为良性肿瘤。取出来的肿块我们将按常规进行病理检查，报告将在三个工作日后发出。到时你可以到外科门诊的候诊室取报告，有什么问题及时和医生取得联系。

Patient: Is the doctor who will operate on me male or female?

病人：为我手术的医生是男还是女？

Nurse: It's a male doctor. But do not worry, we will be at your side during the surgery.

护士：为你手术的是男医生。没关系的，不用害羞，手术时我们会一直陪在你身边。

Patient: Will the tumor recur after surgery?

病人：手术后我还会再生这样的瘤吗？

Nurse: Usually it will not. The tumor is related to your body hormone level. You should eat less food such as chicken, which may contain artificial hormones.

护士：一般不会，因为这与你体内的激素水平有关。你平时应少吃鸡肉等含有激素的食物。

(After the surgery)

（手术结束后）

Nurse: Please come back to the outpatient clinic three days after discharge. The doctor will examine your incision wound. Generally, the stitches will be removed on the seventh day. What will happen and how to deal with the problems you may encounter after the surgery are all listed in the instructions we gave you. Please read them after going back home and contact us at any time if you have any problems. We wish you stay in good health.

护士：请你三天后来门诊让医生替你检查伤口的情况。一般七天拆线，术后可出现的问题及怎么处理，在我刚才给你的健康处方上都有介绍，你回去看看。如有问题，可随时电话联系。祝你健康！

**(2)**

Nurse: Ms. Zhao, you have no appetite these days. It's time to have lunch. Let me give you a pill to stimulate your appetite (helped her take the pill). You'll have an operation in a few days. You should eat more nutritious food.

护士：赵太太，这几天你胃口不好，快开饭了，我给你服些开胃药吧（帮助服药）。过几天你要手术了，要多吃些有营养的食品才是啊。

Patient: I'm afraid of the operation. Look at Ms. Sun at the next bed. Half of her body is bandaged after the operation. It must be very painful and I don't know if her operation is a success.

病人：我害怕极了。看到隔壁这位孙女士手术后，半个身体都被包扎起来了。开刀时一定很痛，也不知效果怎么样！

Nurse: Ms. Zhao, breast tumor is a common disease. It is the second most frequent tumor among women. But if diagnosed and treat early, it has the best prognosis and highest survival rate of all cancers. There will be some pain after the operation. But it will be temporary and can be eased with medication. The most important thing is a successful recovery.

护士：赵太太，乳房肿瘤是一种常见病、多发病，居女性肿瘤疾病的第二位。但只要早期诊断，早期治疗，是肿瘤疾病中预后最好、生存率最高的一种病。手术后会有些疼痛，但这是暂时的，也是有办法解决的。康复才是最为重要的。

Patient: Ms. Zhu over there is going to be discharged from the hospital soon. But she still can't raise her arms. What will happen to her?

病人：对面朱太太手术后都快出院了，可她的手臂还不能抬起来，今后怎么办呢？

Nurse: Here comes your lunch. It looks delicious. You should try to eat all the food and then take a rest after the lunch. I'll come back to teach you how to exercise your arms after the operation. Ms. Zhu will continue her exercises for a few months after she leaves the hospital and her hands will gradually be able to move.

护士：饭菜来了，今天的菜多香啊！你一定要把这些饭菜都吃完啊。饭后休息一会儿，然后我来教你手术后功能恢复的锻炼方法。朱太太出院后，经过几个月的功能锻炼后，她的手也会逐渐抬起来的。

Patient: And...(wishing to ask again).

病人：还有……(想再问问题)。

Nurse: I see. You're afraid that the change of your body will affect your beauty.

护士：我知道了，你是怕手术后由于体态的改变，会影响了你美丽的形象。

Patient: Yes.

病人：是的。

Nurse: Don't worry. The achievements of medical technology research have been applied extensively in the clinic. After you recover from the operation, we can arrange to place an artificial breast for you. The procedure can be done safely and reliably, and the artificial breast will be light, durable, very convincing, and looks real. It will help you keep your original figure. Please eat your lunch now.

护士：这你放心。当代医学工程的成果已在临床上广泛应用。待你康复后，我们可以为你联系安装安全、可靠、轻便、耐用、仿真度高的人工乳房，一定会有助于你保持原有的好体型。快吃饭吧。

Patient: Now I'm not as afraid as before for my surgery. I'll try to eat more. However, if the tumor is malignant, what should I do after the operation?

病人：现在我不太害怕了，我会试着多吃一些的。我要真患的是恶性肿瘤，手术后该怎么办呢？

Nurse: The nature of the tumor will be determined by the pathologist. Please trust our hospital and the doctors. We'll arrange a good plan for you. Your task is to take good care of yourself so that your body is in good condition. Do all you can to make the operation a successful one. Your lunch is getting cold, eat your lunch now. After you've had a rest, I'll chat with you again and tell you what you should do before and after the operation.

护士：肿瘤的性质一般要等病理检查以后才能真正确定。请你相信我们的医院和医生，一切会为你进行周密安排的。你目前的任务就是安心把身体调养到最佳状态，争取手术成功。饭凉了，快吃吧，午休后我再来同你聊聊，告诉你手术前后需要做的事情。

# 56. Mastocarcinoma

# 乳房癌

Patient: Miss Li, I am frightened and don't know how to face this reality. My life will be over if the breast with cancer is not removed as early as possible. If it is excised, on the other hand, how can I live a normal life? How will my husband and my staff look at this situation? It's so cruel.

病人：小李，我很害怕，不知该如何面对这样的事实。如果不尽快地切掉乳房，（癌细胞浸润后）将危及生命，如果切了，那么将如何过正常人的生活，我爱人和同事又将如何接受这一现实，真是太残酷了。

Nurse: Yes, fate often makes fun of people. But it is much easier to overcome the difficulties of losing a breast when compared with the loss of life. The most important thing for you is to live. There will not be much difference on life after the operation. I think you know better than I do about this.

护士：是的，命运常常会捉弄人。可是，比起失去生命，切除乳房后所带来的一切困难要容易克服得多。现在最重要的是要安全地活着。手术对生命几乎没有多大影响，我想，这点你比我更清楚。

Patient: Yes, it is certain that I'll have the operation. I just don't know how to face the fact that I will no longer have a"whole body"after the operation.

病人：是的，接受手术是肯定的。但一想到手术后将要面对不健全的躯体，简直不知所措。

Nurse: I have talked with your husband and he is fully consent to the operation. He hopes that you could live with him the rest of your lives in health. I have also told him about the reality of breast excision and he has indicated that he could face this reality and has prepared in his mind.

护士：我与你爱人谈过了，他完全同意做乳房手术，他希望你能健康地和他共度一生。关于切除乳房的现实我也向他描述过了，他完全能正确地看待这一现实，并做了充分的思想准备。

Patient: really? Thank you very much indeed. I'll receive the operation soon. Could you do something for me?

病人：是吗？真是太谢谢你了。很快我就要做手术了，你能替我办件事吗？

Nurse: Sure. It will be my pleasure.

护士：没问题，你尽管吩咐。

Patient：Please try to buy a padded bra for me. I hope to wear it soon after the operation.

病人：替我想办法买一只假乳罩，好吗？我希望手术后就能戴上。

Nurse：Yes，I will do it and try to let you wear it after your stitches are removed.

护士：好的，我一定尽力去办，争取等你拆线后给你戴。

# 57. Metrectomy

# 子宫切除术

Nurse: Ms. Ge, you will have the operation tomorrow. Now let me do some preoperative preparations for you, OK?

护士：葛女士，你明天要手术，现在我要为你进行一些手术前的准备工作，好吗？

Patient: (showed no expression) Go ahead.

病人：(有气无力地、面无表情地说) 做吧。

Nurse: (Look at her and said with a smile) Are you worrying about tomorrow's operation?

护士：(看了看他的表情，微笑着说) 你是不是为明天的手术担心呢？

Patieent: No, I'm not worried. There are so many myomas in my uterus, the operation is inevitable. Also, I'll have no more menstruation after the operation and my anemia would be corrected.

病人：不，不担心。没什么好担心的。我的子宫上长了这么多的肌瘤，手术是免不了的。而且手术后，就没有月经了，我的贫血就可以改善了。

Nurse: Then you must be worried about how the operation will affect your health and living, right? In fact, uterus is one of the female's most important reproductive organs because it is the cradle of the baby. But you already have a school-aged daughter. You don't have to have another child any more. So, to have it isn't that important to you now.

护士：那你是担心手术后会对你的身体及日后的生活带来什么影响吧？当然，子宫是女性的重要生殖器官之一，因为它是孕育下一代的摇篮。而你已经有了一个女儿，已经上学了，不需要再生育了。所以它存在的意义对你来说已经不那么重要了。

Patient: A woman without uterus isn't a "whole" woman, right?

病人：子宫切除了不就是个不完整的女人了吗？

Nurse: No, what maintains a female character is the female hormone that is secreted from the ovary. Menstruation is uterus endometrium peeling off because of ovarian cycle secretion of estradiol and progesterone. You will only have no menstruation after the removal of your uterus. Nothing else including your sex life will be affected. On the other hand; your anemia will be corrected gradually just as you have said.

护士：不是的，维持女性特征的是女性激素，而女性激素是由卵巢分泌的。月经是由卵巢周期性分泌雌激素和黄体酮激素而引起的子宫内膜的周期性剥落。你子宫切除了，只是没月经，其他不会影响，甚至不会影响你的夫妻生活。相反，正如你说的，你的贫血会慢慢得到改善的。

Patient: Really? I would be affected if one of my ovaries is removed, right?

病人：真的吗？那如果我的一个卵巢也切除了，不就有影响了吗？

Nurse: Even if there is only one or half an ovary, it won't affect the female hormone secretion, because hormone is secreted from the cortex of ovary. Its function of secretion will not change even if only partial cortex exists. If a woman loses both ovaries, she can take estrogen under the instruction of doctors to keep the normal physiological function. My mother had the same operation ten years ago and she is still very healthy today.

护士：即使只剩下一个卵巢，甚至半个卵巢，女性激素的分泌也不会受影响。因为分泌激素的是卵巢的皮质，只要存在部分皮质，它的分泌功能就不会改变。甚至有的病人两个卵巢都切除了，也可以在医生的指导下服用一些雌性激素来保持女性正常的生理功能。我的妈妈在十年前也做了同样的手术，现在很健康。

Patient: Oh, I see. I don't worry any more. OK, please do the preoperative preparations for me.

病人：哦，我现在明白了，不用再担心什么了。来，帮我做准备吧。

# 58. Ovarian Carcinoma

# 卵巢癌

Nurse： Ms. Zhu，what is wrong? Are you OK?

护士： 朱女士，你哪儿不舒服？

Patient： I don't feel well at all. Please take off the tubes.

病人： 我全身都不舒服，帮我把管子都拔掉吧。

Nurse： Your tubes are good. No problem. Today is the first day after your surgery. You may feel abdominal distension，middle back pain and so on. But these can be decreased by change your position. Let me help you.

护士： 你的管子很好，没什么问题。今天是术后的第一天。你可能有腹胀、腰痛等不舒服，但这些通过改变卧位是能够缓解的。来，我协助你翻身。

（The patient is not very cooperative.）

（病人不太配合。）

Patient： Don't give me any more transfusion. It doesn't work.

病人： 不要给我输液了，输了也没用的。

Nurse： You have to have the transfusion because you can't eat anything now. The transfusion fluid contains antibiotics and supportive medications which will help you to recover.

护士： 输液是必要的，你现在不能吃东西，你所输的液体中有抗感染、支持性的药物，会使你的身体慢慢恢复的。

Patient： It isn't effective. I can't be cured. Let me go home.

病人： 恢复不了了，我的病是治不好的，让我回家吧。

Nurse： Why? You see the patients beside you are all recovering very well.

护士： 怎么治不好呢？你看，你边上的病人是不是一个个都恢复得很好。

Patient： It is different. I am different from them. I can't be cured.

病人： 不一样的，我和她们不一样。我的病是治不好的。

（The patient cried even more）

（病人哭得更厉害了）

Nurse： Ms. Zhu，even if you suffer from a bad illness，because medical science has progressed so fast，there are many treatment techniques such as chemotherapy which may be able to cure your illness. The most important thing is for you to have a sanguine mood. Ten years ago，I met a patient with the same illness as yours. She was treated by chemotherapy for six months after her surgery. She joined a Cancer Patient Health

Club at our medical college. Now she has sanguine mood and is doing very well. So, if you have the spirit like hers, and cooperate with us, I think you will recover well. Please try not to worry so much.

护士： 朱女士，即使真的得了什么不好的病，现在医学发展得这么快，对疾病的治疗方法有很多，如术后加化疗，你的病也能治好。重要的是你自己心情一定要开朗些。十年前，我碰到一位和你得同样疾病的病人，她手术后化疗了半年，后来参加了我们医学院的一个肿瘤患者康复俱乐部。心情特别开朗，现在身体仍然非常好。所以，你如果能和她一样开朗，再配合我们的治疗，我想你一定能恢复得很好。因此，你不能太心急。

Patient： I don't worry. But my daughter is still young. What should I do?

病人： 我不着急，可是我的女儿还小，以后怎么办呢？

Nurse： Yes. Your daughter is still young, and she is at school. For your daughter's sake, you should take good care of yourself and cooperate with us. Otherwise, when your daughter sees you in such a condition, she will be sad, right?（The patient cried less）

护士： 是的，你女儿还小，还在上学。为了女儿，你更要积极地配合我们，把身体养得好一点。不然，你的女儿来看你，看见你这个样子，也会难过的，你说是吗（病人的哭泣声小了）

Nurse： You are tired. Close you eyes and take a rest, I will come back to see you later.

护士： 你累了，眼睛闭起来，休息一会儿，我待会儿来看你。

# 59. Sterility

# 不孕症

Nurse: I believe that we all have the same objective which is to assist and cooperate with the doctor to treat Mrs. Yang's pelvic inflammation so that she may become pregnant soon.

护士：我们三个人坐在一起谈话的目的是一致的，就是帮助和配合医生治好病人的盆腔炎症，尽快怀孕。

Patient's Husband: Yes, I think so.（The mother-in-law nodded too.）

病人丈夫：是的，我也这么想。（婆婆同时点点头）

Nurse: You may not fully understand the reasons of not been able to pregnant. In addition to the pelvic inflammation, the major reasons for her not becoming pregnant, are possibly related to mental stress and nervousness. Nervousness can mess up her endocrin system and secretion of female hormones which might suppress the ovulation. What we must do now is to give the patient more care, love and support, and don't keep mentioning about pregnancy. Let's create a relaxed atmosphere for her and at the time let her receive medical treatment. I should say that the pelvic inflammation is curable if we cooperate with the doctor.

护士：对不孕的原因你们二位可能还缺乏认识。现在对病人来说，除了盆腔自身的炎症外，心里紧张和压力也是主要原因，因为任何紧张都可使病人内分泌系统紊乱，女性激素分泌失调，排卵受抑等。所以我们目前需要共同努力的是：多给病人关心爱护和支持，尽可能不提生育之事，让她以完全放松的状态接受药物治疗。盆腔炎不是难治之症，只要好好与医生合作，会治愈的。

Patient's Mother-in-law: Really? How long will it take?

病人婆婆：是吗？那么需要多长时间？

Nurse: No more than three months. If her disease is chronic, and has adhesion, then physiotherapy may be needed for some time after her discharge.

护士：最长三个月。如果是慢性、有粘连的，出院后还要坚持一段时间的理疗。

Patient's Husband: Does physiotherapy has any side effects on pregnancy?

病人丈夫：做理疗对怀孕有副作用吗？

Nurse: Generally speaking, there is no side effect.

护士：一般没有。

Patient's Mother-in-law: Well, from now on, my son and I will not say a word about child-bearing any more. We will help her to receive the treatment with all our hearts.

病人婆婆：好的，从现在起，我和儿子都不再提生育的事，一心一意为她治病。

Patient's Husband: Yes. We'll do our best to reduce her pressure. Thank you, nurse.

病人丈夫：是的，我们会极力帮助她减轻压力的，谢谢你，护士。

# 60. Abortion

# 流产

Patient: I have had some vaginal bleeding for 2 days, together with some pain in the lower abdomen.

病人：我这两天阴道出血并伴着下腹痛。

Nurse: How much did you bleed? When was you last period?

护士：出血多吗？末次月经是什么时候？

Patient: I missed 2 periods. The last one was on May 7.

病人：我已经两个月没来月经了，末次是5月7号。

Nurse: Is your menstruation regular?

护士：您的月经周期准吗？

Patient: It's normal now, but it used to be somewhat late before I was married.

病人：结婚前经常迟来，现在准了。

Nurse: Can you give us some urine for pregnancy test?

护士：您能留点尿液做妊娠试验吗？

Patient: I'll try.

病人：我试试看。

Nurse: The pregnancy test was positive. Where does it hurt and what kind of pain is it?

护士：妊娠测试阳性。什么地方痛？怎样的痛法？

Patient: The pain occurs in the central part of the lower abdomen. It comes in attacks accompanied with vaginal bleeding during the pain.

病人：在下腹正中，一阵阵的痛，痛的时候伴有阴道出血。

Nurse: It seems that you are pregnant, with a threatening miscarriage. You should stay in bed except for eating or going to the toilet.

护士：看来您是怀孕了，有流产先兆。除了吃饭和去厕所，您应当卧床休息。

Patient: OK, I'll do as you said.

病人：好的，我按您说的做。

Nurse: You should go to the emergency room immediately if the bleeding becomes more severe than usual. Come back in a week for a checkup.

护士：如果出血比平时多，您要立刻来看急诊。一周后再来检查。

（Three days later）

（三天后）

Nurse: How are you now?

护士: 您现在感觉是怎么样？

Patient: Not so good. The bleeding is more severe than usual and the attacks of pain reoccur every five to ten minutes.

病人: 不太好，出血增多了。而且有阵发性腹痛，每 5～10 分钟来一次。

Nurse: Let me take a look. Oh, the cervix is already open about four centimeters, And part of the fetus can be seen in the cervix. The fetus will come out soon. I'll prepare the blood for you in case a transfusion is needed. You should be admitted to the hospital immediately.

护士: 让我检查一下。啊！子宫颈口已经开了 4 cm，宫口能看见胚胎，要流产了。我去为您准备血液以备输血，您需要马上住院。

# 61. Instructions for a Woman in Labor

# 产妇指导

Nurse: Hi! Do you need any help?

护士：你好！你有什么需要协助的吗？

Patient: Yes. My last name is Wang.

病人：是的。我姓王。

Nurse: Very nice to meet you. I am nurse Li. You can call me Xiao Li. Do you have any discomfort?

护士：很高兴见到你。我是李护士，你可以叫我小李。你有什么不舒服吗？

Patient: I am 39 weeks pregnant and feel a little distention pain in the lower abdomen today. I thought it may be time to give birth, so I came to the hospital to have it checked out. The doctor at the prenatal clinic suggested hospitalization, that's why I'm here.

病人：我怀孕已经 39 周，今天感到下腹有点胀痛，我想可能要生了，就来医院检查。围产期检查室的医生建议我住院，我就来了。

Nurse: Oh, don't be nervous. I will take you to the delivery room to meet the midwife and have some obstetric examinations.

护士：噢，别着急，我先带你到产房与助产士见面，并且做一些产科方面的检查。

Patient: Good, thank you.

病人：谢谢。

(After introducing Mrs. Wang to the midwife, nurse Li left temporarily. Mrs. Wang had all the tests done. About forty minutes later, the midwife accompanied Mrs. Wang to the nurses' station of the ward. Nurse Li greeted them, and received Mrs. Wang's medical record and test results from the midwife and reviewed them quickly.)

（李护士把王女士介绍给助产士后，暂时离开。王女士在产房做各项检查，40 分钟后，助产士陪同王女士来到病房护士站。李护士边迎面打招呼边从助产士手中接过王女士的病历和检查单，并快速看了一下。）

Nurse: I can tell from your facial expression that the test results must be very good, right? The bed is ready for you. I'll accompany you over there.

护士：从你的面部表情看来，检查结果很不错，是吗？床位都给你准备好了，我陪你过去。

Patient: Great.

病人：太好了。

Nurse: This is your bed. Are you tired?

护士： 这是你的床位。你现在感到累吗？

Patient: A little.

病人： 有点累。

Nurse: Lie down and rest. I'll notify the nutrition department to prepare lunch for you. I will come back in ten minutes and provide the admission imtroduction and also obtain some information from you, OK?

护士： 那就先躺下休息一会儿，我去通知营养室帮你准备午餐。10分钟后我再来给你做入院介绍，并了解一些你的情况，你看如何？

Patient: Good. Nurse Li, the midwife told me to lie on my left side. Why?

病人： 好的，李护士，刚才助产士告诉我睡觉要采取左侧卧位，为什么？

Nurse: Oh, lying on the left side can increase the blood flow between the uterus and the placenta. This is good for the fetus.

护士： 噢，取左侧卧位可增加子宫、胎盘之间的血流，对胎儿较为有利。

Patient: I see. I'll lie on my left side for the sake of my baby.（Nurse Li helped the pregnant woman to lie down slowly, covered her with a quilt and left the room.）

病人： 原来如此，那我为了宝宝一定要坚持左侧卧位。（李护士协助产妇慢慢摆好了体位，盖上被子离开病房。）

（Nurse Li returned to the nurses'station and contacted the nutrition department for Mrs. Wang's lunch, read her medical history, the prenatal record, and the tests results. Then she prepared the guidelines for hospitalization, the introduction list, and expectant mothers'health care manual, and then went to Mrs. Wang's room.）

（李护士回到办公室与营养科联系好了王女士的午餐，翻阅了王女士的门诊病历、围产检查记录和刚才产房内做的检查结果，准备了住院须知、入院介绍单、孕妇保健手册来到王女士床旁。）

Nurse: Mrs.Wang, how do you feel after resting?

护士： 王女士，你休息了一会儿现在感觉怎么样？

Patient: Much better, thanks.

病人： 好多了。

Nurse: I would like to introduce the hospital regulations to you now, OK?

护士： 现在我给你介绍一下医院的规章制度，好吗？

Patient: Sure.

病人： 可以。

（Nurse Li gave Mrs. Wang the introduction one by one, regarding the hospitalization, the regulation for activities, resting, and visitation, the use of equipment in the ward, how to store personal belongings, the use of the signal system, and the doctors in charge of her bed, etc.）

（李护士把住院须知、作息、探访、规章制度、病室内设施的应用、物品的存放、信号系统的使用方法、床位医师等一一做了介绍。）

Nurse: Mrs. Wang, I gave you so much information. Can you remember them?

护士： 王女士，刚才给你介绍了这么多，能记住吗？

Patient: Yes, I can. Thank you very much for the detailed introduction.

病人： 记住了，非常感谢你为我做了如此详细的介绍。

Nurse: I will measure your blood pressure and temperature now. Did you drink any hot water?

护士: 接下来我想帮你量体温和血压。你喝过热水吗?

Patient: No.

病人: 没有。

Nurse: Good, let's begin.

护士: 好的,我们开始吧。

(Nurse Li took Mrs. Wang's body temperature, pulse, blood pressure, and told her that the results were all normal so she would not be worried.)

(李护士分别为王女士量了体温、脉搏、血压、告诉王女士测量的结果在正常范围,让她放心。)

Nurse: I'd also like to obtain some other information about you, OK?

护士: 我还想了解一下你的一般情况,行吗?

Patient: OK.

病人: 好的。

(During the conversation, nurse Li carried out the assessment by following the obstetrics assessment sheet that included life habits, health condition, appetite and sleeping pattern, menstruation history, and previous delivery history, etc.)

(在交谈的过程中,李护士针对产科护理评估单的内容,包括生活习惯、健康状况、食欲睡眠、大小便等情况以及月经史、孕产史等逐一进行了评估。)

Nurse: Mrs. Wang, I can see from the data that you are healthy and your status for giving birth is also good. I think that you can get through the birth smoothly. Since you are having some abdominal distention pain, you are near the delivery time now. You need to stay in the hospital for observation. So don't go out by yourself, OK?

护士: 王女士,从我了解的资料中看出你身体很健康,分娩条件也较好,我想你一定能顺利度过分娩期的。目前你已经临近预产期,而且还有些下腹胀痛的感觉,需要住院观察,不要随便外出,好吗?

Patient: OK. But I am very afraid of giving birth. Giving birth can be very painful, right?

病人: 好的,可我很害怕分娩这一刻的到来。分娩的时候会很疼吗?

Nurse: At the beginning, you will feel a little pain during uterus contractions and cervix dilation. The methods to cope with the pain are building up confidence during your delivery, listening to the midwife's guidance, and resting in between the contractions to maintain your strength. If you still can't tolerate the pain, we can give you anesthesia to ease the pain.

护士: 一开始,子宫收缩、子宫颈扩张的时候会感到疼一点。应对疼痛的方法是首先自己要树立分娩信心,听从助产士的指导,阵痛间隙要充分休息以保持体力。如果你还是不能忍受疼痛的话,我们医院有一种镇痛分娩的方法,可以减轻你的疼痛。

Patient: Is that so? Will the anesthesia have any adverse effects on my baby?

病人: 是吗?这种方法对宝宝会有影响吗?

Nurse: Our hospital does this a lot. Generally speaking, there are on adverse effects. In the process of anesthesia, the midwife will stay at your bedside and monitor you and the baby's conditions. If something abnormal happens, the doctor will take care of it right away.

护士：我们医院已经做过很多次，一般情况下是没有影响的。在镇痛分娩的过程中，助产士会一直守候在你的身边，用监护仪对母亲、胎儿的情况进行持续监护。如发现异常，医生会及时采取措施的。

Patient: Oh, when my husband comes here later, we will discuss the idea of using anesthesia.

病人：噢，那等我先生来了，我们可以商量一下考虑用镇痛分娩。

Nurse: Good. When you have made a decision, please tell me. I will help you contact the midwife. Mrs.Wang, you must have adequate rest, eat properly, be hygienic by keeping your vulva clean, change your underwear often, and note fetal movement. Do you know how to record fetal movement?

护士：好的，有决定了告诉我，我会帮你与助产士联系的。王女士，这几天你要多注意休息，加强营养，注意个人卫生，保持会阴清洁，勤换内裤，注意胎动变化。你会数胎动吗？

Patient: Yes, I do. Last time, at expectant mothers'training, Teacher Chen taught us the method: record fetal movement for an hour every morning, noon, and evening. Each time there must be no less than 3 fetal movements, thus reflecting the fetus is in good condition. Right?

病人：会的，上次在孕妇学校培训时，陈老师已教过数胎动的方法：每天早、中、晚各数一小时胎动，每小时胎动不低于 3 次，反映胎儿情况良好。我说得对吗？

Nurse: Right. You have to continue monitoring fetal movement while in the hospital. You should contact us right away if you feel your abdominal distension pain aggravate, see blood, or your water break, etc.

护士：非常正确。住院期间你要继续注意胎动。你如果感到下腹胀痛加重，或见红、破水等情况，应及时与我们联系。

Patient: Good. Thank you very much.

病人：好的。太感谢你了。

Nurse: What I just told you is in these 2 sheets of paper. If you forget, you can review them again. In the meantime, if you have any problem, you can call me with the signal beacon. I will come right away. Doctor Hu, who is responsible for your delivery, is operating on another pregnant woman now. When she finishes, I'll ask her to see you. Rest now. I will see you again shortly.

护士：我刚才给你说的事项在这两张单子上均有，如果你忘记的话，可以再看看。另外，你如果有什么问题可用信号灯找我，我会马上过来。负责你的胡医生正在为另一位产妇做手术。等她回来我会及时通知她来看你，你放心休息吧。我过一会儿再来看你。

Patient: Thanks for the introduction. I am not nervous anymore. Goodbye!

病人：多谢你的介绍，使我很放心。再见！

Nurse: Bye!

护士：再见！

# 62. Pregnancy Check

# 妊娠检查

Patient: I think I'm pregnant. Would you please give me an examination?

病人：我想我是怀孕了。您可以给我做个检查吗？

Nurse: Take off your shoes. I'll get your weight and height, and then take your blood pressure. When was your last menstruation?

护士：请脱掉鞋子，我们先给您称体重、量身高，再测量血压。您上次月经是什么时候来的？

Patient: It was on August 14, 2009.

病人：2009年8月14日。

Nurse: Are your menstrual cycles regular?

护士：月经周期正常吗？

Patient: Yes, they are.

病人：正常。

Nurse: Then your due date will be May 21, 2010. Have you had morning sickness?

护士：那么，您的预产期是2010年3月21日。您有早孕反应吗？

Patient: I have had a poor appetite, and have been vomiting after meals for more than one month.

病人：胃口不好，有一个多月了吃了饭就吐。

Nurse: Did you have any illness before pregnancy?

护士：怀孕前您得过什么病吗？

Patient: No. I was quiet healthy.

病人：没有，我很健康。

Nurse: What problems have you had during this pregnancy?

护士：这次怀孕过程中有什么不舒服吗？

Patient: I do have some pain in my legs, when I'm tried.

病人：累的时候有点腿痛。

Nurse: Have you had bleeding, watery discharge, or pain in your lower abdomen?

护士：有阴道出血、水样分泌物或下腹痛吗？

Patient: No, I never have such problems.

病人：没有，从来没有出现过这些问题。

Nurse: Did anyone in your family have multiple pregnancy, hypertension, tuberculosis, diabetes or hereditary diseases?

护士： 您家族中有人生过多胞胎吗？患过高血压、结核病、糖尿病或遗传病吗？

Patient： I was one of a pair of twins. My mother and younger sister died during the delivery because of profuse bleeding.

病人： 我是孪生姐妹之一，妈妈和妹妹在分娩中因出血很多死亡了。

Nurse： Let me give you a thorough examination.

护士： 我给您彻底检查一下。

Nurse： You have been pregnant for two months. The findings of the physical examination are all normal. Please come back in one month.

护士： 您怀孕两个月了，身体检查完全正常，请一个月后再来复查。

Patient： All right. Well，what shall I pay more attention to?

病人： 好的，那我应当注意些什么？

Nurse： You should take more nourishment such as eggs，vegetables，fruits，milk，meat，vitamins，iron and so on. You should avoid sexual life in the early three months and the last three months of your pregnancy.

护士： 您应当多吃一些营养品，如鸡蛋、蔬菜、水果、肉类、维生素，铁等。在怀孕的前 3 个月和后 3 个月应尽量避免性生活。

Patient： I think I will. Thank you.

病人： 我会的，谢谢。

# 63. Antenatal Examination

# 产前检查

Nurse：Mrs. White，in order to take good care of you，I need to get some information about your conditions for our nursing records. Would you mind if I ask you some questions?

护士：怀特太太，为了好好照顾你，我需要收集一些关于你情况的资料以便建立护理病历，你介意我问你一些问题吗？

Parturient：No，that's fine.

产妇：不介意，问吧。

Nurse：You are twenty-eight years old and you were hospitalized half an hour ago. Right?

护士：你 28 岁，半小时前入院的，对吗？

Parturient：That's right.

产妇：对。

Nurse：Your education?

护士：你的教育程度呢？

Parturient：I graduated from Tianjin University with a bachelor degree.

产妇：我是天津大学毕业，学士学位。

Nurse：What do you do? Do you have any poison exposure in your daily work?

护士：你做什么工作？日常工作中接触过有毒物质吗？

Parturient：I am a teacher. I never have poison contact.

产妇：我是教师，从来不接触毒物。

Nurse：Have you got any antenatal checks since you were pregnant?

护士：你怀孕以来做过产前检查吗？

Parturient：Yes，I have my antenatal check every month arranged by my obstetric doctor.

产妇：做过，每个月由产科医生安排我做产前检查。

Nurse：Is this your first pregnancy and first baby?

护士：这是你第一次怀孕、第一次生孩子吗？

Parturient：No，I have been pregnant three times since I got married. And I had a boy two years ago.

产妇：不是，我结婚后怀过三次孕，两年前我生了个儿子。

Nurse：When was your last menstrual period（LMP）?

护士：你的末次月经是什么时间？

Parturient: It was on January 7th.

产妇: 1月7日。

Nurse: So your estimated date of deliver (EDD) is on October 14th.

护士: 那么你的预产期是10月14日,是吧?

Parturient: Yes, it is.

产妇: 是的。

Nurse: Next I would like to give you physical and obstetric check-up. You are 165cm and 66kg. What is your blood group?

护士: 接下来我要给你做体检和产科检查。你身高165厘米,体重66公斤。你是什么血型?

Parturient: I was told it was "O" when I delivered my son two years ago.

产妇: 两年前我生儿子时被告知我是O型。

Nurse: Would you please lie down and pull your legs up towards you? I'm going to measure the fundal height and abdominal circumference.

护士: 请你躺下,把腿蜷曲起来好吗?我要量量你的宫底高度和腹围。

Parturient: Are you going to check the heart beat of the baby?

产妇: 你是要听胎心吗?

Nurse: Yes, I am. The heart is beating regularly and strongly. Have you had any pains in your belly before?

护士: 是的。胎心跳动规律有力。你之前有腹疼吗?

Parturient: Yes, they've been on and off during the past four days. They're mild and nor regular.

产妇: 是的,过去4天一直断断续续地腹疼,很轻而且不规则。

Nurse: Do you feel the contractions regular today?

护士: 今天你觉得宫缩规则吗?

Parturient: Yes, they have been regular since five o'clock this morning.

产妇: 从今天早上5点开始规则了。

Nurse: How long is the interval between two contractions? And how many minutes does it last?

护士: 两次宫缩间隔多长时间?宫缩持续几分钟?

Parturient: It is hard to say.

产妇: 说不准。

Nurse: Have you had any watery discharge?

护士: 有水流出来吗?

Parturient: No, I haven't noticed any.

产妇: 没有,我没看到。

Nurse: Why did you come to hospital today?

护士: 今天你为什么来医院呢?

Parturient: I noticed some bloody discharge this morning. But there are still more than nine days before my due date.

产妇：今天早晨我见红了。但距离预产期还有 9 天呢。

Nurse: And the time of your menarche?

护士：你的月经初潮是多大年龄？

Parturient: I got my menarche at the age of twelve.

产妇：我 12 岁初潮。

Nurse: How about the length of your menstrual cycle and length of period?

护士：你的月经周期和持续时间呢？

Parturient: My monthly period comes every twenty-eight days regularly and lasts five to six days.

产妇：我的例假每 28 天来一次，很规律，持续 5～6 天。

Nurse: When did you get married? Have you had any abortions before?

护士：你是什么时候结婚的？之前做过流产吗？

Parturient: I got married three years ago. I had an abortion one year after I bore my son.

产妇：我三年前结婚。我生儿子一年后做过一次流产。

Nurse: Did you deliver your son by caesarean section or episiotomy? Were there any difficulties in the delivery?

护士：你生儿子时做的是剖宫产术还是会阴切开术？分娩有困难吗？

Parturient: By episiotomy. The course of labour was quick，but I bled a lot soon after the baby was born.

产妇：会阴切开。分娩过程很快，但孩子刚出生后我出血很多。

Nurse: Did you receive a blood transfusion at that time?

护士：你当时输血了吗？

Parturient: Yes，they gave me 400 ml of fresh blood.

产妇：输了，他们给我输了 400 毫升鲜血。

Nurse: Do you know what the cause of the bleeding was?

护士：你知道出血的原因吗？

Parturient: I was told that the placenta remained in the uterus for more than thirty minutes.

产妇：我听说是因为胎盘滞留在子宫里超过 30 分钟。

Nurse: Did you suffer from such diseases as hypertension，diabetes or heart problem?

护士：你有过高血压、糖尿病或心脏病吗？

Parturient: Absolutely not. Actually，I have been in a quite good health so far.

产妇：绝对没有。其实我一直很健康。

Nurse: How about your parents?

护士：你的父母呢？

Parturient: My father died of lung cancer，my mother has diabetes.

产妇：我父亲因肺癌去世了，母亲患有糖尿病。

Nurse: Thank you for the information. Don't worry about the bloody discharge. You are now in the preliminary stage of labour. We will observe your conditions. I think labour will start later on.

护士：谢谢你提供的信息。不要顾虑这点出血。这是分娩前兆。我们会观察你的情况。我想不久就会开始临产的。

Parturient: I hope so.

产妇：但愿如此。

# 64. About to Give Birth

# 临产

Nurse: Good morning, Mrs. Byrd. I'm Zhao Jing, your nurse today.

护士：早上好，伯德太太。我叫赵静，今天是你的护士。

Primipara: Good morning.

产妇：早上好。

Nurse: Did you sleep well last night?

护士：昨夜睡得好吗？

Primipara: Not very well. After I was told that my baby would come soon, I was too excited to sleep. You know, this is my first baby.

产妇：睡得不太好。我听说孩子快生了，兴奋得睡不着。你知道吗，这是我的第一个孩子呢。

Nurse: I understand, Mrs. Byrd. Try to relax. You need a good sleep to reserve your energy for the delivery. How are you feeling now?

护士：我理解，伯德太太。尽量放松，你需要好的睡眠以便为分娩养精蓄锐。现在感觉怎么样？

Primipara: I think I'm starting to have labour pains.

产妇：我觉得开始阵痛了。

Nurse: The expected date of delivery is on November 15th, isn't it?

护士：预产期是 11 月 15 日，是吧？

Primipara: Yes, that's right.

产妇：是，对呀。

Nurse: How often do the pains come and how long do they last?

护士：阵痛多长时间一次，每次持续多长时间？

Primipara: About every fifteen minutes and for ten to fifteen seconds.

产妇：大约每 15 分钟一次，持续 10～15 秒钟。

Nurse: Have you got any bloody and watery discharge?

护士：有出血或水样物流出来吗？

Primipara: I've seen a little blood.

产妇：我看到一点点血。

Nurse: From now on you must time your contractions carefully. When they come every five or six minutes and last thirty to forty seconds, ring the bell and call us please.

护士：从现在起，你必须仔细地计算宫缩。当宫缩每 5～6 分钟一次、持续 30～40 秒时，请按铃叫我们。

Primipara：I will. Thank you.

产妇：我会的。谢谢。

※ ※ ※

Nurse：Mrs. Byrd. Have you just rung the bell? Can I help you with something?

护士：伯德太太，你刚才按铃了吗？我能帮你做什么？

Primipara：The cramps are coming more often and lasting longer. They come every five to six minutes now.

产妇：阵痛越来越频繁，持续时间更长了。现在每 5～6 分钟疼一次。

Nurse：Good. We are going to get you prepared for the delivery.

护士：好的。我们要做接生的准备了。

Primipara：What preparations do I need?

产妇：我需要什么准备？

Nurse：I'm going to shave off your public hair. Would you please lie down and open your legs?

护士：我要给你备皮。请你躺下分开双腿好吗？

Primipara：OK.

产妇：好的。

Nurse：If you feel uncomfortable or a cramp comes，please let me know.

护士：如果你感觉不舒服或者阵痛来了，请告诉我。

Primipara：I will.

产妇：我会的。

（Ten minutes later）

（10 分钟后）

Nurse：Mrs. Byrd，I have finished shaving. Let's go to the labour room.

护士：伯德太太，我备完皮了，我们去待产室吧。

Primipara：When will the baby come out?

产妇：孩子什么时候出生啊？

Nurse：It will come out soon. Don't be nervous. Everything will be fine.

护士：孩子很快就会出生的。别紧张。一切都会顺利的。

Primipara：I'll try to relax.

产妇：我会尽量放松。

（In the Labour Room）

（在待产室）

Nurse：Mrs. Byrd，if you feel a contraction coming，please tell me，so I can check the intensity and duration of contractions.

护士：伯德太太。如果你感觉阵痛来了，请告诉我，以便我查宫缩的强度和持续时间。

Primipara：All right.

产妇：好的

Nurse: I'm listening to the baby's heartbeat.

护士：我要听听胎心。

Primipara: How is it?

产妇：怎么样？

Nurse: It is regular and strong. Everything is fine.

护士：规律而有力。一切都很好。

Primipara: I asked the doctor to allow my husband to stay with me during my delivery.

产妇：我要求过医生让我丈夫在我分娩期间陪着我。

Nurse: I know. Your husband is waiting outside the room. I'm going to ask him to come in.

护士：我知道。你丈夫在外边等着呢，我去叫他进来。

Nurse: Mr. Byrd, you have to turn off your cell phone lest it should interfere with the electronic medical equipment.

护士：伯德先生，你得关闭手机以免干扰电子医疗仪器。

Husband: I will do it right away.

丈夫：我立刻就关。

Nurse: Hold your wife's hands and give her support. The delivery will consume a lot of her physical strength and energy. You can feed her some chocolate or water with brown sugar if she is hungry.

护士：握着你太太的手给她鼓劲。生产很消耗体力和精力。如果她饿了，可以喂她一些巧克力或红糖水。

Husband: I see.

丈夫：我明白 .

Nurse: Mrs. Byrd, the doctor has ordered to give you an intravenous drip with oxytocin in it. It will support your labour and the contractions will come more often and stronger.

护士：伯德太太，医生下医嘱给你静脉输催产素，这有助于你分娩，宫缩会来得更频繁更强。

Primipara: Does this mean the pains are getting worse?

产妇：这意思是说会疼得更厉害吗？

Nurse: Yes, but it will speed up the delivery and you will get out of the pains sooner. Now your progress is too slow. You only have a four centimeters dilatation.

护士：是的，但药物会加速分娩，你的疼痛会更快过去。现在你的产程太慢，宫口才开 4cm。

Primipara: Oh, I see. But how many more centimeters do I need?

产妇：噢，我懂了，但我还需要开几厘米呀？

Nurse: Another six centimeters. The baby can't be born until you dilate fully. The medicine will be with you till the placenta is expelled.

护士：再开 6cm，你的宫口开全孩子才能生出来。输液得持续到胎盘娩出。

Primipara: The ache is killing me!

产妇：疼死我了！

Nurse：I'll give you a massage to lessen the pain.

护士：我给你按摩减疼。

Primipara：Thank you.

产妇：谢谢。

Husband：I can do the massage for her if you teach me how to do it.

丈夫：如果你教我怎么做，我可以给她做按摩。

Nurse：Thank you for help.

护士：谢谢你帮忙。

# 65. Delivery

# 分娩

Doctor: Mrs. Byrd，it's time for you to go to the delivery room. Mr. Byrd，let's help her.

医生：伯德太太，你该去产房了。伯德先生，我们来扶她。

Husband: OK.

丈夫：好的。

Primipara: I feel so weak and dizzy.

产妇：我觉得身上没劲，头晕晕乎乎的。

Husband: Come on，sweetheart. We are going to see our baby soon.

丈夫：坚持住，亲爱的。快见到我们的孩子了。

Doctor: Just sit down on the bed.

医生：先坐在床上吧。

Primipara: Ouch!

产妇：哎呦！

Doctor: Is there a cramp coming? Let's wait until passes. Breathe in through your nose and exhale through your mouth slowly at the beginning and the end of each contraction. It can not only make you relaxed，but also provide oxygen to your baby. Are you feeling a bit better?

医生：有阵痛吧？等一下让它过去。在每次宫缩的开始和快结束时，用鼻子吸气，用嘴慢慢呼出。这样不但能让你放松，还能为孩子提供氧气。阵痛缓解了吗？

Primipara: I think so.

产妇：我想是吧。

Doctor: Lie down and move your buttocks towards the edge of the bed with your legs in the stirrups.

医生：你躺下，臀部移到床边，把腿放到脚蹬上。

Primipara: All right.

产妇：好的。

Doctor: When the next cramp comes，you can start to push down. Wait until you can't hold it any longer and then start to push down again，just like when you go to the toilet.

医生：阵痛再来时，你就向下使劲。等到憋不住了，就再向下使劲，就像上厕所那样。

Doctor: Mr. Byrd，when your wife pushes down，grasps her hands and let her feel your strength.

医生：伯德先生，你的太太向下使劲时，你紧握她的手，把你的力量传给她。

Husband: I will.

丈夫：我会的。

Primipara: There's another cramp coming.

产妇：又有阵痛来了。

Doctor: Take a deep breath and push! Push harder! Take another breath and push again! Once more! Is the pain gone?

医生：深呼吸然后使劲！再使点劲！再吸气，再使劲！再来一次！阵痛去了吗？

Primipara: Yes.

产妇：是的。

Doctor: Relax completely. Let's wait for the next one.

医生：彻底放松。让我们等下一次。

Primipara: Oh, here comes another one.

产妇：噢，又来了。

Doctor: Take a deep breath and push down! Come on! Well done. Oh, I see the baby's head.

医生：深呼吸，然后向下使劲！使劲！做得好。噢，我看到孩子的头了。

(The baby is born.)

（孩子出生了。）

Doctor: Congratulations, Mrs. And Mr. Byrd. It's a girl.

医生：恭喜啦，伯德太太，伯德先生，是个女孩。

Primipara: Let me have a look at her.

产妇：让我看看她。

※ ※ ※

Nurse: Good morning, Mrs. Byrd. Did you have a good sleep?

护士：早上好，伯德太太。睡得好吗？

Primipara: Yes, I did. Thank you.

产妇：是的，很好，谢谢。

Nurse: I'd like to check the fundus of your uterus to see how well it has been contracted. Is there much blood?

护士：我想查查你的宫底，看看子宫收缩得好不好。出血多吗？

Primipara: Not too much.

产妇：不太多。

Nurse: Could I have a look at your sanitary pad to see the lochia?

护士：能让我看一眼卫生护垫检查恶露的情况吗？

Primipara: OK.

产妇：好的。

Nurse: Do you know how to clean your perineal area in a right way?

护士：你知道怎么正确清洗阴部吗？

Primipara: I'm afraid not.

产妇：怕是不知道。

Nurse： Each time after you use the toilet，clean from the vaginal opening towards the anus，never do it in the opposite way.

护士： 每次去完厕所，从阴道口向肛门方向擦洗。不能朝反方向。

Primipara： I've got it.

产妇： 我懂了。

Nurse： Have you got milk yet?

护士： 你下奶了吗？

Primipara： Not yet. When will I be able to breast-feed my baby?

产妇： 还没有。我什么时候能给我的宝宝喂奶啊？

Nurse： Don't worry. Your milk will come in one or two days. Let the baby suck from time to time. It will help to bring in your milk.

护士： 别着急，一两天就会有奶的。让孩子多吸吮，这有助于你下奶。

Primipara： I see.

产妇： 我知道了。

Nurse： When you nurse your baby，tickle your baby's lower lip with your nipple. Make sure your baby's mouth is open widely and she takes in part of the darker area around the nipple. If you have any questions，please feel free to ask me.

护士： 你给孩子喂奶时，用乳头轻触开孩子的下唇。一定要把孩子的舌头放在乳头下面，让孩子含住部分乳晕。如果你有任何问题，请随时问我。

Primipara： I will. Thank you very much.

产妇： 我会的。非常感谢。

Nurse： You're welcome.

护士： 不客气。

# 66. Helping a New Father

# 帮助一位新父亲

Nurse: Congratulation! You have a beautiful baby.

护士：祝贺您，您有了一个漂亮的孩子。

New Father: Thank you very much.

新父亲：非常感谢。

Nurse: You look a little nervous. Is this the first time you have held a baby?

护士：您看起来有些紧张。这是您第一次抱孩子吗？

New Father: Yes. I had no experience with babies.

新父亲：是的，我从来没抱过孩子。

Nurse: Don't worry. You won't hurt her by holding her.

护士：您别着急。抱着孩子不会伤着她的。

New Father: She looks so small.

新父亲：她看起来太小了。

Nurse: Yes.The main thing you need to remember is to support her head with your hand. Her muscles are still weak.

护士：是的。重要的是您一定要记住用手托着孩子的头，她的肌肉还太软。

New Father: Can you show me how?

新父亲：您能为我示范一下吗？

Nurse: Sure. First, put a towel on your shoulder. You never know when she may spit. Don't leave anything in your shirt pocket that might hurt her.

护士：当然。首先，在您的肩上放一块毛巾，您不知道她何时会吐口水。不要在衬衫口袋里放任何东西，可能会伤着她。

New Father: Like this pen?

新父亲：像这支笔？

Nurse: Yes. Now, put the baby on your shoulder. Put one hand under her bottom and use the other to support her head. You can walk and talk to her now.

护士：是的。现在，将孩子放在您的肩上，一只手托住她的屁股，用另一只手托着她的头。您现在可以边走边跟她说话了。

New Father: This is good. Thank you.

新父亲：太好了，谢谢您。

Nurse: You'll feel more comfortable with time. She is a cute baby.

护士：您慢慢就会感觉舒服了。她真是个可爱的孩子。

# 67. Breast Feeding

# 母乳喂养

Patient: I am pregnant and will be a mother soon. Could you please tell me some of the advantages of breast feeding?

病人：我怀孕了，快要做妈妈啦。请问母乳喂养究竟有哪些好处？

Nurse: I am sure you would wish your baby to grow very well. The best natural nutrition for an infant is the mother's milk. Because it is not only economic, simple and with proper temperature, but can also increase the baby's immune function, add the baby's anti-disease capability, and promote the growth of the baby's brain cells. At the same time, it can also help your uterus recovery, reduce postpartum bleeding, and reduce the chances of breast and ovarian cancer, and promote bonding between you and your baby.

护士：你一定是希望你的宝宝生长发育得很好，婴儿最理想的天然营养品就是母乳。因为母乳既经济、方便又温度适宜，同时还能提高婴儿免疫功能、增强抗病能力、促进脑细胞发育。对你来说还可以促进子宫复原，减少产后出血，降低乳癌、卵巢癌的发病率，并且还可以增进母子感情。

Patient: With so many advantages, I have decided to breast feed my baby. But what is "pure breast feeding"?

病人：母乳喂养有这么多好处，我决定自己喂哺宝宝。但"纯母乳喂养"又是怎么一回事？

Nurse: Oh, "pure breast feeding" means you feed your baby with nothing but your own breast milk. No other liquid or solid food, nor other woman's breast milk.

护士：噢！所谓"纯母乳喂养"就是母亲用自己的奶喂自己的孩子，不给孩子吃任何其他的液体或固体食品，也不用其他母亲的奶喂自己的孩子。

Patient: When should the baby be fed with pure breast milk?

病人：什么时候应该用纯母乳喂养呢？

Nurse: In the first four to six months after birth when the baby needs the most nutrition for growth.

护士：在产后 4～6 个月内要求用纯母乳喂养，因为这个时期母乳最适合婴儿营养需要、并且能促进婴儿生长。

Patient: I have another question. Should the mother and her infant stay in the same room after birth?

病人： 我再问一下，是否产后都要母婴同室呢？

Nurse: Yes. The mother and her infant should stay in the same room twenty-four hours a day with no more than one hour of separation for medication or nursing of the infant.

护士： 是的。母婴同室就是指母亲、婴儿同住在一个房间内，24 小时都是这样。医疗或给孩子护理操作时，母婴分离不超过一小时。

Patient: Why? I want to know more.

病人： 为什么必须执行母婴同室呢？我想知道得更多一些。

Nurse: Because it will increase the mother's milk secretion，ensure enough milk for the infant，and to help promote mother-infant bonding.

护士： 这是为了能促进乳汁分泌，保证足够的乳汁，保证按需哺乳，还能增进母婴感情。

Patient: What is"early sucking"?

病人： "早吸吮"又是怎么一回事？

Nurse: "Early sucking"means mother-infant skin contact and assisted breast feeding within half an hour after birth. It should last no less than thirty minutes. However the breast feeding can only begin when the mother feels comfortable and the baby shows sign of sucking or mouth reflex movement.

护士： "早吸吮"是指产后半小时内母婴皮肤接触和协助哺乳，时间不得少于 30 分钟。但要母亲舒适，婴儿有准备，并且要在有吃奶表示时，开始喂奶，就是婴儿有觅食反射、吸吮动作等。

Patient: What is the benefit of"early sucking"?

病人： "早吸吮"对婴儿又有哪些好处呢？

Nurse: "Early sucking"can stimulate reflection and increase milk secretion. First milk can increase infant's anti-disease ability，promote peristalsis and removal of fetus stool，reduce infant jaundice，increase the mother's uterine contraction and prevent postpartum hemorrhage.

护士： 及时吸吮能刺激泌乳反射，增加乳汁分泌。尤其是初乳可以增加婴儿抗病能力，促进婴儿肠蠕动，早排胎粪，减少、减轻新生儿黄疸的发生，增加产妇子宫收缩，预防产后出血。

Patient: What is the purpose and meaning of "feeding as needed"?

病人： "按需哺乳"的目的、意义又是什么？

Nurse: "feeding as needed"is to feed the infant when needed without restriction on the frequency and has no fixed time. For example，when the mother feels breast distension，she can feed her infant.

护士： "按需哺乳"就是按照新生儿的需要哺乳，不限次数和时间。如果母亲感到奶胀不舒服，就可以让婴儿吃奶。

Patient: Should all mothers practice"feeding as needed"?

病人： 是否每个产妇都要实行按需哺乳？

Nurse: Yes. Because it can help the mother's milk secretion，help to promote bonding between the mother and her baby，and prevent the mother's breast distension. So why not do it?

护士： 是的。因为按需哺乳能促进乳汁分泌，保证足够的乳汁，增进母婴感情，预防母亲奶胀。那又何乐而不为呢？

Patient：I would like to know，what are the correct postures for breast feeding?

病人：我很想知道母亲正确的哺乳姿势有哪几种？

Nurse：There are three postures：sitting，lying（on back，on side）and holdings the baby.

护士：哺乳有三种体位，就是坐势、卧势（仰卧、侧卧）和环抱式。

Patient：How should the mother breast feed the baby?

病人：哺乳应怎样做呢？

Nurse：The best way is for the mother to sit down and be relaxed and put the baby's face close to her breast. Let the baby's nose next to her nipple，and their bodies form a straight line（chest to chest，belly to belly，chin to the breast），with mother's hand holding baby's buttocks.

护士：最好是母亲放松、舒适、婴儿身体贴近母亲，脸向着乳房，鼻子对着乳头，头与身体成一直线（胸贴胸、腹贴腹、下颏碰到乳房），母亲手托着婴儿臀部。

Patient：How should I let the baby suck the milk correctly?

病人：怎样让婴儿正确地吸吮奶水呢？

Nurse：You can touch the baby's upper lip with your nipple which will induce the baby's desire for feeding. Let the baby's mouth cover your nipple and most of your areola. Allow the baby to suck the milk slowly and deeply，pause from time to time and swallow the milk with action and sound.

护士：你可以用乳头轻轻碰碰婴儿的上嘴唇，诱发其觅食反射。婴儿张大嘴吸入乳头及大部分乳晕，慢而深地吸吮，有时会有暂停，能看见吞咽动作和听见吞咽声音。

Patient：How to hold my breast when feeding?

病人：在喂奶时怎么正确地托好乳房？

Nurse：Put your four fingers together on your chest just bellow the breast and let your forefinger on the bottom and your thumb on the upper part of your breast. The mother's hand should not too close to the nipple.

护士：你把食指到小指四指并拢贴在乳房下的胸壁上，用食指托乳房的底部，拇指放在乳房上方，母亲的手不应离乳头太近。

Patient：What is the proper way to squeeze the milk when I'm not at home or feel distention with milk?

病人：假如我有事外出或奶太胀时应该怎么挤奶？

Nurse：When squeeze your milk you should：First，Wash your hands clean.Second，You can sit or stand，be sure you feel comfortable，then place a container near your breast. Third，Place your thumb on the areola two centimeters above the nipple，and your forefinger on the areola opposite the thumb. Use your other fingers to hold your breast. Use the inner part of your forefinger and your thumb to press your sinus around the nipple gently toward the chest wall for three to five minutes to squeeze the milk out. Do not move the fingers on the skin.

护士：挤奶有几点要注意：①母亲的手必须彻底洗净。②坐立均可，要自己感到舒适，再将容器靠近乳房。③大拇指放在乳头根部上 2cm 的乳晕上，食指放在拇指对侧的乳晕上，其他手指托着乳房。用拇指与食指的内侧向胸壁方向轻轻压挤 3～5 分钟，将乳汁挤出。手指要固定，不要在皮肤上移动。

Patient: How do I know whether my milk is enough for my baby?

病人：我又怎么知道我的奶够不够孩子的需要？

Nurse: This is a good question. You need to know the following: First, Feed the baby at least 8 times a day.Second, Mother has the feeling of breast distention. Third, Hear swallowing sound while feeding.Forth, Change 6 or more diapers for baby every day. Fifth, Baby's weight increases averagely by 18 to 30 g per day or 125 to 210 g per week.Sixth, Baby is quiet between feedings.

护士：这个问题问得好。我告诉你以下 6 点你就知道了：①每天喂奶次数至少 8 次。②母亲有乳胀的感觉。③喂奶时听见吞咽声。④每天可换下婴儿 6 块或更多的湿尿布。⑤婴儿体重平均增加 18～30 克 / 日或 125～210 克 / 周。⑥两次喂奶期间婴儿安静。

Patient: I am afraid that I may not produce enough milk. How can I make sure I'll have enough milk for my baby?

病人：我担心乳汁不够，怎样可以保证有足够的母乳呢？

Nurse: Many young mothers have the same concern. Effective breast feeding needs early sucking, feeding when necessary, correct postures, mother's confidence, pleasant mood, sufficient nutrition and enough rest. Also, don't give the baby other food too early.

护士：这的确是母亲应该关心的问题。要做到充分有效的母乳喂养就要做到早吸吮，按需要哺乳，喂奶姿势正确，鼓励和支持母亲树立信心，保持愉快情绪，营养合理和休息，不给婴儿过早添加辅食。

Patient: What is the common reason for breast distention?

病人：假如乳房肿胀，最常见的原因是什么？

Nurse: The main reason for this is ineffective breast feeding (not feeding when needed) or incorrect posture.

护士：主要是生产后最初几天没有做到充分有效的母乳喂养（未按需哺乳）或姿势不正确。

Patient: What's the reason and how to deal with nipple pain?

病人：假如乳头疼痛，又是什么原因？应该怎样处理？

Nurse: It is because the baby doesn't hold the nipple and areola in the mouth correctly. To prevent nipple pain, you should make sure the baby is sucking the nipple correctly and you should also feed the baby more frequently. Every time when you finish feeding the baby, press a little milk outspread it on your nipple and areola, and wait until dry. Besides, you should wear loose cotton underwear and bra. Don't wash your nipple with alcohol or soap.

护士：乳头疼痛主要是婴儿含接姿势不正确，没有将乳头、乳晕放在婴儿的嘴里。处理的方法就是掌握正确的含接姿势，要将乳头及大部分乳晕含入婴儿口中。坚持频繁的哺乳，每次哺乳结束时，挤出少量乳汁涂在乳头和乳晕上，短暂暴露，使之干燥。此外还要穿戴棉质的、宽松的内衣及胸罩。母亲不要用酒精或肥皂擦洗乳头。

Patient: Could you tell me with what kind of diseases a mother can't breast feed?

病人：你能否告诉我，母亲患哪些疾病不能给孩子喂奶？

Nurse: A mother can't breast feed her baby if she has heart disease, kidney disease, mental illness, epilepsy, acute hepatitis with jaundice, or she is taking medicine such as radiation medicine or anti-hyperthyroidism.

护士：母亲如果患心脏病、肾脏病、精神病、癫痫、甲肝急性期伴有黄疸时，或母亲在使用哺乳期禁止使用的药物，如放射性药物、抗甲状腺药物时，是不宜给孩子喂奶的。

Patient: Thank you very much. I've learned a lot about breast feeding. It's very useful and will benefit both me and my baby. I'll follow your advice.

病人：谢谢你！今天我从你这儿学到很多哺乳方面的新知识，我一定要牢记，并且照做，因为这对孩子的生长和我们做母亲的都有益。

# 68. Vaccination

# 预防接种

Nurse： Good morning，Madam. What can I do for you?

护士： 早上好，女士。我能为您做点什么？

Mother A： Good morning，Miss. My son is more than three months old. I'd like to know what vaccinations he should have.

母亲甲： 早上好，小姐。我儿子三个多月了。我想了解他该接种什么疫苗？

Nurse： You can start him on DPT vaccine.

护士： 您可以开始给他注射白百破疫苗。

Mother A： What is it for?

母亲甲： 白百破是什么病？

Nurse： DPT stands for diphtheria，pertussis and tetanus. There are three shots altogether.

护士： 白百破就是白喉、百日咳和破伤风。这个疫苗共有三针。

Mother A： When should I bring him back for the second shot if he gets the first one today?

母亲甲： 如果今天给他打第一针，我什么时候带他来打第二针？

Nurse： One month from now on and the same interval for the third shot.

护士： 一个月后，第三针是同样的间隔。

Mother A： Will there be any reaction after the shot?

母亲甲： 打完针有什么反应吗？

Nurse： Some children have a slight fever one or two days after the injection.

护士： 有的孩子打针一两天后有点发烧。

Mother A： I see.

母亲甲： 我明白了。

Nurse： Has your son got polio vaccine yet?

护士： 您的儿子接种脊髓灰质炎疫苗了吗？

Mother A： I'm afraid not.

母亲甲： 恐怕没有。

Nurse： I'll give him the polio vaccine today. There are three types. This red sugar pill is type I.

护士： 今天我给他脊髓灰质炎疫苗。一共三型。这粒红色糖丸是I型。

Mother A： Can he have two vaccines at the same time?

母亲甲： 他能同时接种两种疫苗吗？

Nurse： No problem with DPT and polio vaccines.

护士： 白百破和脊髓灰质炎这两种同时接种没问题。

Mother A： When should I give the sugar pill to him?

母亲甲： 我什么时候给他吃糖丸呢？

Nurse： The pill does not keep at room temperature，so you must give it to him as soon as you get home. Don't let him take any warm water or food until one hour after taking the pill.

护士： 这糖丸不能在室温保存。所以您一到家就给他吃。吃后一小时不能喝热水和吃热东西。

Mother A： Will there be any reaction?

母亲甲： 有什么反应吗？

Nurse： No reaction in most cases. There's nothing to worry about. Come back one month from now on for the sugar pill types II and III.

护士： 大多数情况下没反应。不用担心。一个月后请来取II型和III型糖丸。

Mother A： I see.

母亲甲： 我知道了。

Nurse： Here is the vaccination schedule for babies. Please read it carefully. It lists the kinds of vaccinations your baby should have and the timings.

护士： 给您一份孩子预防接种时间表。请仔细阅读，上面列着您的宝宝需要接种的疫苗种类和时间安排。

Mother A： Thank you for your help.

母亲甲： 非常感谢您的帮助。

Nurse： It's my pleasure.

护士： 很高兴为您服务。

（Another mother comes in.）

（另一位母亲进来。）

Nurse： Good morning，Madam. Can I help you with something?

护士： 早上好，女士。要我帮您做什么吗？

Mother B： My daughter had three shots of DPT vaccine last year. Does she need this year?

母亲乙： 我女儿去年打过三针白百破疫苗。今年还用打吗？

Nurse： How old is she?

护士： 她多大了？

Mother B： One and a half years old.

母亲乙： 一岁半。

Nurse： Then she should have a booster one this year. One injection is enough.

护士： 那么她今年需要加强一次，只打一针就够了。

Mother B： Anything else?

母亲乙： 还有其他什么吗？

Nurse： She has to start on MMR vaccine—that is for measles，mumps and rubella. By the way，have you got the vaccination schedule?

护士： 她得开始接种麻风腮疫苗——就是预防麻疹、风疹和流行性腮腺炎的疫苗。顺便问问，您有接种疫苗时间表吗？

Mother B： Yes，I have. I just came to make sure. Thank you for the information.

母亲乙： 是的，我有。我只是来确定一下。谢谢您提供的信息。

Nurse： You're welcome

护士： 不客气。

（The third mother comes in.）

（第三位母亲进来。）

Nurse： Good morning. Can I help you?

护士： 早上好，女士。要我帮忙吗？

Mother C： Yes. My baby son was vaccinated against varicella seven days ago.Yesterday he began to run a fever and I saw some little red spots on his back，just like mosquito bites.

母亲丙： 是的，我的宝贝儿子一周前种了水痘疫苗。昨天开始发烧，而且我看到他的背上有些小红点，像蚊子咬的一样。

Nurse： Are they rashes or herpes?

护士： 是皮疹还是疱疹？

Mother C： They are rashes.

母亲丙： 是皮疹。

Nurse： He is having a reaction to the varicella vaccination. Don't worry. He will get better in about one or two weeks.

护士： 这是水痘疫苗的反应。别着急，一两周左右就能好。

Mother C： Can I bathe him now?

母亲丙： 现在我可以给他洗澡吗？

Nurse： You'd better not to do it until the rashes are gone.

护士： 最好等皮疹消退再给他洗澡。

Mother C： I've got it. Thanks a lot.

母亲丙： 我知道了。多谢。

Nurse： My pleasure.

护士： 很高兴为您服务。

# 69. A Child with Pneumonia

# 肺炎患儿

## (1)

Nurse： Mrs.Li，is your baby getting any better?

护士： 李太太，今天宝宝好一点了吗？

Child's Parent： No，she seems to be getting worse. She has had the intravenous transfusion for three to four days without any improvement.

患儿家长： 没好！反而更厉害了。输了三四天的液一点效果都没有。

Nurse： Is her coughing better?

护士： 咳嗽是不是感到轻松一点了。

Child's Parent： Yes.

患儿家长： 是的。

Nurse： Some baby patients have dry paroxysmal cough at the early stage of pneumonia. As time goes on，the disintegrated and dead bacteria and virus become sputum，which will stimulate the bronchi and result in paroxysmal cough and sputum. It is like a battle field where lays many dead enemy soldiers，sputum is the waste product that is being cleaned from the body's respiratory system. There is a disease development process. You should not worry too much. We are giving the baby a very effective treatment，but it takes time for the drugs to take effects. Let's try to be a little more patient，OK?

护士： 有的孩子肺炎初期只是阵发性干咳。但随着时间的推移，崩解的粒细胞及被杀死的细菌、病毒形成痰液，刺激支气管引起阵发性咳嗽、咳痰。就像战场上打仗，会留下许多敌人的尸体。其实痰液就是清理战场的产物，是疾病发展的自然过程。你不要太着急，我们正在积极治疗。药物发挥作用也要一段时间，再观察观察好吗？

Child's Parent： We are very worried for our only baby since she has been ill for more than ten days.

患儿家长： 都10多天了，现在就一个孩子，我们心里急啊。

Nurse： I can understand how you feel. However，your worries cannot solve any problems. Rather，it will affect your own immune system. You should take better care of yourself otherwise you'll get sick，which in turn will affect your baby's health. So you should get more rest and eat more nutritious foods to increase your resistance to diseases.

护士：我理解你的心情但着急解决不了问题，反而影响你自身的抵抗力。到时候不要孩子好了，你倒下了，反过来再传染给孩子，那就更不合算了。你也要注意多休息，多吃营养丰富的食物，以增强抵抗力。

Child's Parent：Then what should I pay attention to?

患儿家长：那我平时要注意些什么？

Nurse：At home you should open the windows often to keep the air fresh. When your baby coughs，pat her back softly to help her cough up the sputum. When patting，you should close your five fingers of your hand and pat on the baby's back with only the edge of the hand. Pat her softly and let the vibration from the patting to help the baby cough up her sputum（Demonstrated how to pat）.Since your baby is too young to spit，she can only swallow it. When you find some mucus in her stool，it's the sputum she had swallowed.

护士：平时你要注意保持室内空气新鲜，经常开窗通风。宝宝咳嗽的时候，及时拍背帮助她把痰液咳出来。拍背时注意五指并拢内屈，使手掌边缘同时接触孩子的背，引起振动，借振动作用帮助痰液排出（示范拍背的方法）。像你的孩子不会吐痰，一般都咽到肚子里去了，所以有时你会看到大便中有黏冻样的东西，那就是痰液。

Child's Parent：Oh，now I see. I thought it was the bad food she ate.

患儿家长：是啊，我还以为吃坏了呢。

Nurse：Sometimes because the sputum stimulates the gastrointestinal track or due to the virus's effect，some babies will have diarrhea. But you need not worry too much because not every baby has diarrhea. Since your baby has a fever，we'll take her temperature every four hours. Please call us to measure her temperature at any time if you feel she has a fever. If her temperature is too high，the doctor will give her an antipyretic drug. Please don't give her any medicine yourself. Feed your baby more water and change her clothes when she is perspiring too much. You may put a dry towel on her back to prevent her from catching cold. I will come around some time later. You may press the call button to call us if you need us.

护士：是的，有的孩子由于痰液刺激胃肠道或者是病毒本身的作用，有时还会拉肚子呢！不过你不要太紧张，并不是每一个孩子都会拉肚子。现在你的宝宝还有点发烧，我们会每 4 小时给她量一次体温。你如觉得宝宝身体烫，随时叫我们来量体温，假如体温过高，医生会让宝宝吃退烧药的，但你不要自己觉得她发烧了就随便给她吃药。平时多给宝宝喝点水，出汗多时要更换衣服，或在背上垫一块干的毛巾，防止着凉。我过一会儿再来看宝宝，你有事请按铃。

## （2）

Nurse：Hello，Mrs.Li，your baby has diarrhea. Please let me check his buttocks to see if it is red.

护士：李太太，你好。宝宝有点拉肚子，请让我看看他的屁股红不红。

Patient's Mother: You don't need to check. There is nothing wrong with his buttocks. But his pneumonia has become more serious. I wonder if the drug he took is adequate. You see，the baby is coughing and vomiting，having diarrhea，and has lost weight. If he was your baby，would you let him be like this?

患儿妈妈：不要看了，屁股没什么，倒是这肺炎，是不是用的药不对？怎么越来越重？你看宝宝，又咳又吐，还拉肚子，都瘦了！如果是你的孩子，能让他这样吗？

Nurse: Yes. I would be worried if my baby is sick like that.

护士：是的，如果我看到自己的孩子这样也会急的。

Patient's Mother: （Bursting into tears）Gosh. I am so worried about his disease.

患儿妈妈：（流泪）就是啊，我都担心死了。

Nurse: （Holding her shoulder）Mrs.Li，your baby's symptoms are common for the recovery period of pneumonia. You see，his temperature is lower than before，isn't it?

护士：（扶着她的肩膀）李太太，像你宝宝这情况是婴儿肺炎恢复期常见的症状。你看宝宝的烧，是不是退了？

Patient's Mother: （Became calmer）Yes，his temperature is lower. The doctor also said his lung was much better. But you see the baby still has vomiting and diarrhea.

患儿妈妈：（情绪稍平稳）体温倒是退了，医生也说肺好多了。但你看宝宝，又吐又拉。

Nurse: Yes，I know. I have seen these symptoms. You see what he is vomiting is white and sticky sputum. The baby's stomach and esophagus are different from adults. It can be stimulated to vomit easily. Most of his stools also contain sputum，which was swallowed by the baby. The sputum can stimulate the movement of the intestine. So the baby relieves the stool more times than usual.

护士：是的，这吐和拉我都看见了。你看宝宝吐的东西，白白黏黏的，这都是痰。小孩的胃、食管和大人不一样，容易受刺激呕吐。还有这拉肚子，你看，也是痰，这是小孩咽下去后拉出来的。而且痰咽到肚子里会刺激肠子动得快，所以宝宝大便次数也多了。

Patient's Mother: Then，it is good for him，isn't it?

患儿妈妈：那这是好事啦。

Nurse: Of course. The doctor has said that your baby can go home in a couple of days when the sputum production is reduced.

护士：是呀，医生说了，宝宝再住两天，痰少点就可以回家了。

Patient's Mother: （Wiped her tears）I see. I feel much better now. Thank you.

患儿妈妈：（擦干眼泪）是这样啊。那我就放心了，谢谢你。

Nurse: You are welcome. It is my job.

护士：不用谢。这是我的工作。

# 70. A Child with Asthmatic Pneumonia

# 喘息性肺炎患儿

Nurse： Hello，Mr.Wang，it's time to do the nebulization for your baby.

护士： 你好，王先生，现在要给你的宝宝做喷雾治疗了。

Patient's parent： No.

患儿家长： 不做！

Nurse： （Looked at the baby）what is the matter?

护士： （低头问）怎么啦？

Patient's parent： My baby will cry loudly as soon as he is given the nebulization. Since his hospitalization，he has been deviled. His head has been punctured with needles so many times; it looks like a beehive.

患儿家长： 一做喷雾治疗我的孩子就拼命哭。你看这孩子到医院给你们折腾的，这头上扎得像蜂窝似的。

Nurse： Sorry. We have the same feelings as you. We all love the baby and wish him cured sooner. Nebulization is the best way to treat asthmatic pneumonia and it can also prevent the disease from changing to asthma. How about if we do the nebulization when he is asleep? It's more effective when he is sleeping than when he is crying.

护士： 对不起，我们的感受和你是一样的。都希望孩子早点好。喷雾治疗是治疗喘息性肺炎最好的方法，还可以预防其转变为哮喘。要不等他睡着了再做？睡着了做效果比哭闹时好。

Patient's parent： OK. Go ahead to give him the fluid transfusion first.

患儿家长： 也好，先输上液再说。

（After beginning of the transfusion）

（输液开始后）

Patient's parent： Nurse，my baby has been crying non-stop since you gave him the transfusion. Are there any problems with the drug you are using? Have you made a mistake? I think he has got more diseases since he came to the hospital. You have given him the fluid transfusion for two days，yet he is still screaming severely.

患儿家长： 护士，输上液后我的孩子哭得没停过。是不是所输的液体有问题？你们有没有加错药？看病看病，越看越多，输了两天液，孩子还是哭得这么厉害。

(After examining the baby and the transfusion carefully.)
(护士仔细检查了输液及孩子的情况后。)

Nurse: The transfusion is OK. Maybe there are some other reasons for his crying.
护士: 输液不错，孩子哭可能有其他原因。

Patient's parent: I'm sure there are some problems with the fluid you use today. He did not cry when you gave him the transfusion yesterday. Why is he crying today?
患儿家长: 肯定今天输的液有问题，昨天输就不哭，怎么今天会哭呢？

Nurse: The drug we used has to be checked twice by two nurses. Let me ask a doctor to examine the baby.
护士: 输液中的药我们要两人核对后才能加进去。我去请医生来帮孩子检查一下吧。

Patient's parent: Hurry up! What are you waiting for? He is not your baby, so you just do not care about him. What kind of attitude is this?!
患儿家长: 快去，快去，还磨蹭什么？不是你的孩子不知道心疼。什么态度?!

Nurse: I'm sorry. The doctor is coming right away.
护士: 对不起，医生会马上来。

(After examination, the doctor believed the reason for the baby's irritation was wheezing.)
(医生检查过后，认为还是喘憋引起的烦躁。)

Nurse: The baby feels uncomfortable and is crying because of wheezing. Let's give him some calmative drug and provide the nebulization as soon as possible. He will feel much better after the nebulization. The drug he inhales can release the bronchus spasm.
护士: 孩子是因为喘了不舒服才哭的。给他用点睡觉的药，尽快将喷雾治疗做了就会好的。喷雾中有缓解气道痉挛的药。

Patient's parent: Is this drug toxic? Does it have any side effects for children? Is it addictive? Does he need to inhale the drug every time he coughs? My company is not doing well and my salary is not very good. The drug is too expensive for me.
患儿家长: 这个药有毒吗？对小孩的副作用大吗？吸了会上瘾吗？是不是每次咳嗽都需要吸药？我们单位效益不好，我挣钱也不多，这费用哪吃得消啊？

Nurse: This drug is not toxic and it isn't addictive. The side effect is also small. When your baby is discharged, all you need to do is to avoid its attack again.
护士: 这些药没有毒，无太大副作用，也不会上瘾。回去后做好预防工作，控制住不发作也就好了。

Patient's parent: When my child is sick, I don't know what to do. I wish it was me who is sick, not my baby.
患儿家长: 小孩一生病，我这心里就乱了，恨自己不能代替他。

Nurse: I understand. Now, your baby is sleeping. Let's give him the nebulization.
护士: 我能理解，孩子睡着了，给他做喷雾治疗吧。

# 71. A Child with Diarrhea

# 腹泻患儿

Nurse: Good morning, Ms.Zhang, does the baby defecate a bit less today?

护士：张太太，宝宝今天大便次数少一点了吗？

Patient's Mother: No, still a lot. Are the drugs you used for my child correct?

患儿妈妈：少什么少？还是这么多。你们给我家小孩用的药对不对？

Nurse: We are responsible for every patient. There are certain principles to the treatment of every disease. The dosage of the drug was calculated according to the baby's age and weight. Please do not worry.

护士：我们对每一位病人都是负责的。每种疾病的治疗都有一定的原则。药物的剂量是根据宝宝的年龄和体重计算的，请你放心！

Patient's Mother: How could I not worry! What I'm concerned about the most is that you might have delayed her treatment.

患儿妈妈：呵，我怎么能放得下心！我最不放心的就是怕你们把病给耽误了！

Nurse: I can understand how you feel. Please believe me for what I said to you was from my heart. People used to say"To recover from an illness is like reeling off raw silk from the cocoons."It will take certain process for the disease to become better. What your baby got is viral enteritis, and in general, a virus infected disease needs about one week or more to recover.

护士：我能理解你的心情，请相信我对你说的都是心里话。俗话说"病去如抽丝"，疾病好转都有一个过程。你宝宝得的是病毒性肠炎。一般来说，病毒感染的疾病要一周左右的时间，才会好转。

Patient's Mother: Look, the child has diarrhea again. Call the doctor quickly.(The baby is crying)

患儿妈妈：呦，你看，小孩又拉了，快去喊医生过来。(孩子哭)

Nurse: OK, don't worry. I will call the doctor right the way.

护士：好，你别急！我马上去喊医生。

(After examine the baby, the doctor thinks the water content in the stool has decreased, the illness has taken a favorable turn.)

(医生检查后，认为粪便中的水分减少了，病情有好转。)

Patient's Mother: You keep saying the illness is getting better. I know you do not care about my child.

患儿妈妈： 又说好！我就知道你们不心疼孩子。

Nurse： The doctors here are all very experienced. The doctor who exami-ned your child also tested the acid-base concentration of her excrement. The situation is really much better.

护士： 这里的医生都是很有经验的。刚才医生还用试剂测试了一下粪便的酸碱度，情况确实是好多了。

（The baby's mother prepared to change the diaper for the child.）

（家属准备给孩子换尿布）

Nurse： Ms. Zhang let me help you.

护士： 张太太，我来帮你。

（The nurse washed the buttock of the baby with warm water and put on a clean diaper.）

（护士用温水给孩子清洗臀部，换上干净的尿布。）

Nurse： Ms. Zhang，the baby's stool is much better. But she still should be fed with lactose free milk powder. It is easy to digest and is good for the intestines mucous membrane to repair. Also，your diet should also be light at the present time，so that there will be less fat in your breast milk. In addition，you should give more water to the baby to supplement the baby's water need.

护士： 张太太，宝宝的大便情况好多了。不过，还是要继续喂去乳糖奶粉。这样容易消化，有利于肠黏膜的修复。你最近阶段的饮食要清淡，这样奶水中的脂肪含量也能少一些。另外，你要给宝宝多喂水，补充宝宝所需的水分。

Patient's Mother： Your attitude is not too bad.

患儿妈妈： 你的态度还算是不错。

Nurse： Thank you. The baby is about to sleep. I will come to see her later.

护士： 谢谢，宝宝好像是要睡觉了，待会儿我再来看宝宝。

（Two hours later，the nurse came back a second time to her bedside.）

（两个小时后，护士第二次来到床边。）

Patient's Mother： Thank you very much. My baby has not had a bowel movement for two hours. I feel much better now.

患儿妈妈： 宝宝已经两个小时没拉了。我现在放心多了，谢谢。

# 72. A Child with Febrile Convulsion

# 高热惊厥患儿

Nurse： Mrs. Xu，your daughter has sleep for an hour after taking the sedative. Is she having any discomfort now?

护士： 徐太太，你的女儿用了镇静剂后睡了一个小时了。现在有没有不舒服的表现？

Patient's Mother： Discomfort? She must be in discomfort. When she was twitching a while ago，her eyes were rolled up and her four limbs were stiff. How could she be comfortable? Take my child's temperature again.

病儿妈妈： 不舒服？她肯定不舒服，刚才抽搐时两眼上翻，四肢僵硬，怎么会舒服呢？再给我孩子量量体温吧。

Nurse： Her body temperature is normal now. It was 37.2℃ when I took it five minutes ago. I will take her temperature again later.

护士： 她现在体温是正常的，我五分钟前给她量的体温是37.2℃。过一会我再给她量吧。

Patient's Mother： How come your attitude is so bad? You are unwilling to take her body temperature when I asked you to. Look at her，her face is all red. She must have a fever.

病儿妈妈： 你这个护士服务态度怎么这么差？叫你量个体温你也不愿意。你看她脸红红的，肯定又发烧了。

Nurse： I am sorry Mrs. Xu. I made you angry. Don't worry，I will take her temperature at once and will also send for a doctor.

护士： 徐太太，对不起，惹你生气了，别着急，我马上再给她量一下，并请医生来检查一下。

（The nurse took Up Xu Jing's temperature. It was 37.0℃. After finishing checking the patient; the doctor thought the infant's condition was stable and did not need special treatment at that moment，except continuing observation.）

（护士给徐晶量了体温，是37.0℃。医生检查完后认为患儿病情稳定，暂时不需要特殊处理，需继续观察。）

Nurse： Mrs. Xu，the doctor has examined your child and thought that everything is turning to normal. We should try not to disturb her now and let her have a good rest. We will observe her condition closely.

护士：大姐，医生给你的孩子检查过了，一切在恢复过程中。现在尽量不要打扰她，让她好好休息吧，我们会密切观察她的病情的。

Patient's Mother：Observation，observation，always observation. Is this your pretext? What is the use of observation? You just don't care because she is not your child.

病儿妈妈：又是观察，这就是你们的托辞吗？观察有什么用？你们当然不着急，又不是你们的孩子。

Nurse：Don't worry，Mrs. Xu. We pay attention to all the children. We will use medicine in time according to her condition.

护士：徐太太，你放心，我们对每个孩子都是很重视的。我们会根据她的病情及时用药的。

Patient's Mother：Use medicine. Do you know how much money I have already spent on medicines?

病儿妈妈：又是用药，你知道我已经花了多少医药费了吗？

Patient：Mom，I want to drink some water.

病儿：妈妈，我要喝水。

Nurse：（Patting the child gently while voluntarily feeding her water，saying something else deliberately to change the conversation）Her complexion is much better. The most important thing for us to do now is to cure the child's disease together.

护士：（主动为孩子喂水，并轻轻拍孩子，岔开话题）孩子脸色好多了。现在我们共同把孩子的病治好是最重要的。

Patient：Thank you auntie nurse.（Lied down quietly.）

病儿：谢谢护士阿姨。（安静地躺下。）

Patient's Mother：（Tears falling down）Do you know how much I worry about her? She has been in the hospital for the third time. She twitches every time she has a fever. I am really afraid that there is something wrong with her brain. What should I do?

病儿妈妈：（眼泪掉下来）你知道我有多着急吗？她已是第三次住院了。一发热就抽搐，我真怕她脑子抽坏了，以后可怎么办？

Nurse：Mrs. Xu，don't worry. There is no organic pathological change in your child's brain. Her illness is Febrile Convulsion. This illness does not have serious consequences and will slowly get better after she grows up. You need not be too upset，and should try your best to cooperate with us. Otherwise it is not good for her treatment.

护士：徐太太，不要着急，你的孩子看来大脑并没有器质性病变。现在诊断是高热惊厥，这种病没有严重的后遗症，等她长大后会慢慢好转的。你不能太烦躁，应尽量配合我们的工作，不然对孩子的治疗也是不利的。

Patient's Mother：Thank you. My attitude was pretty bad. I am sorry.

病儿妈妈：谢谢你，刚才我的态度很不好，对不起。

Nurse： It's O.K. I understand how you feel. You are tired. Take a rest and I will see Xu Jing after a while. Please call me if you need me.

护士： 没关系，我理解你的心情，你累了，休息会儿吧。我过会儿再来看徐晶，有事请呼我。

# 73. A Child with an Acute Asthma Attack

# 哮喘急性发作患儿

Nurse： Shen Min，do you feel better after being nebulized?

护士： 沈敏，你刚才做了喷雾治疗感觉舒服一点了吗？

Patient Child： Auntie Nurse，I feel bad.（Crying）

患儿： 护士阿姨，我难受。（哭）

Nurse： （putting the girl into a semi-reclining position）Shen Min，you are a big girl now. Don't cry any more. Crying will increase the oxygen consumption which will make you feel even worse. I love you very much. Have a good rest，OK?

护士： （给孩子靠在床头半卧位）沈敏，你是大孩子了，乖，不要哭了，哭了会增加耗氧量，你就更不舒服了。听话，阿姨最喜欢你了，好好睡一觉，好吗？

Patient Parent： She has taken so many medicines，why is she still wheezing?

患儿家长： 已经用了这么多药了，怎么还喘啊？

Nurse： We just gave her a bronchodilator. It will relieve the bronchial spasm. Your child will feel better after a while，and the wheezing will be relieved too.

护士： 刚才我们用的是支气管扩张剂，可以解除支气管痉挛。过一会儿你的孩子会感觉舒服一点的，喘息也会慢慢缓解。

Patient Child： Auntie Nurse，I still feel bad，and don't want to sleep.

患儿： 护士阿姨，我还是难受，不想睡觉。

Nurse： I will call for a doctor，OK?

护士： 阿姨去请医生来看你，好吗？

（After examination，the doctor asked the nurse to give the patient a sedative and oxygen inhalation.）

（医生检查后给予镇静剂和吸氧。）

Nurse： I will let you inhale some oxygen and give you a sedative drug via intramuscular injection on your buttock. This will help you sleep and you will feel much better when you wake up.

护士： 阿姨给你吸点氧，再在屁股上打一针睡觉的药。这能帮助你好好睡一觉，醒来的时候你会感觉舒服多了。

Patient Parent： Does the sedative have any side effects?

患儿家长： 打睡觉针会有什么副作用吗？

Nurse： Your child is restless now; this will cause bronchial spasms more easily aggravate the breathing problem. Giving her a sedative will decrease the oxygen consumption and improve her hypoxia.

护士： 现在患儿烦躁，容易使支气管痉挛，加重呼吸困难。给她镇静剂后，可以降低耗氧量，改善缺氧症状。

Patient Parent: My child often has acute attacks. You should cure her completely this time.

患儿家长： 我孩子经常哮喘急性发作，这次一定要给我们治好。

Nurse: The treatment of asthma is a long-term process. It needs the parents' cooperation. You should keep fresh air circulating in your home，avoid allergens and irritating odors，improve her nutrition，and avoid food which may induce asthma attack，such as fish，shrimp，milk，and so on. She needs to continue take the medicine even after she feels better. We'll tell you the details at that time. If you have any questions，you may ask me. I will come back shortly. You may press the call button if there is something urgent.

护士： 哮喘治疗是一个长期的过程，也需要你们家长积极配合。要保持屋里新鲜空气流通，避免容易引起过敏的物品及刺激性气味。加强营养，但应该避免诱发哮喘的食物，如鱼、虾、牛奶等。等你孩子病好一点还要继续用药，到时候我们会详细给你讲解的。你有什么疑问也可以直接问我。我过一会儿再来。你有什么事情按铃。

（Two hours later）

（两小时后）

Nurse: Shen Min，how do you feel? Are you feeling any better?

护士： 沈敏，怎样，感觉好一点了吗？

Patient Child: Auntie nurse，I feel much better now. I can sleep lying flat on the bed.

患儿： 护士阿姨，我好多了，都能平躺着睡觉了。

Nurse: You are better now. After you go home，you should continue taking the medicine，do some exercises，and don't be too naughty. You should avoid going to public places if possible. Watch your clothing to prevent from catching cold. This will help you to prevent an asthma attack like this time.

护士： 这次你是好多了。以后一定要坚持用药，适当进行体育锻炼，不能太调皮，少去公共场所，及时增减衣服，预防感冒。这样就不会像今天这样发作了。

# 74. A Child with Congenital Heart Disease and Infection

# 先天性心脏病合并感染患儿

Nurse: Hello, Feng-Feng's mom. How is your baby doing? I'm here to take his body temperature. (Taking the baby's rectal temperature)

护士：枫枫妈妈，你好。现在小孩怎样？我来给他测量体温。（护士给小孩测量肛温）

Patient's Mother: What is his temperature?

患儿妈妈：体温多少？

Nurse: 39.2℃.

护士：39.2℃。

Patient's Mother: What's the matter? Our child has been in the hospital for two to three days. Why hasn't his fever gone down?

患儿妈妈：怎么回事？我们家孩子已经住院两三天了，为什么体温一直反反复复不退？

Nurse: Don't worry too much. Your child's body immunity is poor. The fever will be down after his infection is under control.

护士：不要太着急，你孩子身体抵抗力相对较差。等感染控制住，体温会慢慢退下来的。

Patient's Mother: He is not your baby so you don't have to worry. He's having such a high fever, how can we not worry.

患儿妈妈：不是你家的孩子你当然不着急。孩子烧成这样，我们家长都急死了。

Nurse: It's the great love of parents all over the world. I can understand how you feel and I also hope your baby will recover quickly.

护士：可怜天下父母心，我能理解你们的心情，我们也希望孩子快点好。

Patient's Mother: You only say the things we like to hear. So far we have spent more than 1, 000 Yuan, but the baby's fever is still the same. He cries and screams non-stop. It is not getting any better at all. It must be due to the poor treatment and medicine you gave him. Where is the doctor? I want to see him.

患儿妈妈：你们只会拣好听的说。我们一千多块钱花进去了，连个发烧都退不下来。小孩哭闹不停，一点都不见好，一定是你们的治疗措施不当，用药不当。医生呢？我要见医生。

Nurse: I am just about to ask the doctor to come to have a look on your baby. Please wait a moment. I will call him at once.

护士：我正要请医生来看看。你们稍等，我马上去请医生。

（After examining the baby，the doctor prescribed medicines to lower the baby's temperature. The doctor also ordered an enema for him.）

（医生看过患儿之后，给予药物降温，并开出灌肠的医嘱。）

Nurse：After examining your baby，the doctor has prescribed the new antipyretic drug for him. I will give him the medicine and then wipe his body with warm water. His body temperature should go down shortly. The baby will quiet down after I give him the enema.

护士：医生检查过后，开了新的退热药，我现在就给他用上，再给他用温水擦个身。等一会儿体温会降下来的，接下来马上给你的孩子灌肠，孩子就安静了。

Patient's Mother：You always give him medicine when his temperature is high and apply enema when he cries. But his symptoms have recurred again and again. Don't you have other methods to treat him?

患儿妈妈：发烧就开药，过一阵子又会升上去，孩子哭闹了就灌肠，难道你们就没有其他办法？

Nurse：Feng-Feng's mom，I am sorry for letting you worry. We first need to reduce the baby's temperature to quiet him down，and then alleviate his discomfort. At the same time，we are treating the cause of his disease. Your baby has a congenital heart disease and his immunity to diseases is low.

护士：枫枫妈妈，对不起，让你着急了。目前我们先把孩子的体温退下来，让小孩安静，尽量减少他的一些痛苦。同时，我们也在给他进行病因治疗。你的孩子有先天性心脏病，抗病能力差一些。

Patient's Mother：The child coughs endlessly and breathes heavily. Are these all related to his congenital heart disease too?（Her tone begins to relax.）

患儿妈妈：现在小孩不停地咳嗽，还喘呢，这也和先天性心脏病有关？（语气开始缓和。）

Nurse：Yes. A child with congenital heart disease has relatively poor immunity and may be slower in his overall development than healthy children. It is easy for him to develop a lung infection when suffering from colds，and a lung infection can aggravate his heart problem. This is what your baby has，a complicated bronchus pneumonia. We have treated his symptoms with oxygen inhalation，aerosol spray，and intravenous medicines. But，it takes time to recover. In the course of the treatment，in order to obtain better and faster results，I hope you would cooperate with us and support our work. Your baby has cough with sputum. Turn him，pat his back，and provide water for him to drink. This will help him to cough up the sputum.

护士：是这样的，患有先天性心脏病的孩子抵抗力相对较差。有的发育落后于其他孩子，一旦受凉或被感染易并发肺部感染，而肺部感染就会加重心脏症状。这次你的孩子就是合并了支气管肺炎。针对孩子的气喘与咳嗽我们已经对症处理了，如吸氧、雾化，还有静脉用药。但发挥明显的作用还要有个过程。在治疗过程中，为了取得更好更快的疗效，希望你们尽可能配合和支持我们的工作。咳嗽会有痰，你们应经常给孩子翻身拍背，多给孩子喝水，有助于痰液排出。

Patient's Mother: Really? Could you teach me how to pat him?

患儿妈妈：真的呀，能教我吗？

Nurse: Pat him like this.（The nurse demonstrated.）

护士：这样拍。（护士做示范。）

Patient's Mother: Is this right?（Turned over the baby and patted his back.）

患儿妈妈：这个样子对吗？（为患儿翻身拍背。）

Nurse: Right, but make your hand into a hollow form.（Demonstrated again.）

护士：对的，但是应注意将手拱成空心状。（再次做示范。）

Nurse: I'll give the child an enema first. It is not good that he keeps crying and screaming.

护士：我先给孩子灌肠吧，这样一直哭闹对孩子的病是不好的。

Patient's Mother: OK.（Adjusting the baby's body posture to go with the nurse's enema procedure）

患儿妈妈：好的。（调整患儿体位，配合护士灌肠。）

（The baby fell asleep. The nurse came to his bedside again.）

（小孩安静入睡了，护士再次来到床边。）

Patient's Mother: Nurse, is there any method of curing our baby's heart disease?

患儿妈妈：护士小姐，我们小孩的心脏病，有治好的办法吗？

Nurse: Yes! I have read your child's clinical data. He has the ventricular septal defect about 0.5 cm. There is no need to have an operation. We can use an interventional method to block it which has very little trauma to him. He can be discharged from the hospital within 2 to 3 days. There are many children cured using this method in our department. As matter of fact, there are two of them right now in the next room.

护士：有的！我看过你小孩的临床资料，是室间隔缺损，缺口比较小，大约 0.5 cm。解剖部位也还好，以后不用开刀。做介入封堵就可以把缺口补好，损伤小，两三天就可以出院。现在我们病区做这类封堵术的小孩挺多的，隔壁房间就有两个。

Patient's Mother: Can our baby be treated with this procedure now?

患儿妈妈：我们小孩现在能做吗？

Nurse: It is better to do it at about three to five years old when the child's tolerance is better. At that age the child is not yet attending school, therefore it will not interfere with his study. At the present time, you should make sure that your child will not catch cold, prevent him from strong stimulation, and don't take him to crowded places. Pay attention to his nutrition and keep his bowel movement smooth. We will give you a brochure with health guidelines before you leave the hospital.

护士： 最好3～5岁时做，小孩那时候的耐受力比较好，也不影响学习。现在应注意避免受凉感冒，避免强烈刺激，少到人群集中的地方，注意加强营养，保持大便通畅。等到出院前，还会给你发健康教育指导处方的。

Patient's Mother: Thank you. Because I was so worried, I might have talked to you very rudely. Please forgive me. Frankly, I feel the service here is quite good. I do not worry any more about my baby staying here.

患儿妈妈： 谢谢你，我实在太着急、太紧张，说话有些激动，请原谅。说句老实话，我感觉这里服务态度蛮好的。小孩住在这里我也放心了。

Nurse: Thank you for supporting our work. From now on, we should communicate with each other more often.

护士： 感谢你对我们工作的支持，以后我们彼此多交流多沟通。

# 75. A Child with Allergic Rhinitis

# 过敏性鼻炎患儿

Nurse： You child has allergic rhinitis. Please take him to have an allergen test to find out what he is allergic to.

护士： 你的孩子患了过敏性鼻炎，请去检查一下过敏原，看是什么原因引起的过敏。

Child's Parent： Does this examination have any side effects?

患儿家长： 做这个检查有没有副作用？

Nurse： Don't worry. It is just like a skin test and has no side effects.

护士： 请放心，就像做皮试一样，没有副作用。

Child's Parent： Why did you give so many punctures on his arm?

患儿家长： 那要刺那么多的点是做什么的？

Nurse： （Pointed to the liquid antigen）This is the antigen extracted from animals and plants which may cause allergic reactions. If he is allergic to it，we shall see the result fifteen minutes after he is exposed to it.

护士： （指着抗原液）这是从各种容易产生过敏的动植物中提炼出来的抗原。孩子若有过敏的话，一接触过 15 分钟就可以看得出结果。

Child's Parent： Is the antigen toxic?

患儿家长： 抗原有没有毒？

Nurse： No. We have examined many patients. It is safe.

护士： 没有的，我们已做了很多病人，很安全的。

（After the examination）

（检查后）

Nurse： Here are the results. Your child is allergic to dust mites with three（+）and to fungus with two（+）.

护士： 结果出来了，你的孩子是对尘螨过敏，有三个（+），还有霉菌是两个（+）。

Child's Parent： What? Have you injected mites and fungus to my child's body? I asked if it was toxic and you said no. You are hurting him! I'll sue you. You must pay for what you did. I will not forgive you if my child is infected by the fungus.

患儿家长： 什么？你把什么虫和霉菌扎进我孩子的身体里了？我问你有没有毒，你说没有，你这不是害人么！我要告你，要你赔偿。将来我孩子有霉菌感染，我和你没完。

Nurse： You have misunderstood. This is a reagent which is not toxic. The dose is very small, and any excess antigen has been absorbed by the cotton tips right away. It is definitely safe for him. We have done it on thousands of patients. The examination is similar to an immunization shots and the dose we used is much less than that. So you need not to worry.

护士：你搞错了，这是试剂，没有毒的。我们的用量极其少，而且刺完马上用棉签吸掉余量，对孩子是绝对安全的。我们已经做过上千例了，这和预防针相似，但比预防针用量小得多。所以你不要担心。

Child's Parent: Is it really safe?

患儿家长：真的不会有事？

Nurse: Please trust me. I love your baby and hope he is safe and healthy just like you. The test results are here. Now, we can try to help him overcome his allergies and treat his illness?

护士：请你相信我。我同你一样爱你的宝宝，同你一样希望他安全、健康。现在结果出来了，我们一起来想办法帮助宝宝脱敏、帮助宝宝把病治好，好吗？

# 76. A Child with a Bone Marrow Transplant

# 骨髓移植患儿

（The child painfully crouched in the bed. The nurse wiped the child's tears with a disinfected tissue paper and massaged her back gently.）

（患儿表情痛苦地蜷缩着身体卧于床上。护士俯下身体，用消毒纸巾轻轻擦去孩子眼角的泪水，并用手轻轻地抚摸着她的脊背。）

Nurse： Is the pain in your abdomen?

护士： 是不是肚子疼？

（The child cried silently without verbal response. The nurse moved her hand slowly to the child's abdomen and pressed it lightly. The child moved the nurse's hand to the lower part of her abdomen.）

（患儿无言，默默地流泪，护士慢慢地将手移至患儿腹部并试探着轻轻按压。孩子扳着护士的手下移至下腹部。）

Nurse： Is the pain here?

护士： 是不是这儿疼？

Patient： Yes，but I feel a little better now.

患儿： 是的，不过现在好一点了。

Nurse： Does it hurt all the time?

护士： 是不是一直在疼？

Patient： No，but often. I really want to see my mother when I have severe pain.

患儿： 不，但疼的时候多。疼得厉害时我就想妈妈。

Nurse： You can go out to see your mother after you have recovered. But now，you can call me when you feel pain. OK? Later I will ask the doctor to give you some medicine which will make you feel better.

护士： 等你病好了，就能出去看你妈妈了。现在要是疼了叫阿姨好吗？待会儿，阿姨请医生给你用点药，用了药就会不疼了。

（The child nodded and held the nurse's hand.）

（患儿拉着护士的手，点点头。）

# 77. Care for a Child's Fear

# 患儿恐惧心理护理

Nurse： Hello，Lili. Did you sleep well last night?（Holding her hands gently with a smile.）

护士： 喂！莉莉。你来啦，昨晚睡得好吗？（拉着莉莉的手，面带微笑。）

Patient's Child： I'm afraid of the operation. I couldn't fall asleep. I don't want the operation.

患儿： 我怕开刀，睡不着，我不要开刀。

Nurse： How is that? Lili，are you scared of the pain? Have you got an injection in the unit?

护士： 怎么啦，莉莉，是不是怕开刀时痛呀？刚才在病房里打针了吗？

Patient's Child： Yea，it hurts so much where they gave me the injection. I don't want the operation（crying as she spoke）.

患儿： 打了，我打针的地方好痛，我不要开刀（边哭边讲）。

Nurse： That injection will make you calm. The doctor in the operation room will inject you some sleeping drugs which will make you fall to sleep. When you wake up，the operation will be over. It's magic，right?（Chatted while fondling the child's forehead.）

护士： 刚才打的可是镇静针哦。等一会儿，让麻醉师给你打一点睡觉的药，等你一觉醒来，已经开好刀了，而且又把昨天的觉补回来了。多神奇呀！

（边交谈边抚摸孩子的额头。）

（The girl stopped crying but kept silent.）

（患儿停止哭闹，沉默。）

Nurse： Look at her. She is the anesthetist，a great magician. She has helped many patients younger than you to have no pain during their operation. If you want no pain，then you must cooperate with her.

护士： 你看，这是魔术麻醉师，她的本领可大了，有许多比你小的小朋友开刀也一点不痛呀。不过你要配合她哦！

Patient's Child： （nodding）I will cooperate with you.

患儿： （点头）我一定配合你们。

# 78. Dietary Instruction for an Elder

# 老年人饮食指导

Nurse：Grandma Yin，I am the nurse in charge of your treatment. Is your abdomen pain getting better?

护士：殷婆婆，我是你的床位护士，你现在肚子痛好点了吗？

Patient：Oh，it's much better now. Thank you.

病人：好多了，谢谢你。

Nurse：Did you have your supper in a restaurant last night? What kind of food did you have?

护士：你昨天晚上是不是在外面饭馆吃的晚饭？能告诉我你吃了些什么吗？

Patient：Yes，I had my dinner last night in a restaurant. I had shrimps，fried nuts，fried radish cake and some vegetables.

病人：我是在外面吃的晚饭，主要吃了点虾、油炸三果、萝卜丝饼，还有蔬菜。

Nurse：Did you eat more food last night than usual?

护士：你吃得比平时多吗？

Patient：Yes，I ate more than usual. I felt so full. The flavor of the restaurant food was wonderful.

病人：是的，比我平时吃得多，我都感到有点撑了。饭店的菜味道很好。

Nurse：Was the shrimp poached?

护士：虾是水煮的吗？

Patient：No，the shrimps were fried.

病人：不，是椒盐炸虾。

Nurse：What time do you usually have your supper?

护士：你平时几点钟吃晚饭？

Patient：About 5：30 to 6：00 pm.

病人：大约下午5：30～6：00吧。

Nurse：Were you tired yesterday?

护士：昨天你是不是累了？

Patient：Yes. A few of my younger colleagues invited me to discuss things with them. I was busy with them the whole day. Then they invited me to have supper with them at the restaurant.

病人：是的，昨天单位里有几个年轻人问我些问题，我就去了，结果折腾了一天，然后他们就请我一起到餐馆吃晚饭。

Nurse： Have you suffered from cholecystitis before? If so，were the episodes related to inappropriate diet and rest?

护士： 你的胆囊炎以前发作过吗？如有发作，是不是与饮食不当与休息不好有关。

Patient： There were two episodes. Both happened after eating a bowl of smoldered meat noodles.

病人： 有过两次，都是吃了一碗焖肉面后发作的。

Nurse： Grandma Yin，I have some dietary suggestions for the elders，especially for those who are suffering from chronic cholecystitis or pancreatitis.

护士： 殷婆婆，我有些建议，是针对老年人吃饭方面的，尤其是有胆囊和胰腺疾病的老年人。

Patient： What suggestions?

病人： 是哪些建议呢？

Nurse： It's helpful for the elders not to eat a full meal every time，preferable 80% full. Have light meal，avoid fried or oily food. The fried nuts，radish cake and fried shrimps you had last night are not good for your chronic cholecystitis. Since you like to go to bed early，the time of your supper should be earlier，no later than 7：00 pm. Also，you should not eat too fast and you should cut the food into smaller pieces，and make them softer. This way is better for your health.

护士： 老年人每餐应吃得少一点，大约八分饱就行。饮食宜清淡一点，少吃或不吃油腻和油炸食品，你昨晚吃的油炸三果、萝卜丝饼和椒盐虾都对你的胆囊炎不利。晚饭吃得早一点，不要晚于晚上 7 点，尤其是你喜欢早睡。另外吃饭的速度不能太快，食物切得小一点，做得烂一点，这样有利于你的健康。

Patient： How much vegetable should I eat every day?

病人： 我一天要吃多少蔬菜好呢？

Nurse： You should have 1/2 pound to 1 pound vegetable each day. Vegetables are cleaners for the human body. Adequate dietary fiber is one of the most important factors for bowel function.

护士： 一天的蔬菜应达到 0.5～1 磅。因为蔬菜是人体的清道夫，使你的大便保持通畅。

# 79. Preventing an Elder from Choking

# 老年人哈噎的预防

Nurse： Grandma Yang，how are you feeling now? Any discomfort?

护士： 杨婆婆，你感觉怎样？有什么不舒服吗？

Patient： My goodness. Am I in a hospital? I have a sharp pain in my chest.

病人： 哎呀，我在医院里吗？胸口怎么这么痛啊！

Nurse： Grandma Yang，take it easy and calm down. You had an accident a little while ago and we had to press your chest to save your life. That's why you are having this chest pain.

护士： 杨婆婆，不要紧张，刚刚你发生了点意外。我们抢救你的时候，按压了你的胸部，所以你现在胸部会疼痛。

Patient： I remember I was in a family party in my house welcoming my granddaug-hter who had just come back from America. I cooked some sticky rice balls，and we were celebrating. But how did this accident happen?

病人： 我记得刚刚还在家里，我的孙女从美国回来，家里人都团圆了。于是我们就做了糯米食物汤圆，庆祝一下。哪知会出现这种事。

Nurse： Oh，older people like you should be more careful when you eat foods made of sticky rice. It is better you don't eat them at all.

护士： 哦，老年人吃糯米食物的时候要注意一点，最好不要吃。

Patient： But sticky rice such as rice balls and pastries is my favorite food.

病人： 可我就喜欢吃糯米食物的，像团子、糕点等。

Nurse： If you like them so much and have to have some，then you should make the balls as small as possible，or cut the pastries into smaller pieces and eat them one by one in a slow pace.

护士： 既然你喜欢吃，那就要将团子做得小一点，将糕点切成小块，吃的速度慢一点，一口一口地吃。

Patient： I see. I should make smaller balls，cut the pastries into smaller pieces and eat them slowly，right?

病人： 我知道了。团子做得小点，糕切得小点，吃的速度慢一点，是吗？

Nurse： Yes. Before eating，you should sit in a comfortable upright position or inclining forward your body a little bit. Lying down in bed isn't a good position for eating this kind of food.

护士： 是的。而且，吃饭之前把身体位置调整好，人坐直或略向前俯，尽量不要躺着吃糯米食物。

Patient: Oh, I almost forgot. Today when I ate the sticky rice balls I was reclining on my chair.

病人：对了，今天我吃的时候是靠在藤椅上的。

Nurse: What were you feelings when the accident happened?

护士：刚刚发生意外的时候，你有什么感觉？

Patient: Nothing special. It seemed as if a curtain was put down slowly in front of a window before I was going to bed.

病人：没有什么感觉，就好像睡前有一扇窗户的窗帘慢慢地在放下来。

Nurse: Any other uncomfortable feeling?

护士：没什么其他不舒服吗？

Patient: Nothing else.

病人：没有。

Nurse: That is good. It'll be all right for you to have sticky rice foods, but make sure pay a little more attention to it.

护士：那好。你下次吃糯米食物的时候注意一下就行了。

Patient: Thank you.

病人：谢谢。

# 80. Preventing an Elder from Falling

## 老年人跌倒的预防

Nurse: Teacher Wang, what's the matter with you?

护士：王老师，你怎么啦？

Patient: Ah, Miss Zhang. I fell from the steps when I came downstairs and felt a sharp pain on my left ankle and also felt nausea.

病人：哦，是张护士啊。我刚刚下楼时不小心踩空了，当时左脚踝部痛得不得了，还有点儿恶心。

Nurse: Oh, I'm sorry to hear that. Let me take a look.

护士：真不巧啊。让我帮你检查一下。

Patient: Please tell me, is there any fracture? The pain is a bit less now.

病人：我是不是骨折了？你告诉我呀。不过现在疼痛已好了点。

Nurse: Teacher Wang, your injury is not very severe. There does not seem to be a fracture. But you should take an X-ray to be sure if you just have some soft tissue injury or also have hairline fracture.

护士：王老师，你的情况不算严重，从我检查的结果来看没有骨折。但是要确定你是单纯的软组织损伤还是伴有骨裂，通过拍片后才能确定。

Paint: How long would it take to heal if I have a hairline fracture?

病人：如果我有骨裂的话，需要多长时间才能好？

Nurse: You should not bear any weight during the first three weeks. You might need a cast to immobilize your injured ankle joint. You can use a crutch to help you walk and you should monitor the local extremity circulation. You should also do some partial exercise to prevent muscle atrophy and joint stiffness.

护士：你三周内不能负重。可能要用石膏托固定受伤踝关节，同时观察局部的血液循环，另外配制一副拐杖，局部进行锻炼，以防关节僵硬及肌肉萎缩。

Patient: OK.

病人：好的。

Nurse: How do you feel now? Let me help you up and sit down on the bench for a while, we will then monitor the injured ankle a little bit more, OK?

护士：你现在怎么样了？我现在扶你起来，在边上的凳子上坐一会儿。我们再观察一下好吗？

Patient: All right. I have been nearsighted seriously since I was young, and now my eye doctor told me that I have cataracts.

病人：好的。我眼睛从年轻时就不好，严重近视，听医生说，现在又有点白内障。

Nurse: An elder person like you usually suffers decreased visual acuity, decreased accommodation in the eyes, decreased peripheral visions and is more sensible to glares. Since you have severe myopia and some cataract, you should be especially careful when going downstairs and walk slowly.

护士：噢，那你更应该小心。老年人本来视敏度、调节能力和视野就下降，对强光又不适应，加上又有白内障，上下楼梯尤其是下楼梯时更应小心，走路速度要慢。

Patient: I am very impatient. In addition, I select the out-of-the-way place for my exercise because don't like people watching me when I exercise.

病人：我有心急的毛病。另外，我锻炼时不愿人家在旁边看着我，所以我就选择在人少的地方锻炼。

Nurse: Teacher Wang, you should ask your husband to accompany you when you exercise so you can take care of each other. Also, the time for you to exercise should be early in the evening before dark. It is easer to fall if there is not enough light.

护士：王老师，今后你锻炼时，最好由你的老伴陪着你，这样你们可以互相照应。还有锻炼时间最好早一点。如果路上光线不好，很容易跌倒的。

Patient: Okay. Also, I exercised a bit longer today than usual and I was tired. Does this have something to do with my fall?

病人：好的。另外告诉你，我今天多锻炼了一点时间，有点累，这是不是与我跌倒有关？

Nurse: Maybe. I think there are several factors that caused your fall.

护士：可能有关，我认为引起你今天跌倒的原因有好几个呢！

Patient: I will be more careful next time. My sore is much better. I want to go home now.

病人：好的，我会注意的。我现在疼痛好多了，我想回家了。

Nurse: Let me accompany you home.

护士：那我扶你回家。

Patient: Thanks.

病人：谢谢。

# 81. Nursing Care for an Elder with Osteoporosis

## 老年人骨质疏松的护理

Patient: Miss Zhang, could you tell me why my bones are so fragile? They fractured as I moved only a few flowerpots.

病人：张护士，请你告诉我，我的骨头为什么这么不结实呢？我不就搬了一下花盆吗？怎么就断了呢？

Nurse: Grandma Tang, this is an age-related bone demineralization called osteoporosis. As people grow older they will lose their bone mass, which makes their bones porous and fragile.

护士：汤婆婆，你年纪大了骨质减少了，骨头里有许多小孔，所以不坚实。医学上称为骨质疏松。

Patient: My appetite is good and I have my normal diet. Why should I lose bone mass?

病人：我平时胃口挺好的，一天三顿饭吃得好好的，怎么会骨质减少呢？

Nurse: What kind of foods do you usually eat?

护士：你平时吃些什么？

Patient: Porridge, rice, vegetables, fish, eggs and so on.

病人：粥、饭、蔬菜、鱼、蛋等。

Nurse: Do you take milk, small shrimps, fried little fish, and sparerib soup?

护士：你喝不喝牛奶，吃不吃小虾米、炸小鱼和排骨汤之类的食物？

Patient: I do not like the smell of milk and feel nauseous when I smell it. I also seldom eat small shrimps, little fried fish, and sparerib soup because my teeth are not very good.

病人：我平时不吃这些食物。我不能闻牛奶的味道，闻到就恶心。由于我牙不好，也不常吃小虾米、炸小鱼和排骨汤之类的食物。

Nurse: Do you take calcium pills?

护士：你吃不吃钙片？

Patient: Oh, once a doctor told me to take calcium pills because my bones were aching. I took the calcium pills and vitamin D for about half a month. I stopped taking them after the pain reduced, because I thought these pills were medicines and should not be taken for too long.

病人：哦，有一次我感到骨头痛，去医院看病，医生曾叫我吃钙片，我就吃了半个月左右的钙片和维生素D。后来骨痛好了点，就不吃了。我想这是药片，不能多吃的。

Nurse: When was that?

护士：　这是什么时候的事？

Patient:　About three years ago.

病人：　大约三年前的事。

Nurse：　You are suffering from severe calcium deficiency now which causes your bones to fracture easier. I suggest that you drink one to two bottles of milk a day，soup with small shrimps，green vegetables，seafood，bean products and peanuts. If you do not like milk，you can take calcium pills instead. I think your osteoporosis will get better if you follow my suggestions.

护士：　现在你缺钙比较严重，以至于容易骨折。我建议你今后每天喝 1～2 瓶牛奶，菜汤里加点虾米。平时也可以多吃点深绿色蔬菜、海产品、豆制品和花生。如你实在不喜欢牛奶，那就吃钙片。这样你的骨质疏松就会好得多。

Patient:　Okay.

病人：　好的。

Nurse：　In addition，exercise more everyday because bones usually grow stronger when they bear more weight.

护士：　另外你平时应多锻炼身体，骨头承受压力后才能变得结实。

Patient:　What kind of exercises should I do?

病人：　那我参加哪些活动呢？

Nurse：　You may take a walk，shadowbox，or ride bicycles，etc. What kind of exercises do you like the best?

护士：　可以散步，也可以做操或打拳，或者骑自行车等。你喜欢哪一种锻炼方法？

Patient:　Shadowboxing will embarrass me. I prefer taking a walk or riding the bike.

病人：　我是不会学打拳的，我怕难为情。散步和骑车都可以。

Nurse：　Try to maintain a half-an-hour to one-hour walk everyday.

护士：　那你就坚持每天散步 0.5～1 小时。

Patient:　OK，I'll do that.

病人：　好的。

# 82. Senile Dementia

# 老年性痴呆

Patient: Miss Zhang, my memory is getting worse. I keep forgetting things. I almost forgot my nephew's name the other day. My doctor told me that I have early stage Alzheimer's disease. I have heard that people who suffer from Alzheimer's disease will become a fool. It is terrible.

病人：张护士，我的记忆力越来越坏，近来老是遗忘，有时连我外甥的名字都叫不出来。医生说我得了早期老年性痴呆。听说得了这个毛病最后会变傻的。实在可怕！

Nurse: Mr. Liu, I understand what you are thinking. Don't be nervous. Could you tell me what your daily life is like?

护士：刘先生，我理解你的想法，但是你先别紧张。你能告诉我你日常的生活吗？

Patient: I usually get up at 6 am. After brushing my teeth and washing my face, I will have breakfast. Then I enjoy Suzhou Pin Tan for half an hour and watch TV for about one hour. I talk with my wife for some time, and then it will be time for lunch. I usually take a nap for about half an hour (I don't want a long nap because I am afraid it will affect the quality of night sleep). Then I usually go downstairs for a walk, find a chair to sit down and chat with my neighbors. After that I'll have my supper. I usually go to bed at about 8 pm.

病人：我早晨一般 6 点起床，洗漱后吃早饭，听半小时苏州评弹，看大约一小时电视，和老伴聊聊，就吃中饭。下午打半小时瞌睡（我不敢多睡，怕影响晚上睡觉），就下楼走一圈，再找个椅子坐会儿，与其他人聊聊天，就回来吃晚饭。晚上大约 8 点左右就睡觉了。

Nurse: Do you usually eat enough vegetables and fruits?

护士：平时蔬菜和水果吃得多吗？

Patient: Yes, I do but not too much. My wife and I eat about half a pound of vegetables every day. I am old and my teeth are not very good.

病人：吃的，但不多，我老伴和我一天大约吃半磅左右蔬菜吧。我年纪大了，牙齿不好。

Nurse: What kind of cookware do you use?

护士：你家烧饭用的是什么锅子？

Patient: Originally we use aluminum cookware. Lately, we changed to iron pans because we have heard that aluminum cookware is not good for health. But the electric rice cooker is still made of aluminum. Is it bad to use aluminum cookwares?

病人：我家原来用的是铝锅。后来听说铝锅烧饭对身体不好，就将炒菜锅换成铁锅了，但是电饭煲还是铝的。是不是用铝锅不好？

Nurse: Some researches have found that taking excessive aluminum can cause Alzheimer's disease.

护士：有研究发现，吃的食物中含铝太多，会导致老年性痴呆。

Patient: Really? I need to tell my son to change an electric rice cooker for me.

病人：真的吗？那要叫我儿子给我换个电饭煲了。

Nurse: Mr. Liu，in order to delay your disease process，you should exercise more. It is not enough just to take a little walk. Since you live near a large park，you could take a walk there or take up shadowboxing to increase your total activity to two hours a day. Make sure you pay attention to safety. Try to exercise your brain also. Do some simple calculations such as helping your wife record daily spending，or play mahjong for about one hour. Since your teeth are not very good，you should cut the vegetables and fruits into smaller pieces before eating them.

护士：刘先生，为了延缓你的病情发展，你平时要多活动。一天只在院子里走一圈是不够的。公园离你家比较近，你可以打打太极拳，散散步，一天活动的时间增加到两小时左右，但要注意安全。还有要多动脑子，可以帮你的夫人记记日常开支的账，也可以搓麻将，时间大约一小时左右。既然你的牙齿不好，可将蔬菜和水果切得小一点再吃。

Patient: Thank you. Is there anything else I should pay attention to?

病人：谢谢你，那我还有其他需要注意的事吗？

Nurse: You can eat more fish，less starchy foods，and helping your wife with household chores is good for you，too.

护士：你平时可多吃些鱼，少吃淀粉类食物。帮你夫人干点家务活，这对你的病也是有好处的。

Patient: I like eating salty fish. Can I eat them often?

病人：我平时喜欢吃咸鱼，可不可以经常吃？

Nurse: You should try to avoid salty food. Do you smoke?

护士：你最好少吃咸鱼，你抽烟吗？

Patient: Yes. Sometimes. But I am not addicted to smoking.

病人：有时候抽，但没有瘾。

Nurse: That is good. You should quit smoking all together.

护士：那还好，你应该戒烟。

Patient: OK，Thanks.

病人：好的，谢谢。

# 83. Nursing Intervention for Abuse of Medication by the Elderly

# 老年人滥用药物的护理

Nurse: Hello, Mr. Wu. I'm the nurse in charge of your treatment. My last name is Zhang, so you can call me Xiao Zhang. Well, how do you feel now?

护士：吴先生，你好，我是你的床位护士，我姓张，你叫我小张吧。你现在有什么不舒服吗？

Patient: I'm all right except feeling fatigue all over my body.

病人：就是觉得全身没力，其他没什么。

Nurse: I've heard from your daughter that you have diabetes mellitus. Is that true?

护士：听你女儿说，你有糖尿病，是吗？

Patient: Two years ago my doctor told me that I had mild diabetes. He said that my blood sugar would be controlled if I took a restricted diet and exercised more often. However, I caught a cold a few days ago and had my blood sugar level checked at the hospital, the level was high. The doctor told me to take some medicine to lower my blood sugar.

病人：两年前医生就说我有轻度糖尿病，要我饭吃得少一点，平时多活动，血糖就能控制住了。但几天前我有点感冒，来医院验血后发现血糖挺高的，医生要我吃药，说是可以降血糖的。

Nurse: Did you buy those drugs the doctor prescribed for you from the hospital pharmacy?

护士：你在医院里买医生给你开的药了吗？

Patient: No, I didn't. I heard that the price of drugs in the hospital was a little higher than the drug stores outside, so I did not buy them in the hospital. I wanted to save some money because I have to pay all my medical expenses by myself.

病人：没有。听说医院里的药要比外面药店里的药贵一点，我就没在医院里买，我是自费的，想省点钱。

Nurse: What happened to you then?

护士：后来呢？

Patient: Yesterday, I bought the drugs as prescribed by my doctor from a drug store near my home. As my doctor told me that the level of my blood sugar was considerably high, I took one pill this morning. I soon felt palpitations and became unconscious.

病人：昨天我拿着医生的处方去我家附近的药店买了药。今天早晨，我想医生说我血糖蛮高的，我就吃了一粒降糖药。没多长时间我就觉得心慌，后来就迷迷糊糊了。

Nurse: Were you sweating at that time?

护士：你当时出汗吗？

Patient: I had cold sweat all over then. Ms. Zhang, could you tell me what my disease is?

病人：我出了一身冷汗。张护士，你能告诉我，我生了什么病？

Nurse: Mr. Yang, this happened to you because you took excessive dose of drugs that lowered your blood sugar too much.

护士：杨先生，你吃的降糖药的量多了一点，使你的血糖降得太低了，就出现了这种情况。

Patient: Oh, then I should take less drug the next time, right?

病人：哦，那我下次少吃点，行吗？

Nurse: No. You should follow your doctor's advices. He will adjust the dosage according to your blood sugar level. Moreover, you need to carry some biscuits or candy with you all the time.

护士：不行，你得听医生的，医生要根据你的血糖水平调整药物用量。另外，你以后身边带点饼干或糖果之类的东西。

Patient: Why should I carry these foods? Didn't my doctor suggest me to cut this kind of food from my diet?

病人：带这些吃的东西干吗？医生不是要我少吃这些东西吗？

Nurse: If you have symptoms like palpitation, hand trembling, cold sweat and dizziness, you can eat some biscuits or candy first and then see a doctor.

护士：你如果有心慌，手抖、出冷汗、头晕等症状，就吃点饼干或糖果，然后再看医生。

Patient: I see. Thank you, Ms. Zhang.

病人：我知道了，谢谢张护士。

# 84. Home Visit

## 家庭访问

Nurse: Good morning, Mr. Lee. How are you feeling these days?
护士：早上好，李先生。这些天您感觉怎么样？
Resident: Not too bad.
居民：还不错。
Nurse: Would you please put the thermometer under your armpit?
护士：请您把体温计放在腋下好吗？
Resident: OK.
居民：好的。
Nurse: Let me have a look at the refrigerator. There is so much food in it. Have you been following the recipe I gave you?
护士：让我看看冰箱。里面有这么多食物啊。您按照我给您的食谱吃东西了吗？
Resident: Yes, I have.
居民：是的，我按食谱吃的。
Nurse: How many times does the assistant nurse deliver meals?
护士：护理员每天送几次饭？
Resident: Twice a day.
居民：每天两次。
Nurse: How many times has she come this week to help you to buy food, have a bath, and do the cleaning and laundry? Are you satisfied with her job?
护士：这星期她来过几次帮您买食物、洗澡、做清洁和洗衣服？您对她的服务满意吗？
Resident: She's come here twice to do all these for me. She is a very good girl.
居民：她来了两次，帮我做所有的事。她是个很好的姑娘。
Nurse: Can I have the thermometer now? Your temperature is 36℃. Let me listen to your heart and lungs, and take your blood pressure.
护士：把体温计给我吧。您的体温是36℃。我给您听心肺和测血压。
Resident: Anything wrong?
居民：有什么问题吗？
Nurse: Your heart and lungs are quite normal. Your blood pressure is one hundred and twenty over eighty mmHg. I'm going to give you an examination. Well, your right leg has a little edema. Have you found a dark red spot on your right knee? Did you

fall recently?

护士： 您的心肺都很正常。您的血压是120/80mmHg。我给您做个检查。哦，您的右腿有点水肿。您发现了右膝有块暗红的地方吗？您最近摔倒过吗？

Resident: I didn't fall, but my right knee hurts sometimes.

居民： 我没摔倒过，但有时右膝盖痛。

Nurse: I will call your doctor and he will come to see you soon.

护士： 我会打电话给您的医生，他很快会来看看。

Resident: That's fine.

居民： 那就好。

Nurse: I'm going to collect a drop of blood from one of your fingers to test your blood glucose levels. Which hand do you prefer?

护士： 我要采一滴血测您的血糖。您想用哪只手？

Resident: This one please.

居民： 用这只吧。

Nurse: It's done.

护士： 采完了。

Resident: Is my blood sugar still high?

居民： 我的血糖还是很高吗？

Nurse: Yes, it is. Here are the medications for you for the next week. There are seven containers for seven days and four small boxes for morning, noon, afternoon and evening of each day. Make sure of the day and time on the labels before you take the medicines.

护士： 是的，还是很高。这些是您下周的药。7天7个药盒，每天分早晨、中午、下午和晚上四个小药盒。请看清标签上的日期和时间再服药。

Resident: Yes, I will.

居民： 好的，我会的。

Nurse: Here are the insulin shots with disposable syringes for seven days. I have put them in the refrigerator. You know how to do the injection by your-self, don't you?

护士： 这是7天的胰岛素针剂和一次性注射器。我放在冰箱里了。您会自己注射，对吧？

Resident: Yes, I do.

居民： 是的，我会。

Nurse: Don't forget to do the injection 30 minutes before each meal.

护士： 别忘了在饭前30分钟注射。

Resident: I'II remember it.

居民： 我会记住的。

Nurse: I know you like to have preserved vegetable with congee, But preserved vegetable has too much salt in it, That's why your leg has edema.

护士： 我知道您喜欢吃腌菜就米粥。但腌菜含盐太多。这就是您的腿水肿的原因。

Resident: I see. I'II try to have more fresh vegetables instead.

居民：我明白了。我会尽量多吃新鲜蔬菜。

Nurse：Your shoes are kind of tight for your feet. Do you need special shoes which are looser，softer and more comfortable?

护士：您的鞋对您的脚来说有点紧。您需要更宽松、柔软、舒适的特制鞋吗？

Resident：Sounds like a good idea. Where can I get them?

居民：这主意听起来不错。在哪里可以买到呢？

Nurse：I'II tell the footwear shop your size，and they can deliver a pair to you tomorrow.

护士：我会把您的鞋号通知鞋店，明天他们会给您送一双来。

Resident：Great. Thank you for everything.

居民：太好了！谢谢您为我做的一切。

Nurse：It's my pleasure. If you have any questions or problems，please feel free to call me. See you next time.

护士：这是我的荣幸。如果您有任何疑问或问题，请随时给我打电话。下次见。

Resident：See you.

居民：再见。

# 85. Anxious Syndrome

# 焦虑综合征

Patient: My doctor plans to reduce the dose of my medicine. If I don't take enough medicine, I can't sleep well and my illness will get worse. Could you help me ask the doctor not to reduce the dose of my medication?

病人：我的医生要给我减药。这样我晚上肯定睡不好，毛病就会加重。这样肯定不行。你帮我跟医生讲讲，不要减药，行吗？

Nurse: I understand how you feel. But the whole treatment process consists of many stages. At some point the dosage of the medicine will need to be reduced.

护士：你的心情我理解。但是，治疗是一个完整的过程，总有减药的时间。

Patient: I see. But it is not the right time, yet.

病人：我知道，但现在肯定不行。

Nurse: Your doctor knows about your condition very well. He adjusts your medicine according to your condition. You should trust your doctor.

护士：医生对你的病情很了解。这是根据你的病情进行的用药调整，你应该信任你的床位医生。

Patient: I do trust my doctor. But I don't know what to do if I cannot sleep well at night.

病人：我不是不相信医生，可万一减了药真的睡不着，那该怎么办？

Nurse: Don't worry, the nurse on duty at night will look after you. She will call the doctor on duty to give you medication if you can't fall a sleep. And she will report your situation to your doctor in detail the following morning. So what you should do now is to relax. As you know, your anxiety and nervousness will affect your sleep.

护士：你放心，晚上我们的值班护士会定时巡视病房。如果你真的睡不着，她会联系值班医生给你酌情用药，第二天护士也会向你的床位医生做详细汇报。所以，现在你要做的是放松自己。要知道，你紧张焦虑的情绪反而会严重影响你晚上的睡眠。

Patient: I feel a little better now after your explanation.

病人：听你这么一解释，我现在放心一点了。

Nurse: Great. Let's take a walk to relax some.

护士：那太好了。我带你出去散步，放松一下。

Patient: OK and thanks.

病人：好的。谢谢你。

# 86. Sleep Pattern Disturbance

# 睡眠型态紊乱

Nurse: You look very sad. I know there are no words that can comfort you. Since we are alone, may be you'd like to tell me what happened. This may make you feel better.

护士：看得出，你现在很伤心。我知道此时任何安慰的话都是多余的。现在只有我们两个人，你可以把你的伤心事说出来，这样也许会舒服一点。

Patient: I feel very sad. We have been married for more than ten years and I never thought he would do such a thing. I have decided to get a divorce. But it is not what I really want. I have done so much for our family.

病人：我真的很伤心，十多年的夫妻，想不到他会这么对我，我决定离婚。但我还是不甘心，我为这个家付出的太多了。

Nurse: Anyone would feel sad if they were in the same situation as you. But it is useless to be sad. The key is what you decide to do.

护士：遇到这样的事情，每个人都会难过。但事情已经发生了，伤心也于事无补。关键是你如何做决定。

Patient: We have a 12-year-old daughter. I can't stand to be separated from her. I hope I'll be granted the right to bring her up.

病人：我有一个 12 岁的女儿，我舍不得离开她，我想争取女儿的抚养权。

Nurse: Do you think you have the ability to bring your daughter up by yourself now?

护士：那你觉得像你现在的情况，有能力抚养女儿吗？

(The patient was silent.)

（病人沉默。）

Nurse: So you must brace up for your daughter. Since you have decided to divorce your husband, you should make a plan for your future. But above all, you should have good health and a stable job. Do you agree?

护士：所以，为了女儿，你一定要振作起来。既然你已经做出了离婚的决定，我觉得现在你该静下心来计划一下未来的日子。但前提是你要有一个健康的身体，有一份稳定的工作。你说对吗？

Patient: Yes. For my daughter's sake, I must step out of the shadow as quickly as possible.

病人：你说得对，为了女儿，我也该尽快从这个阴影中走出来。

Nurse: The first thing you should do now is to have a good sleep. Would you like to have some medicine to help you sleep?

护士： 你现在首先要做的就是睡个好觉。要不要服一些药帮助你睡眠？

Patient: No. I feel much better after talking with you. I will try to sleep by myself without the medicine. Thank you.

病人： 经你这么一讲，我觉得好多了。我想自己试着睡，谢谢你。

# 87. Anorexia Nervosa

# 神经性厌食

Patient: What's wrong with me?

病人：我到底得了什么病？

Nurse: You are suffering from Anorexia Nervosa?

护士：你患的是"神经性厌食症"。

Patient: Can I recover from this disease?

病人：这病能治好么？

Nurse: Sure. But we need your cooperation.

护士：当然能看好，但需要你的配合。

Patient: I'm so regretful now. In order to keep my pretty figure, I reduced my eating intentionally. Sometimes I even induced vomiting after I ate. Gradually I did not want to eat anything, and had an upset stomach when I see the food. Now my menstruation has stopped. I can't even look after myself. It is my own fault.

病人：现在我真的很后悔。当初为了保持自己漂亮的身材，每天都刻意减少自己的进食量，有时甚至在饭后采用自我催吐法将食物呕出。慢慢的就开始吃不下东西了，而且见到吃的东西就难受。现在甚至出现了闭经，生活都不能自理，都怨我自己。

Nurse: Everybody loves a beautiful figure. You have stepped in a vicious circle just like lots of other girls who try to limit their eating to reduce their weight. But now you are aware of the importance of health. Actually, you can depend on exercises to keep your figure. Exercise is good for both your health and your figure. Restricting eating alone will not keep your beautiful figure effectively and it will ruin your health. It is not worth while.

护士："爱美之心，人皆有之"，像你这样拼命节食减肥的女孩不少。你像其他人一样，步入了减肥的误区。现在你已经意识到了健康的重要性，为时不晚呀。实际上要保持良好的身材，可以通过运动来达到，这样既锻炼了身体，又保持了健美的体型。如果只是一味地采取极端节食的话，不仅不能有效地保持自己健美的体型，反而还会损害自己的健康，得不偿失。

Patient: Right. Now I worry about my health very much. I forced myself to eat more. But it didn't work. What should I do?

病人：是啊，我现在最担心的就是自己的健康，强迫自己多吃点，但是吃不下去。我该怎么办呢？

Nurse: First, you should be optimistic and accept the various treatments from your doctor.

Second, you are in severe malnutrition now, it is not good for you to eat large amount of food suddenly because your gastrointestinal function has been disturbed due to long period of restricted eating. So take it easy. You should gradually increase the amount of food, eat less each time but eat more frequently. Third, gradually increase the amount of exercise, for example, from lifting your legs on the bed to having a short walk. In a word, be patient and trust yourself. I'm sure you will recover from your illness. Do you agree with me?

护士：首先你要保持良好的心态，积极配合医生的各项治疗。其次，目前你严重营养不良，而且因为长期过度节食，造成了你胃肠功能紊乱，如果突然之间大量进食，肯定会适得其反。所以千万不可操之过急，只能循序渐进，少食多餐，逐步增加进食量。在此基础上，再逐步增加运动量，如从在床上做简单运动伸伸腿开始，再到床下走动等。总之，不要着急，要慢慢来，对自己要有信心。我相信你会慢慢地康复起来。你自己觉得呢？

Patient: I'll try my best.

病人：我听你的，我会努力的。

# 88. Impaired Social Interaction

# 社交障碍

Nurse： I sense you are very nervous and anxious now. You are looking down and rubbing your hands.

护士： 从你现在低垂的眼神和不停搓手的举动中，我能感觉到你面对我时的紧张不安。

Patient： (still looking down) I don't know. I'm afraid of communicating with women, especially young ladies. I have palpitations, dyspnea, and choking. I dare not look at you.

病人： (没抬眼)我也不知道。反正特别怕与女性接触，特别是年轻的，我会心慌、胸闷、透不过气来，我不敢看你。

Nurse： I can understand your pain and struggle. If I were you, I probably would have the same feelings. I have a son who is not much younger than you. Can you try looking at me so we can get acquainted better?

护士： 你内心的痛苦和挣扎我能理解。如果我是你，处在这样的境况下，可能也会和你一样的。我的孩子比你小不了几岁。你能看一看我，彼此熟悉一下吗？

(The patient looked at the nurse quickly, and then looked down again.)

(病人眼神在护士身上很快掠过，又低垂了下去。)

Nurse： How do you feel?

护士： 感觉怎么样？

Patient： Nervous. I am afraid to look at you.

病人： 紧张，不敢看。

Nurse： I'm your nurse. You will see me everyday. I'm glad you took the first step for treatment today. We can communicate with each other in an orderly way, step by step. Don't worry. This strategy should not make you very uncomfortable. Every day, you should find that you have made some progress. Do you have the will to fight your condition with us?

护士： 我是你的床位护士，以后你每天都会见到我。事实上，今天你已经勇敢地跨出了第一步，我很高兴我们可以试着采用循序渐进的接触方式。请放心，这种接触方式不会使你太难受。每次只要像今天这样进步一点点就行。我想知道你愿意和我们一起与病魔做斗争吗？

Patient： I trust you. I know you want to help me. I hope I can learn to communicate with women just like other men. But I'm not sure if I will succeed.

病人：我信任你们，知道你们是在帮助我。我也非常希望自己能够正常地与异性交往。但是我担心我做不到。

Nurse: Don't worry. We will make a plan for you according to the principles of systematic desensitization therapy. It will not be very hard for you. I hope you can accept my suggestion.

护士：不用担心，我们将按照"系统脱敏"的原则，为你制订相应的计划。相信不会有太大的难度，希望你能接受我的建议。

Patient: OK. I will cooperate.

病人：好吧，我会好好配合的。

# 89. Counseling an Agitated Patient

# 急躁病人的疏导

Nurse: Mr. Zhang, you've been using the oxygen for two hours. Are you feeling any better?

护士：张先生，你已经吸了两小时的氧气，感觉舒服一点吗？

Patient: No. I still feel suffocated and uncomfortable. The main reason is that the flow rate of the oxygen is too low, and you are not willing to let me increase it.

病人：不舒服。仍然感觉到憋气、难受。主要是你氧气流量开得太小了，是你们舍不得给我吸氧吧。

Nurse: Mr. Zhang, the flow rate of the oxygen is right for you. You are an elderly person. If the oxygen flows too fast, it might cause carbon dioxide retention. You see, the color of your lips and fingers has turned pink and your respiration is calm. It seems you're better now.

护士：张先生，开得正合适啊。你年纪大了，氧气流量开得太大后要引起二氧化碳潴留的。你的嘴唇和指甲红润多了，呼吸也平稳了，看上去好多了。

Patient: Who's sick here? You or I? When I say I don't feel well, I don't feel well. Go and find a doctor. Your attitude is very poor.

病人：是谁生病？你还是我？我感觉不好就是不好。快去找医生来。你的服务态度真不好。

Nurse: Mr. Zhang, I'm sorry I made you angry. I'll ask the doctor to come over at once.

护士：张先生，对不起，惹你生气了。你别着急，我马上去请医生来。

(After examining the patient, the doctor determined that his condition was stable. Because of the nervous and irritable state of the patient, the nurse suggested to give him a placebo.)

（医生检查后，认为病情已趋向稳定。鉴于病人的紧张、急躁状态，护士建议给予其安慰剂。）

Nurse: Mr. Zhang, the doctor has examined you. He thinks you're better now even though you still don't feel well. Please take this medicine to alleviate your symptoms.

护士：张先生，医生检查了，觉得你虽然还感觉不舒服，但已有好转。请你再服下这些药，使胸闷的情况得到改善。

Patient: More medicine? My medical bill will increase.

病人：又服药，医药费又增加了。

Nurse: (helped him to take the pills and changed the subject) you are eating and sleeping better these days.

护士：（帮助服药，有意岔开题）这几天你胃口好多了，晚上睡眠也好。

Patient: It makes no difference. My illness keeps coming back. It won't go away.

病人：好有什么用。这病还不是过一阵子又发，好不了。

Nurse: Please don't worry. Being stressed is bad for your recovery. Getting angry or upset will stimulate the vague nerve and cause your bronchial muscles to contract, which will increase the resistance of the air flow. It might cause your illness to recur.

护士：不要着急，心情烦躁对治疗不利。生气、发脾气会使迷走神经兴奋，使支气管平滑肌收缩而增加气流阻力。这样容易使疾病复发。

Patient: Are you implying I have a bad temper?

病人：你是说我脾气不好？

Nurse: I'm saying that your attitude is pessimistic and you don't have confidence in your treatment. When you get better and are discharged from the hospital, you should begin exercising to strengthen your immune system, avoid catching cold, and comply with your treatment. All of these will help you to prevent the recurrence of your disease.

护士：我是说你有些悲观，对自己的治疗缺乏信心。等这次病愈出院后，你一定要进行适当的体育锻炼，增强体质，预防感冒，坚持治疗。这样才能有效地防止再次发病。

Patient: It's no use.(Sighing)

病人：没用的(唉)!

Nurse: You look tired. Have some rest. I'll come back later. Please call me whenever you do not feel well.

护士：你累了，休息会儿吧。我过一会儿再来看你。有事请呼我。

# 90. Re-establishing Self-confidence (Traffic Accident)

# 信心重建(车祸)

Nurse: How are you? We understand how you feel and are very sorry.

护士: 你的心情我们非常理解，也为你的意外遭遇感到痛心。

(Patient was crying, silent, in a very sad mood.)

(病人哭泣、无语、沉浸在悲痛中。)

Nurse: (firmly holding the patient's right hand) You must take good care of yourself. We have arranged everything for your family and all you need to do is stay here for the treatment.

护士: (紧紧握住病人的右手)你一定要保重。家里的事情大家都安排好了，你尽管在这里安心治疗。

Patient: What meaning does my life have? (Rushed toward the window madly.)

病人: 我活着还有什么意思！(疯一样地向窗口冲去。)

Nurse: Hold her! (The patient was held back to her bed.) Don't do that. Be calm, close your eyes, and try to relax. You need to be brave. If you end your life, what will happen to your husband? He needs you.

护士: 赶快抱住她！(大家一起把病人抱回了床上。)不要这样，你先安静一下，闭上眼睛放松一会儿。事已至此，你一定要勇敢地面对现实。如果你不想活下去了，那你的丈夫怎么办呢？他还等你去照顾呢！

(The patient weeping.)

(病人默默地流泪。)

Nurse: You must be strong, cooperate with the treatment, and try to recover soon. We will arrange for you to visit your husband when his condition permits.

护士: 所以你一定要坚强点，好好地配合治疗，争取早日康复。等你丈夫病情允许了，我们会安排你去看看他的。

Patient: (getting up again) I need to go to the toilet.

病人: (又一次起床)我要上厕所。

Nurse: (worrying that she may have an accident in the restroom) This is the bedpan; you can use it on your bed.

护士: (担心她在厕所发生意外)我给你便盆，你就在床上解吧。

Patient: No, I can't urinate on the bed. Let me go to the toilet.

病人: 不行，我解不出来，我要上厕所。

Nurse: Don't worry.(turning towards her visiting relatives and friends) Everybody, please wait outside the room. Let me help you.(The nurse helped her loosen her trousers and the patient sat on the bedpan.) Don't rush. I will let you listen to the sound of running water. I am sure you can do it yourself. Since you will have to use bedpan after the operation, this is a good opportunity for you to practice it now.(A few minutes later, the patient had used bedpan successfully.) Well done, you must follow our guidance and cooperate with us.

护士: 别着急。(对来访的亲戚和朋友说)请大家到病房外面等候。我来帮助你。(帮病人解裤子,病人坐上便盆)慢慢来,我给你听流水的声音,你一定会自己解出来的。你手术后也要在床上大小便的,所以现在正好练习一下。(几分钟后病人在床上顺利解了小便。)不是很好吗?你一定要和我们合作。

Patient: I want to see my husband.

病人: 我想去看看我丈夫。

Nurse: Don't worry about him. The doctors in the ICU will do their best to help him. Besides, you cannot get there by yourself.

护士: 你放心,ICU的医生会尽力帮助他的。而且你现在这样去行吗?

(The patient looked at her wounds and said nothing.)

(病人看看自己的伤,不语。)

Nurse: You were also hurt and have bone fractures. Only after surgery and recovery from your wounds can you accompany your husband.

护士: 你也受伤了,骨头都断了。只有早日康复,才能陪伴你的丈夫。

Patient: (Calmed down) OK, II will cooperate with you.

病人: (平静了许多)好吧,我会配合的。

Nurse: OK, now let me begin the preoperative preparations for you.

护士: 那么我来给你做手术前准备吧。

# 91. Rehabilitation (Traffic Accident)

# 康复(车祸)

Nurse： Miss Shen, you are recovering so fast, how come you are unhappy? (The patient kept silent, both her eyes still closed. The trembling upper eyelids indicated that she had heard the words of the nurse.)

护士： 小沈，你恢复得很快，为什么不开心呢？（病人沉默，双眼继续合着。抖动的眼皮表明她已经听到了护士的话。）

Nurse： Can you tell me the reason why you are not happy today? Maybe I can help you solve the problem. Depression is not good to your health, and will affect your recovery. (The nurse goes on asking with gentle voice.)

护士： 你能告诉我今天不开心的原因吗？或许阿姨能帮你解决问题。闷在心里不利于健康，更会影响你的恢复。（继续轻声问。）

(The patient opened her eyes. The nurse held her hands tightly to encourage her and to build up her confidence. Miss Shen signaled her father to bring the paper and pen, and wrote down the following with her trembling hand, "Did I have a car accident? Why I can not say a word? I will fall behind on my school work.")

（病人半信半疑地睁开眼睛，护士紧紧握了一下小沈的手，以传递更多的力量，给她树立信心。小沈示意爸爸拿来了纸和笔，用颤抖的手虚弱地写下：我是不是发生车祸了？我为什么不能发出声音了？我的学习要跟不上了！）

Nurse： Yes, you had a car accident. But because of your strong will, your life has not suffered too much. You cannot say a word, because we just removed the trachea tube. Once you overcome the psychological barrier and stop refusing to talk, your voice will become louder day by day if you continue to practice talking. You are a smart girl. You don't need to worry about your study. A healthy body is the foundation for study. You can do more things if you are healthy. Therefore, you'd better dispel any misgivings now, have a good rest. And try to be discharged from the hospital early.

护士： 是的，你是经历了一次车祸，但因为你的坚强，你的生命没有受到什么影响。你说话暂时不能发出声音是因为我们刚为你拔除了气管套管，只要你能克服因无声而拒绝说话的心理障碍，坚持每天说话你会发现声音会一天比一天响亮。你是个聪明的孩子，所以学习更不用担心了，健康是学习的资本，有了健康的身体才能做更多的事情。所以现在你要抛开一切顾虑，把身体养好，争取早日出院。

Patient: (grinned, put down the paper and pen, and managed to say) Thanks!

病人：(咧开嘴笑了，她丢下纸和笔，使劲地说)谢谢。

# 92. Gingivitis

# 牙龈炎

Patient: Nurse, my gums bleed when I brush my teeth. I don't know why.

病人：护士，我刷牙时牙龈出血，不知道是什么原因。

Nurse: How long has it been like this?

护士：这种情况有多长时间了？

Patient: For about five months.

病人：大约有5个月了。

Nurse: Open your mouth. Let me have a look. There are a lot of dental calculus and odontolith on your teeth. They can stimulate the edge of the gums and cause inflammation and bleeding of the gums.

护士：张开嘴，让我看看。您的牙齿上有很多牙垢和牙石，它们会刺激牙龈的边缘而引起牙龈发炎和出血。

Patient: What are dental calculus and odontolith?

病人：什么是牙垢和牙石？

Nurse: The dental calculus is the soft calculus on the surface of teeth or at the edge of gums. It appears yellow or grey. It's soft and easy to remove. The odontolith is the hard calcified or calcifying lump which is mainly formed by dental plaque. It's difficult to remove.

护士：牙垢是附在牙齿表面和根缘处的软垢，呈黄色或灰白色，较软，易除去。牙石是附在牙面上的钙化或正在钙化的牙菌斑为基质的团块，不易除去。

Patient: How do you remove the dental calculus and odontolith?

病人：怎样除去牙垢和牙石呢？

Nurse: The dentists can do it. They remove them with a special instrument or an ultrasonic scaler.

护士：牙医可以做到。他们用一种特殊的器具或超声波洁牙器来除去牙垢和牙石。

Patient: That's wonderful. Could you please tell me more about ultrasonic scaler.

病人：那太好了。您能再告诉我一些超声波洁牙的知识吗？

Nurse: Ultrasonic curettage is an effective method of debridement of the soft tissue walls of periodontal pockets. Histological studies of tissue excised after curettage have shown that healing occurs by epithelialization of the sulculus surface and resolution of inflammation in the gingival corium. The ultrasonic technique is equally as effective as conventional hand instrumentation in calculus removal, but less effective in stain removal. Of course it is more rapid than hand instrumentation.

护士：超声波刮治术是一种清扫牙周袋软组织壁的有效方法。刮治后的组织学研究表明：龈沟和牙龈真皮内炎症得到消除。超声波技术清除牙石的作用与常规的手持器械同样有效，但除去色斑的效能较差，当然速度快得多。

Patient: Have you found any side effects?

病人：你们发现它有副作用吗？

Nurse: No.

护士：没有。

Patient: Can we prevent dental calculus and odontolith?

病人：牙垢和牙石可以预防吗？

Nurse: The most important thing is to pay more attention to dental hygiene. Especially you should learn to brush your teeth correctly.

护士：最重要的是注意口腔卫生，尤其是学会正确地刷牙。

Patient: I brush them horizontally.

病人：我横着刷牙。

Nurse: That's a wrong way. The correct way is to brush them up and down. To brush them horizontally may rub all the natural enamel off. I think it is also very important to select a suitable toothbrush, The head of the toothbrush should not be too long or too short. For adults, the length of the head of the brush is not more than 35 mm, and the width is not more than 13 mm. For children, the length is not more than 28 mm; the width is not more than 11 mm. For infants, the length is ont more than 25 mm; the width is not more than 8 mm.

护士：那是错误的方法。正确的方法是上下刷。横着刷可能破坏珐琅质。我认为选择一把合适的牙刷也是很重要的。牙刷头不可过长或过短。成年人刷头长度不超过 35 毫米，宽不超过 13 毫米。儿童，长度不超过 28 毫米，宽不超过 11 毫米。幼儿，长度不超 25 毫米，宽不超过 8 毫米。

Patient: I have learned a lot. Thank you very much.

病人：我知道许多知识。谢谢您。

Nurse: Not at all.

护士：不客气。

Patient: I want to have my teeth cleaned. Could you make an appoinment for me?

病人：我想洗牙，您能给我约个时间吗？

Nurse: A11 right. The dentist has got rather a full day tomorrow; you can come here at 10 a.m. the day after tomorrow.

护士：好吧。医生明天已经排满了。您可以后天上午 10 点来。

Patient: All right. Good bye.

病人：好吧，再见。

Nurse: Good bye.

护士：再见。

# 93. Epistaxis

# 鼻出血

Patient: My nose is bleeding.

病人: 我的鼻子出血了。

Nurse: Does it bleed often?

护士: 是否常常出血?

Patient: Several times a day.

病人: 一天要出几次。

Nurse: What have you done about it?

护士: 你是怎样处理的?

Patient: I came to see the doctor yesterday. He inserted a little cotton ball in my nose. It stopped the bleeding then. But when I went home, it started all over again.

病人: 我昨天来看过医生。他给我塞了一点棉球,后来就停止了,但我回家以后,又出血了。

Nurse: I see. Did the doctor take your blood pressure?

护士: 医生给你量过血压吗?

Patient: Yes. He told me it was normal.

病人: 量过。他告诉我我的血压正常。

Nurse: The doctor would likely want to have your blood tested and then examine your nose to find out the cause of the bleeding. After that he will prescribe some treatment for you.

护士: 医生希望你查查血,然后给你检查鼻子,找出出血原因后再给你处理。

# 94. Glaucoma

# 青光眼

Patient: Miss Wang, I will be discharged soon. You have helped me applying eye drops in the hospital. What shall I go back home?

病人：护士长，我要出院了。在医院里都是你们帮我滴眼药水，回去后我应该怎么做？

Nurse: Don't worry. I'm just about to talk to you about that. In general, the eye drops such as Pilocarpine and Timolol are used to reduce the intra-ocular pressure. When you use them, you should wash your hands first, and then check the eye drop. You should then use a cotton swab to pull open your lower eyelid gently and drip one to two drops of the eye medication into the lower vault, then use the dry cotton swab to wipe away the overflowed drops. When using the Pilocarpine, you need to press the area of dacryocyst two to three minutes after dropping to avoid the eye drops flow into the nasal cavity by the lacrimal duct and causing toxic effects. In addition, there should be an interval of five to ten minutes between applying the two kinds of eye drops.

护士：你不要着急，我正要和你谈谈呢。一般降眼压的药水有皮罗卡品眼液、噻吗心胺眼液。你滴的时候要先洗手，检查眼液，用棉签轻轻拉开下眼睑将药液滴入下穹隆一两滴，然后用干棉签拭去溢出的药液，如果滴皮罗卡品，滴完后用干棉签按压泪囊区两三分钟，以免药液经泪道流入鼻腔吸收引起中毒。另外，滴完一种眼液应间隔 5～10 分钟后再滴另一种眼液。

Patient: Oh, I see. I used to apply all the eye drops into my eyes at once. No wonder a lot of the eye drops overflowed every time.

病人：哦，原来要这样做，以前我都是一下子把所有药水全滴进去，难怪每次滴药液都要流出很多。

Nurse: Yes, because your left eye has not been operated, you should continue to use the eye drops. When you get back home, you should keep in a cheerful mood. Bad temper can induce glaucoma. So you must overcome it.

护士：是的，而且你的左眼还没手术，所以也要坚持用药。回去后要保持心情愉快。你的脾气太急，容易诱发青光眼发作，应该要克制。

Patient: I know that, but it is difficult for me to control my temper. What else should I pay attention to?

病人：这我也知道，但就是改不了。还要注意什么？

Nurse: About diet, you should eat more vegetables and fruits and maintain the free movement of the bowels. Do not drink more than 300 ml of water each time and don't drink strong tea or coffee. All these can prevent high intra-ocular pressure. In addition, you should come to the hospital to check your intra-ocular pressure regularly.

护士：饮食方面呢，要多吃蔬菜水果，保持大便通畅，每次喝水不超过 300ml，少喝浓茶和咖啡，这都是防止眼压升高的措施。另外要定期到医院来查眼压。

Patient: Now I know what I should do after your instruction. Thank you.

病人：听你这么一说，我知道应该怎么做了，谢谢你。

# 95. Retinal Detachment

# 视网膜脱离

Nurse: Good morning, Mr. Ni. The operation will be tomorrow. I will go over with you a few things to prepare for the operation and to tell you what you need to know after the operation.

护士：倪先生，你好！明天就要做手术了，现在我要为你做术前准备，并告诉你手术后的一些注意事项。

Patient: Oh, that's fine. Thank you. The doctor had told me about the procedures of the surgery when making his round this morning. He said the operation will have certain difficulties and risks, so I am worried about the operation.

病人：哦，好的，谢谢你。今天早晨查房时医生已告诉我手术的方法，而且说手术有一定的难度和风险，所以我很担心手术后的效果。

Nurse: It is right for the doctor to inform you of the difficulties and risks about this operation. Although the operation is more complicated, may lasts a little longer, and only a few hospitals can do it, you don't have to worry. Our department has been doing this operation for some time. A lot of patients have had this operation and the results were very good. However, it is intently interrelated to you whether the operation will be successful of not.

护士：医生和你讲清楚手术的难度和风险是对的。这种手术比较复杂，手术时间也较长，开展这种手术的医院也不是很多。但是你放心，我们科开展这种手术已有一段时间，手术做得较多，效果也不错。只是手术的成败与你密切相关。

Patient: Oh, what should I do?

病人：噢，那我该怎么做呢？

Nurse: The doctor will inject some special kind of oil into your eye during the operation. This will reduce your retina problem. You should maintain on the "prone position" or the "lowering your head sit-up position" for about two weeks after the operation. It will be very tiring to keep this position continually. So you may want to practice now to get used to it.

护士：手术的时候，医生会往你的眼睛里注射一种特殊的油，这种油注射后使你的视网膜能够复位。手术后要采取俯卧或低头坐位持续两周，一直保持这样的位置是很累的，所以，你现在可以先试着感受一下，有一个适应的过程。

Patient: I used to sleep on my side. It will be hard for me to sleep on prone position for two weeks. But I'll try it because it is for me to recover my vision early. I will do my best.

病人： 平时我习惯侧睡，现在要我趴在床上睡两个星期真的很难受的。我可以先试着练练，想到这是为了视力早点恢复，我会尽力适应的。

Nurse： Great fellow. We will assist you to the best of our ability. In addition，you need to eat more vegetables and fruits that have more coarse fibers，drink more water but small amount each time，maintain the free bowel movement，and do not push too hard when you go.

护士： 真是好样的，我们会尽量帮助你的。另外，术后要多吃粗纤维的蔬菜和水果，少量多次饮水，保持大便通畅，不能用力屏气。

Patient： Oh，are these all related to the recovery too?

病人： 哦，这也与治病有关系吗？

Nurse： Yes，it is very important. After the operation，your detached retina is slowly recovering. However，if you push too hard while having a bowel movement，the retina will become detached again. This will make the operation in vain.

护士： 关系大着呢。术后你脱下的视网膜正慢慢恢复，你大便时太用力，视网膜就会再次脱落，那样手术就白做了。

Patient： Oh，I see. Are there any other things I need to pay attention to?

病人： 原来是这样。那还有要注意的吗？

Nurse： After the operation，you should talk as little as possible and don't laugh too hard. In addition，you can't do any sports or heavy physical labor. So you must give up playing your favored soccer game for a while.

护士： 手术后尽量少讲话，也不要大笑。另外出院后，一段时间内也不能运动或做重体力劳动，更不能踢足球，所以你的足球瘾要戒了。

Patient： It seems that I have to stop doing what I love to do for my eye. I know now what I should do after the operation. Thanks for your instruction.

病人： 看来为了眼睛我只能忍痛割爱了。听你这么一讲我知道手术后应该怎么做了。

Nurse： Okay，now I will help you to cut your eyelash. If you have any questions，please ask me at any time.

护士： 好的，现在我来帮你剪掉睫毛。如果你还有什么问题随时问我。

# 96. Foreign Body in Trachea

# 气管异物

Nurse: Bingbing, what are you eating? Can I have a look?

护士：兵兵，在吃什么好东西呀，给阿姨看看。

Patient: Auntie, I am eating peanuts. It is delicious.

患儿：阿姨，我在吃花生，可好吃呢。

Nurse: (to Banging's mother) your son just had the operation yesterday. He should eat some soft foods. Don't you remember what caused his suffocation accident? It's the peanuts. Why do you let him eat peanuts again?

护士：(对兵兵的妈妈)孩子昨天刚刚手术，今天应该吃一点软的食品。而且他就是因为花生呛住了而手术，你为什么还要给他吃花生呢？

Patient's Mother: Kids in our village are all fond of peanuts. He will keep crying if he does not get some.

患儿妈妈：我们农村的小孩都喜欢吃花生米，不给他吃，他要闹的。

Nurse: Your child is too young to eat hard foods such as peanuts, beans and melon seeds. Children younger than five year old, their laryngeal protection reflex is still under development. They are more likely to swallow the hard things into trachea than adults. Yesterday, your child would have been in great danger if you had come to the hospital later.

护士：孩子太小，像花生、豆子、瓜子一类的硬物不能给他吃。因为五岁以下的儿童喉的防御反射功能还不全，容易将硬的食物吸入气管。你们昨天幸亏及时来医院看病，要晚一点就会有危险了。

Patient's Mother: Really?! We didn't suppose it was so serious.

患儿妈妈：真的?！我们也没感觉到有什么危险。

Nurse: If the peanuts stuck in the trachea any longer, they would swell and stimulate the trachea, resulting in dyspnea and fever, even death when the trachea was blocked completely. We have seen a child already dead when he was brought to the hospital.

护士：花生在气管里的时间一长，就会膨胀，刺激气管引起呼吸困难、发热、严重堵塞气管时就有生命危险。以前我们就碰到过孩子送到医院已经死亡了。

Patient's Mother: It seems I should not give him peanuts any more.

患儿妈妈：看来以后不能给他吃花生了。

Nurse：Correct，but that is not enough. Laughing or crying should be avoided at meal time because it is more likely for the kids to swallow foreign objects into the trachea accidentally. In addition，they should not have small objects in their mouths，like pen cap，nails，and so on while playing.

护士：不光是不能吃花生一类东西，在吃饭的时候也不能逗笑或哭闹，因为哭闹的时候深吸气容易将异物吸入气管。另外小孩玩耍的时候嘴里也不能含小物品，像笔套、钉子等。

Patient's Mother：We had no idea about these things before. We always let the kids do as they wish. With your instruction，I will pay more attention from now on.

患儿妈妈：以前我们也不懂，孩子要怎样就怎样，听你这么一说以后要重视了。

Nurse：I hope you will tell other people in your village to avoid giving these dangerous foods to their kids，and to prevent the kids from laughing and crying at meal time. Here are some health education materials. You can read and scatter them to the people around you.

护士：你们回去后还要告诉周围的人，不要随便给小孩吃花生、瓜子等食物，也不要在吃饭的时候让孩子哭闹。我这里有一些宣传材料给你带回去。

Patient's Mother：Great. It's so nice of you for telling me so many things. Thank you very much.

患儿妈妈：好的，谢谢你告诉了我这么多知识。

Nurse：You are welcome.（To Bingbing）Bingbing，can you give the thing in your hands to your Mum? I will bring a big apple for you.

护士：不用谢。（对兵兵）兵兵，阿姨给你去拿苹果吃，把手里的东西给妈妈好吗？

Patient：Okay.

患儿：好的。

# 97. Laryngocarcinoma

# 喉癌

Nurse： Mr. Ma，the doctors have prepared your operation plan based on the results of your fiber-optic laryngoscope and biopsy. They believe that a total laryngectomy is the best option because recurrence and metastasis are likely to happen if only a partial laryngectomy is carried out.

护士： 马先生，你的手术方案是医生根据纤维喉镜及病理报告的情况来决定的。如果不做全喉切除，只单纯做半喉切除的话，容易复发和转移。

Patient： But after the operation，I will not be able to talk any more. How can I stand to be a mute person?

病人： 可是手术后我不能讲话，从此变成一个哑巴，这我怎么能接受？

Nurse： Yes. I can understand what losing vocal ability means to you. But it's necessary in order to save your life. I wish you can accept this fact. I will do my best to help you.

护士： 是的，我能想象手术后将永远丧失语言功能对你意味着什么。但是，这项手术是保全生命必须的。希望你能够接受这一现实，我会尽力帮助你的。

Patient： I'm not against the operation. I am a broad-minded man and a director in the factory enjoying talking to people. How can I work and live if I cannot talk any more?

病人： 我不是不愿手术。平时我是一个性格开朗的人，喜欢说话，在单位又是一个领导，不能说话你让我怎么生活、工作呢？

Nurse： We've treated many patients like you. They all live very well after their operations. And we have gathered plenty of experiences on post-operation communication. Before the operation，you should study to express yourself with sign language and get used to putting your thoughts on paper. After the operation，you should eat more nutritious foods to speed up healing the incision. Then you can receive the training of speaking with your esophagus or artificial larynx.

护士： 我们曾经遇到过许多和你一样的病人，他们现在都生活得很好。我们积累了一套完整的术后交流经验。手术之前，你先训练用固定的手势来代替说话，习惯把你的想法写在纸上。手术后要注意营养，让伤口尽快恢复。以后可以训练用食管发音或用人工喉发音。

Patient： Really?（Spoke with a smile and hopes appeared in his eyes.）

病人： 真的？（很惊喜，眼中有了一点希望。）

Nurse： Of course it's real. Do you know Li Wenhua，the Chinese cross-talk partner of Mr.

Jiang Kun? He suffered laryngocarcinoma, but after his operation, he mastered the esophageal vocal ability and went back to the stage.

护士：是真的，以前和姜昆一起说相声的李文华老师得的也是喉癌。手术后练习用食管发音，不照样能够重新登上舞台表演吗？

Patient: Oh, he also had this operation. I could see some hope after hearing your story.

病人：原来他也做过手术，听你这么一说，我倒有点希望了。

Nurse: What you should do is eating more and growing stronger to recover faster from the operation.

护士：你现在的问题是要多进食，把身体养好，使手术后的伤口尽快恢复。

Patient: Right, I will try my best to cooperate with you. Thank you.

病人：对对，我一定要好好配合你们，谢谢。

# 98. Systemic Lupus Erythematosus

# 系统性红斑狼疮

Nurse： Miss Zhang，how do you do? You seem depressed these days. I don't know what you are thinking. Can you tell me why? Let me share some of your pain.

护士： 小张，你好，这几天看你闷闷不乐，不知道你有什么想法，告诉我，让我来分担你的痛苦好吗？

（Miss Zhang kept silent.）

（小张保持沉默。）

Nurse： Miss Zhang，please think it over. You parents are so worried about you because you keep silent and refuse to eat anything. It is too much for them. In addition，you know one's mood will affect his immune function. Having bad mood for a long period of time will result in dysfunction of one's immune system. It might worsen your condition. Only when you can face your illness，can you recover quickly. Miss Zhang，please take your time and tell me about your feelings.

护士： 小张，你想一想，如今你整日不说话，什么也不吃，你的爹妈非常着急。这样不是让他们太操心了吗？再说，一个人的情绪会影响其免疫功能，长期不良的情绪会导致机体免疫功能紊乱，从而加重病情。你只有正确面对疾病，才能早日康复。小张，你能慢慢地将自己的想法告诉我吗？

Patient： OK. I have heard that persons with systemic lupus erythematosus must avoid sunlight，cannot get married nor bear children. Moreover this disease has no cure. It is like a fatal disease. That is why I am so sad.

病人： 那好，我听说得了系统性红斑狼疮，就不能见阳光，还不能结婚、生育，而且这病又治不好，等于得了绝症。你说我能不难过吗？

Nurse： I can understand your feelings. But systemic lupus erythematosus is not so terrible. Your disease is in the early stage and has not affected other organs. If you follow the doctor's order，take the medicines consistently，the disease will be controlled. You can get married; bear children，work and study like any other women. We have many patients with this kind of disease and some of them have had it for more than 20 years. They are fine now. So please believe us. As for avoiding the sunlight，it is because this disease is very sensitive to the light. You should try to avoid ultraviolet light，avoid exposing under the sun for too long; you can put on shirt，trousers，wear sunglasses and use an umbrella especially when you are out in the summer. Do not use alkaline soap and other chemicals such as hair-color agent and hair spray. Try not to eat mushrooms and celery, and so on.

护士： 你的想法我理解，但是系统性红斑狼疮并非如此可怕，而且你处于疾病早期，没有任何脏器的功能损害。只要你按照医嘱用药，等病情完全稳定以后，在医生的指导下，可以正常地生活，包括结婚、生育、工作和学习。我们以前收治过很多得这种病的病人，有的已经有20年左右的时间了，现在他们生活得都很好，因此你尽管相信我们。至于不能见阳光，主要是这种病对光敏感，只要避免紫外线的照射，避免长时间的接触阳光，尤其在夏天外出时，穿上长袖衫、长裤，戴上墨镜，用伞遮阳就可以了。在平时不用碱性肥皂、染发剂、头发定型剂等。饮食方面避免食用香菇、芹菜等。

Patient: Oh, I have also heard that taking Prednisone will make me fat.Is that true? If it is true, then I don't want to take it.

病人： 噢，那么我听说用泼尼松龙治疗以后人体会变得很胖、很难看，是吗？如果是真的，我不想用它。

Nurse: No. This steroid medication is the main drug for the treatment of systemic lupus erythematosus. Because you'd like to have children some day, we can not give you other immunosuppressive agents. The doctor will adjust your dosage of the Prednisone according to your condition. The side effect of the Prednisone, like moon face, is a temporary phenomenon. After reducing the dosage, the side effect will disappear gradually. You should not stop the medication or reduce the dosage by yourself for the concern of how you may look. Otherwise all your previous efforts will be wasted.

护士： 那可不行，激素是用来治疗系统性红斑狼疮的主要药物，考虑到你今后还要生育，所以不能用其他免疫控制剂。医生会根据你的病情逐步调整泼尼松龙的用量，用药以后出现的圆脸只是暂时现象，待减量后情况会逐渐好转。你可千万不能为了自己的容貌而自行减药或减量，否则会前功尽弃的。

Patient: I see. Thank you for your instructions.

病人： 知道了，谢谢你的指导。

Nurse: You are welcome. If you have any other questions, we can have another talk at any time.

护士： 没关系，以后你如果还有问题的话，我们随时进行交谈好吗？

Patient: Thanks again.

病人： 再次谢谢。

# 99. Thumb Reconstruction

# 拇指再造术

Head Nurse： What's the matter，Miss Chen? You have expected to have the operation as soon as possible，haven't you?

护士长： 小陈，你怎么啦？你不是一直希望早点动手术吗？

（Patient glimpsed the head nurse sadly，still kept silent.）

（病人还是未说话，只是用忧愁的眼睛看了一下护士长。）

Head Nurse： If there is something disturbing you，just tell me. Maybe I can give you a hand. If you don't tell me，then I can't help you.

护士长： 有什么烦心事说出来让我听听，或许我能帮助你。你要不说，我又怎么帮你呢？

Patient： I...（Hesitantly）

病人： 我……。（欲言又止）

Head Nurse： （watching her encouragingly）It is OK. Just think I am your big sister. Tell me what you are thinking，OK?

护士长： （用鼓励的目光看了看小陈）没关系，你就把我当你大姐，有什么说什么，好吗？

Patient： （nodding）I am so scared and worried about tomorrow's operation. I don't feel like doing it.

病人： （点了点头）想到明天真要做手术，我既害怕又担忧，所以我不想做了。

Head Nurse： I understand. What we should do now is to eliminate these psycholog-ical influences，not to avoid the surgery，so you can go home as soon as possible.

护士长： 我非常理解你此刻的心情，只是我们现在要做的是消除这些心理影响而不是逃避手术。这样你才能早日出院。

Patient： But，I still don't want to have this operation.

病人： 可是，我还是不想做手术。

Head Nurse： You must have the operation. Let me tell you the importance of your thumb.

护士长： 手术是肯定要做的。你可能还不知道人拇指的重要性吧？让我来跟你说说。

Patient： Oh.

病人： 哦。

Head Nurse： The thumb carries 50% of the functions of your hand. Without your thumb you can not grasp，pinch，and hold. You are still a young girl. You can not work，study well and live a happy life without your thumb. This is especially true since you are a right hand dominant person.

护士长：人的五个手指中，拇指的功能约占全手功能的一半以上，缺失了拇指将严重影响手的抓、捏、握功能。你还年轻，以后的工作、学习、生活都离不开手，何况，这还是你的右手呢！

Patient: (thinking, nodding, and relaxing a little bit) Will missing one toe affect walking after the operation?

病人：（若有所思地点了点头，表情有所舒展）那手术后少了一个脚趾头会不会影响走路呢？

Head Nurse: Don't worry. Walking relies mainly on the thenar and the heel. It should not have much effect on your walk without the second toe. Do you still have any worries?

护士长：这你不用担心，因为走路的着力点是在足底和足跟，没有第二足趾对行走是影响不大的。你还有什么担心吗？

Patient: I am afraid my operation will fail and I can not image the shape and the function of the constructed "thumb".

病人：我还担心手术会不会失败？手术后手指外形怎么样？功能又怎样？

Head Nurse: Take it easy. The success rate of this operation is more than 99% in our hospital and the chief surgeon will perform the operation for you. As to the shape and function of the reconstructed thumb, I can show you the other patients who have received this operation and will be discharged soon.

护士长：你别急。这类手术的成功率在我院是99%以上，而且手术是主任亲自为你做，你可以放心。至于外形和功能，请你起来，我带你到其他病房去看看那些就要出院病人的手指，你更会放心了。

Patient: (gladly) really?

病人：（一脸惊喜）真的吗？

Head Nurse: Of course.

护士长：当然。

(The head nurse talked with Miss Chen while walking. After twenty minutes, they came back to the ward.)

（一路上，护士长边走边和小陈谈心，20分钟后返回病房。）

Head Nurse: Can I do anything else for you?

护士长：小陈，现在还需要什么帮助吗？

Patient: (shyly) Nothing else. Thank you so much for your help.

病人：（害羞地）不需要了，真谢谢你的帮助。

Head Nurse: You are welcome. This is my duty. How do you feel now?

护士长：没关系，这是我应该做的。现在你心情怎么样？

Patient: (sincerely) Big sister, I feel much better. I really appreciate what you have done for me. Thank you very much. I feel confident about tomorrow's operation. I will listen to you to prepare well for the operation. I will eat and sleep well, and bravely accept tomorrow's surgery.

病人：（由衷地）大姐，好多了。真的非常感谢你。现在我对明天的手术充满了信心，我一定听你的话做好手术前准备，吃好睡好，勇敢地接受明天的手术。

Head Nurse：I hope you have a successful operation. I will come back to give you rehabilitation instructions after your operation.

护士长：祝你手术成功！手术后我还会来为你做术后康复指导的。

Patient：Thank you.

病人：谢谢你！

# 100. Coronary Artery Bypass Grafting

# 冠状动脉搭桥术

Nurse: Ms. Zhao, it has been six days since you had the operation. You have recovered well (smiling). But, it seems you have no bowel movement for several days. Do you feel uncomfortable?

护士：赵太太，你开刀到现在已经有6天了，恢复得挺好(微笑)。对了，你好像很多天没大便了，有什么不舒服吗？

Patient: Yes, I really want to go to the toilet. I've tried but failed because I'm afraid my incision might become ruptured.

病人：是的，我很想上厕所，可我试过，没成功，因为我怕伤口裂开。

Nurse: Ms. Zhao, CABG operation is the most effective method for the coronary artery disease. As for patients who have gone through the operation, you need to have a good rest and increased nutritional intake. At the same time you should maintain free bowel movement. When you go to the toilet, you should avoid pushing too hard because it can increase the burden on your heart. I can understand your misgivings. Your incision will heal completely in twelve days. Since it has been six days now and this morning we saw that your incision is healing very well, I think it will not be affected by normal defecate.

护士：赵太太，对于冠心病的治疗来说，冠状动脉搭桥术是效果最好的一种手术方式。手术以后病人需要做的就是好好休息，增加营养。另外也要保持大便通畅，防止大便时用力，因为这样会增加心脏负担。你的顾虑我能理解，不过这种伤口一般术后12天就能全部愈合。今天已经是第6天了，而且早上我们看过你的伤口，长得挺好的，我想它应该不会影响正常的排便。

Patient: That's good. But I have not been to the toilet for some days, I'm afraid I can not do it successfully.

病人：这样我就放心了，但我已经好几天没上厕所了，估计还是不能很顺利地解出。

Nurse: Don't worry, I can help you. How about letting me massage your abdomen now? It can stimulate the intestine's movement and promote defecating.

护士：别担心，让我来帮你，我先来给你按摩腹部好吗？它可以刺激肠蠕动，促进排便。

Patient: All right. Thank you.

病人：好的，谢谢。

Nurse: You haven't eaten vegetables and fruits these days, haven't you? (Speaking with a smile while massaging the patient.）

护士：你这些天不太敢吃蔬菜和水果是吗？（一边按摩一边微笑着说。）

Patient：Yes，how do you know? I used to eat many fruits and have regular bowel movement. But since the operation I dare not eat anything but rice and fish soup.

病人：是啊，你怎么知道的？以前我每天都是吃很多水果的，排便一直很正常。但是开完刀后就什么都不敢吃，每天都吃点米饭和鱼汤啊什么的。

Nurse：No wonder your skin is so nice. There are lots of vitamins and fiber in fruits and vegetables. Vitamin is beneficial to your body and skin，and fiber is beneficial for bowel movement. The heart operation has nothing to do with your gastrointestinal tract. So don't worry. How about having a banana now?

护士：难怪你的皮肤这么好！很多水果和蔬菜都含有很多的维生素和纤维素。维生素对身体包括皮肤都有好处，纤维素则可以帮助排便。比如：香蕉、芹菜、竹笋等。心脏手术跟胃肠道没什么关系，不用担心，现在吃根香蕉好不好？

Patient：OK（smiling）.Thanks.

病人：好（开心地笑），谢谢你。

Nurse：It's my pleasure（peeling a banana）.In order to keep free bowel movement，besides eating more fruits and vegetables rich of fiber，and massaging your abdomen，you should try to go to the toilet at same time every day to make it a habit. In addition，you need to come down from the bed and move around little more. It's good for your recovery.

护士：没关系。（给病人剥好香蕉。）为了保持排便通畅，除了多吃纤维素含量多的水果、蔬菜，按摩腹部之外，你还可以每天定时去厕所，养成习惯。另外，你也要适当下床活动，这对你的康复也是有好处的。

Patient：I see. I don't worry any more after your explanation. Thanks a lot.

病人：我知道了，听你这么一解释，我放心多了。谢谢你。

Nurse：You are welcome. I need to see another patient now，but I will see you later. You can ring me any time if you need me，and I will be right over.

护士：不用谢。现在我需要去看另一位病人，待会儿我再来看你，你如果有事就打铃，我会立刻过来的。

（Half an hour later，the nurse came to the bedside again.）

（半小时后护士再次来到床边）

Nurse：Ms. Zhao，how do your feel now?

护士：赵太太，现在感觉怎么样？

Patient：I just went to the toilet and had bowel movement. Your method is very effective.

病人：我刚刚去过卫生间了，你的方法真的很有效。

Nurse：Your gastrointestinal tract is pretty good and you are willing to cooperate with us，that is the reason you have achieved such a good result. You see，your temperature have been normal all this time，and other conditions are also stable. I believe you will recover soon.

护士：你的胃肠道本来就很好，而且你也很愿意配合，所以才会取得这么好的效果。你看，到现在你的体温一直正常，其他情况也都很稳定，一定很快就会康复的。

Patient：Thank you very much，Miss Liu.

病人：太谢谢你了，小刘。

# 101. Heart Valve Replacement

# 换瓣术

Nurse: Teacher Ma，did you sleep well last night?

护士：马老师，昨晚睡得好吗？

Patient: Don't even mention it! I don't feel well at night these days，and I always hear the"dong，dong"sound of my heart. Is there something wrong with my new valve?

病人：哎，别提了！这几天晚上，我一直感觉不好，总是听到咚咚的心跳声。是不是我新换的瓣膜出了什么问题？

Nurse: Teacher Ma，you don't need to worry too much about that. Your new valve is a mechanical one from abroad. The sounds you heard are from the metal sound of heart beat which is normal. You'll become used to it.

护士：马老师，你多虑了。因为你换的是机械瓣，而且是进口的，这种声音是心跳时发出的金属碰撞声，是正常现象，不必介意。你会慢慢适应的。

Patient: Oh，I see，I feel much better after your explanation. I'll leave the hospital the day after tomorrow. Is there anything else I should pay attention to after I leave the hospital?

病人：噢，原来这样。听你这么一说，我感觉放心多了。后天我就要出院了，回家后，我还应注意些什么？

Nurse: Teacher Ma，after leaving the hospital，make sure that whenever you feel your heart is beating irregularly or you get a new health problem，you should rest and see a doctor nearby right away to find out the cause and to get the proper treatment. It's rare that the artificial valve becomes dysfunctional. But as soon as the valve dysfunction is confirmed，please call us immediate so we can figure out the proper treatment plan for you. Our department telephone number is 65223637-8110.

护士：马老师，出院后，你自己要经常注意：当你发现自己的心跳不整齐或突然出现新的健康问题时，应马上休息，就近就医，寻找原因，对症治疗。一般瓣膜失灵是极少见的，但也要提高警惕，一旦证实为失灵，应及时与我科联系，研究治疗方案。我科的电话号码是65223637-8110。

Patient: When can I return to my job?

病人：那我什么时候可以恢复工作？

Nurse: In general，three moths after the operation，depending on your physical condition，you can get some indoor and outdoor exercises. You should，according to your capability，proceed in an orderly way and step by step so that you do not feel palpitation and short of breath. Between three to six months after the operation, according to your heart function and physical condition, you can do some light work for half a day, and rest for half a day.After six months you can resume to full-time work, gradually from light work to normal work.

护士：一般手术后 3 个月内，根据你的体力情况，可适当进行室内和室外活动，量力而行、循序渐进，以自己不感到心慌、气短为度。术后 3～6 个月，可根据你的心功能、体力等考虑半天轻工作，半天休息。术后 6 个月，可以恢复全天工作，由轻工作逐步过渡到正常工作。

Patient: In addition to these, do I need to pay attention to my diet?

病人：除了注意这些外，在饮食上要不要忌口？

Nurse: After the heart valve replacement operation, your have to take anticoagulant drugs such us Warfarin the rest of your life. Some foods such as spinach, cabbage, cauliflower, carrot, tomato, potato, pork liver and so on, which have high content of vitamin K, may reduce the effect of this drug, so you should eat these foods as little as possible.

护士：行置换机械瓣膜者需终身服用抗凝药物，如华法林。有些食物可减低药效，如维生素 K 含量较高的菠菜、白菜、菜花、胡萝卜、番茄、土豆、猪肝等，应尽量少吃，以免影响抗凝效果。

Patient: Thanks Miss Wang. I'll be careful after leaving the hospital. By the way, how often should I have my blood tested? Is it all right to have the test done in a local hospital?

病人：王护士，谢谢你。回家后，我一定多加注意。另外想问一下，我出院后查血要间隔多长时间，可以当地医院化验吗？

Nurse: Teacher Ma, you should have your blood tested every two weeks to make sure that your PT ranges from 24 seconds to 30 seconds and the activity of prothrombin is about 35%. Your doctor will adjust the dose of the anticoagulant according to your blood test result. You can have the test done in a local hospital if they are equipped. If your test result is abnormal, please contact us anytime, and we will adjust your dose according.

护士：噢，马老师，每隔两周还需到医院抽血化验凝血酶原时间及活动度，一般凝血酶原时间应保持在 24～30 秒，凝血酶原活动度在 35% 左右。医生会根据你每一次的化验结果适当调整抗凝药物的用量。当地医院如有条件的话，可以在当地化验。如果结果有不正常，请随时与我们联系，我们将为你进行抗凝药物量的调整。

Patient: I understand and thank you very much, Miss Wang.

病人：我明白了，十分感谢你，王护士。

Nurse: You are welcome. Whenever you have any questions, please call us any time, and we will follow you up by phone as well. I hope you have an early recovery.

护士：不用谢，平时你遇到问题可随时来电话咨询，我们也会打电话对你进行随访的，祝你早日康复。

# 102. Kidney Transplantation

# 肾移植

(1)

Nurse： Mr. Chen，congratulations on the successful operation.

护士： 小陈，祝贺你手术取得了成功。

（Mr. Chen tried to open his eyes.）

（小陈试着睁了一下双眼。）

Nurse： The operation is only the first step to the success of the transplantation. We will need your cooperation in the following steps，could you do that?

护士： 手术的成功只是移植的第一步。接下来的每一步，都需要得到你的配合，能做到吗？

Patient： Yes，I can.

病人： 能。

Nurse： Now，please extend your right leg and keep in the straight position.（The nurse helped Mr. Chen in placing his right leg.）Good，keep it like this. Please relax.

护士： 现在，请你右下肢保持外展伸直位。（护士扶着小陈的右腿）对，就这样，请放松。

Patient： Should I keep it in this position all the time?

病人： 需要一直保持这个姿势吗？

Nurse： No. But you should keep his position for two days. When you feel tired，you may move the leg，but you should avoid bending your thigh to prevent disturbing the blood supply to the transplanted kidney.

护士： 不。最好能坚持两天。如果累了，可以移动，但尽可能不要让大腿屈曲，以免影响移植肾的血液供应。

（During the first few hours after the operation，nurse Wu helped Mr.Chen to turn his body and bent his right lower limbs. His vital signs and other monitored parameters all appeared normal.）

（术后几小时内，护士小吴帮助小陈翻身，右小腿屈曲。病人生命体征各项监护指标都正常。）

(2)

Nurse： Good morning，I appreciate your cooperation. Have you passed any gas yet?

护士： 你好，非常感谢你的配合，你感觉肛门排气了吗？

Patient： Yes，I did. I feel hungry and I want something to eat.

病人： 是的。肚子里咕噜咕噜地在叫，很饿，想吃东西。

Nurse： You may eat now，but take it easy. Have some warm water first.（Mr.Chen drank 100 ml of water.）

护士： 现在可以进食了，但要慢慢地来，先喝口温开水。（小陈一口气喝了100ml。）

Patient： I have not drunk water like this since the beginning of the hemodialysis.

病人： 进行血液透析以来，我还没有这样畅快地喝过水。

Nurse： If you don’t feel any discomfort，you may start with a liquid diet form now on. Please do not take milk，sweet drinks or high fat liquid to avoid abdominal distension or diarrhea.

护士： 如果没有不适，就可以进流质饮食了。但请不要马上进牛奶、甜的及含油量高的流质，以免胀气与腹泻。

**（3）**

Nurse： Mr. Chen，you are recovering very well after the operation. You may go home in a few days.

护士： 小陈，手术后你恢复得很好。再过几天，你就可以回家了。

Patient： May I go home?

病人： 可以回家了？

Nurse： Yes. But you should keep taking your medicine，and continue cooperate with us on your diet，daily activities，and self-monitoring.

护士： 是的，但回家后，希望你能坚持服药，并在饮食、活动及自我监测等方面与我们配合。

Patient： I will keep taking the medicine. Just let me know which ones I should take.

病人： 服药能做到，你只要告诉我该服哪些药就行。

Nurse： I know you can do it well. You should also respect the timing for medication，come back to the hospital for the follow-up checks，monitor the drug level on a regular basis，and follow the instructions from the specialist to adjust the dosage of the immunosuppressive medication. Please be careful and never stop medication or take other medicines by yourself. You will also need to monitor you body temperature，blood pressure，urine quantity by yourself. Please see a doctor without any delay when you have temperature higher than 38℃，or a rising of the blood pressure，or an abrupt decrease of the urine.

护士： 我知道你行。但服药一定要遵守时间，并定期来院检查，定期监测药物浓度，听从专科医师的嘱咐调节免疫抑制剂的剂量，万万不能随便服药与停药。回家后需要你学会自己检测体温、血压、尿量。当体温高于38℃、血压增高或尿量突然减少，请及时就诊。

Patient： I don’t know how to measure blood pressure. What should I do?

病人： 我不会测血压，怎么办？

Nurse： Don’t worry. I am going to teach you now.

护士： 没关系，现在我来教你。

# 103. Lung Transplantation

# 肺移植

## （1）

Patient：I want to drink some water.

病人：我想喝水。

Nurse：Yes，I know how thirsty you are now. This is a normal phenomenon after the surgery and is also a required therapy. We're controlling the amount of fluid in your body，because the less water in your body，the lesser pulmonary edema and the better respiration.

护士：是的，我知道你现在很口渴，这是术后的正常现象，也正是治疗所需要的。我们在控制你体内的液体，水分越少，你的肺水肿程度就越轻，呼吸就会越好，越省力。

Patient：But I am so thirsty. My mouth is so dry.

病人：可是我真的很渴，嘴巴很干。

Nurse：OK，I will give you some water. You must follow a recovered patient，Mr. XX's example.（This person had the same lung transplantation surgery.）He endured the extreme thirst and recovered，because he believed his doctor who told him that the thirstier is the better for his recovery. I'm sure that you will put up with this difficulty too，right?

护士：我能让你喝一点点，但你一定要坚强，你应该像已经康复的XX病人那样（一个肺移植存活病人）。医生说了越干越好，他坚持了，康复了。我相信你也能克服这一点小小的困难，对不对？

Patient：Well，OK.

病人：嗯，好吧。

Nurse：Good，here is 20ml of water. Wet your mouth and lips.

护士：来喝下这20ml水，慢慢湿润你的嘴巴。

Patient：Thank you.

病人：谢谢。

Nurse：For a speedy recovery，you have to endure the difficulty for now. We have faith in you.

护士：忍耐暂时的痛苦，争取最快最好的康复，我们相信你。

Patient：I'll do my best.

病人： 我会好好配合。

**（2）**

Patient: I don't like to rinse my mouth again. The fluid tastes terrible.

病人： 我不想漱口，它的味道很不好。

Nurse: Well, that is Nystatin, I know it tastes bad, but it is very effective to control the mycete.

护士： 哦！这制霉菌素的确有些味道，但它对于霉菌的抑制作用是很好的。

Patient: But why do I have to rinse out every few hours? I didn't eat anything.

病人： 隔几个小时就漱口一次，我根本就没吃东西。

Nurse: Bacteria breed easily and quickly in the oral cavity and the trachea is close to the opening of the esophagus. It will cause lung infection if the bacteria in the mouth cavity enter the lungs. Therefore oral hygiene is very important.

护士： 我们的口腔很容易滋生细菌。气管与食管的开口很接近，如果口腔里的细菌进入肺部，就会引发肺部感染，所以口腔卫生是非常重要的。

Patient: Oh, I see.

病人： 哦。

Nurse: Don't worry. The other two gargle liquids aren't as bad as the Nystatin.　Try it, OK?

护士： 你放心，三种漱口液，只有制霉菌素味道不好，其他都不难闻，试试看。

Patient: It's sweet and has mint flavor.

病人： 是甜的，还有点儿薄荷味道。

**（3）**

Nurse: Mr. XX, the mask is used to help you breathe. You may experience some discomfort. You may feel that your nose and mouth are blocked from the outside air. But don't worry. The respirator will provide enough oxygen to you and it is absolutely safe.

护士： ××先生，现在我们使用面罩来帮助你呼吸，有些不舒服，你可能会觉得鼻子、嘴巴和外界空气隔开了，放心，呼吸机能够提供你足够的氧气，绝对保障你的安全。

（The patient nodded.）

（病人点头示意。）

Nurse: It is a great progress from the use of trachea incubation to the use of mask. Your condition has become better and better every day. Now you should work with the respirator and close your mouth during inhalation to avoid air from getting into your abdomen. Try it, OK?

护士： 从插管到使用面罩是一个很大的进步，情况一天比一天好，一定要有信心。现在你要配合好呼吸机，吸气时闭上嘴巴，这样空气就不会进入你的胃内，试试看！

（The patient tried.）

（病人试做。）

Nurse: Very good. The mask is tight, isn't it? This is because we want to make sure that the respirator will supply the most effective air flow to you. Certainly, we'll loose it intermittently.

护士： 很好！面罩很紧是吗？这是为了不漏气，保证呼吸机给你最有效的呼吸支持，当然我们会给你间断松开的。

（The patient nodded.）

（病人点头。）

Nurse： Please make gestures to show your need，OK? There's a bell next to your right hand. Fell it! You can ring it when you feel uncomfortable.

护士： 有什么需要做手势告诉我们，好吗？右手边有个铃铛，摸摸看！感觉不舒服就按响这个铃铛，好吗？

# 104. Earning Patients' Trust

# 获得病人信任

Patient's Grandma: Xiao Yan, you have a high fever and your parents are not here. I am so worried.

患儿奶奶：小燕呀，你的体温这么高，爸妈又不在，我都快急死了。

Nurse: Xiao Yan, what a beautiful name! Granny, I am nurse Wang. I am here to give Xiao Yan an intravenous transfusion.

护士：小燕，多美的名字啊！老奶奶，我是小王。我来给小燕输液。

Patient Child: I do not want to have an injection.

患儿：我不要打针！

Patient's Grandma: (Looking at nurse Wang up and down) you've only worked a short time, right?

患儿奶奶：（上下打量）你才工作的吧？

Nurse: I've already worked for more than a year.

护士：我工作一年多了。

Patient's Grandma: It's very difficult to give a child a transfusion. Are you sure you can do it?

患儿奶奶：给孩子打针很难的，你行吗？

Patient Child: It will hurt. I do not want an injection.

患儿：打针痛，我不要打针。

Nurse: Xiao Yan, I know a story about a brave swallow. Do you want to hear it?

护士：小燕，阿姨知道一只勇敢的小燕子的故事，讲给你听好吗？

Patient Child: Sure.

患儿：好的。

(While looking for Xiao Yan's vein, the nurse told the child the story "A brave swallow". Then she got a razor.)

（护士一边寻找静脉，一边讲"勇敢小燕子"的故事，然后拿起剃刀。）

Patient's Grandma: What are you doing? Is it necessary to use a razor to give someone a transfusion?

患儿奶奶：干什么，输液还要剃刀？

Patient Child: No, No!

患儿：不要，不要！

Nurse: Granny, the veins on her arms are very thin. I've decided to use the vein on her head. It will be easier to find the vein there and it won't affect Xiao Yan's body movements. I am going to shave a little hair off her head. It will grow back soon.

护士：老奶奶，小燕手上的静脉细，我决定给她打头皮静脉。头皮静脉清晰易见，打好后容易固定，并且可以不影响燕子身体的活动，只是要剃掉一点点头发，你放心，我尽量少剃一些。头发也会很快长出来的。

Patient's Grandma：Are you sure what you are doing? Shall we get a more experien-ced nurse!

患儿奶奶：你知道你在干什么吗？要不换个经验多点的护士来打吧！

Nurse：Granny，although I am young，I'll put my heart and soul into every injection I give. Trust me.（Turned to the other patients）There was a brave swallow in the story. Look! Here's another brave swallow in our ward too.（Succeeded in inserting the needle.）

护士：老奶奶尽管我年轻，但我会用心去打好每一针的，请相信我。（对其他病人）刚才故事里有一只勇敢的小燕子，大家看啊，我们病房里也飞来了一只勇敢的小燕子。（进针成功。）

Patient's Grandma：Thank Goodness.

病儿奶奶：谢天谢地。

Nurse：Granny，you may be tired now. Why don't you take a rest? I'll finish the story about the brave Swallow. XiaoYan，OK?

护士：奶奶，你老累了，去休息会儿。我把"勇敢小燕子"的故事给小燕讲完，小燕，好吗？

Patient Child：Yes!（Fell asleep while listening to the story）

患儿：好的。（听着故事，渐入梦乡。）

Patient's Grandma：I am so sorry，I was...

患儿奶奶：姑娘，不好意思啊，刚才我……。

Nurse：Never mind. You were just anxious. We will give you some medication to take home. Take half a pill three times a day of this medicine，and take one measure twice a day of this liquid. Have I made it clear?

护士：奶奶，别说了，你这是急的呀。待会儿输液结束后，还有带回去治疗的药，这是药片一日三次，每次半片；这是药水，一日两次，每次一格，我讲清楚了吗？

Patient's Grandma：Yes，I see. You're a very good nurse.

病儿奶奶：讲清楚了，我听明白了，你真是位好护士。

# 105. Dialogue with a Dying Patient

# 与濒死的病人交谈

Patient: Nurse, do you have a few minutes? I'd like to talk to you.

病人： 护士，能给我几分钟吗？我想跟您聊聊。

Nurse: You have been very quiet lately. Is anything bothering you?

护士： 您最近很静，有什么事情使您烦恼吗？

Patient: Yes, I don't feel I am getting any better. But my family still says everything is fine.

病人： 是的，我没感觉有如何好转，但我的家人总是说一切都好。

Nurse: Do you fell everything is fine?

护士： 您觉得一切都好吗？

Patient: No. Few people want to talk to me.The doctors and nurses won't answer my questions. I am sure something is wrong.

病人： 不。没有人愿意跟我说话，医生和护士都不回答我的问题。我肯定哪儿出毛病了。

Nurse: I see.

护士： 我明白。

Patient: I can tell something is wrong. When I first came into the hospital, everyone came and visited and talked. Now few come, and they act differently.

病人： 我能知道确实有问题。我刚住进医院的时候，每个人都来看望我，跟我说话。现在很少有人来了，而且他们跟以前都不一样。

Nurse: I see.

护士： 我明白。

Patient: And another thing.When I ask the doctor and my family when I can go home, they just look at each other.Then they say"in a little while". I am not blind.I can tell they are not telling me something.

病人： 还有一件事，当我问医生和我的家人我何时能回家时，他们只是彼此互相看着对方，然后说"过几天"。我不是瞎子，我能看出有些事他们不告诉我。

Nurse: Have you talked to them about how you are feeling?

护士： 您跟他们说过您的感觉吗？

Patient: Maybe I will today. I need to know what is happening.

病人： 也许我今天会跟他们说。我要知道到底发生什么了。

# 106. Hospice Care

# 安宁照护

Superintendent of Nursing Department：You would like to take a bath very much，right? You haven't had a shower for one month. If I were you，I also couldn't bear it.（turning to Mrs.Jiang）You wanted to give him a bath，didn't you，Madam?

护理部主任：您很想洗澡，是吗？一个月没冲淋了，如果是我也会熬不住的。（转向蒋夫人）夫人也想帮他洗是吗？

Mrs.Jiang：Yes，but I dare not.

蒋夫人：是的，就是不敢。

Superintendent：Please ask the doctor in charge to come to help，get the resuscitation cart，oxygen unit and suction ready.（turning to Mrs. Jiang）Mrs. Jiang，we are going to assist you in bathing your husband and we need you to sign here because there might be risks of hematemesis or shock during the bathing process.We will shoulder the responsibility together.Is that acceptable?

护理部主任：请床位医生护驾，准备好抢救车和氧气装置，还有吸引器。（转向蒋夫人）蒋夫人，我们准备和您一起帮他洗澡，需要您签个字，洗澡的过程可能存在呕血、休克等危险，我们将共同承担责任，可以吗？

Mrs.Jiang：（She nodded and signed on her husband's chart.）

蒋夫人：（点点头，在病历上签了字。）

Superintendent：Madam，the head nurse，the nurse in charge and I are going to give him a bath. Since he is rather weak，he can only bathe for ten minutes. We need to place all the protective devices such as a chair in the bathtub. Mr. Jiang，all of us are your younger sisters，so I hope you wouldn't mind our giving you a bath. Your wife will bathe the lower half of your body and we will take care of the upper half. What do you think?

护理部主任：护士长、床位护士和我还有夫人，我们共同帮他洗澡。由于患者较虚弱，只有 10 分钟时间，我们需要在浴缸内放好椅子等所有保护设备。蒋先生，我们都是你的妹妹，你不介意我们帮您洗澡吧？您夫人替您洗下半身，我们替您洗上半身，如何？

Mr.Jiang：（nodding）Thank you!

蒋先生：（点头）谢谢你了！

Superintendent：Well，let's regulate the water temperature and room temperature and get started! Mr. Jiang, I am going to wet your hair with the nozzle first.The water temperature is just right. Would you like to feel it?(using shampoo to knead his hair with the help of the head nurse and the nurse in charge) Is this too hard? If you feel any discomfort, please feel free to tell me, OK?

护理部主任：好了，让我们调好水温和室温，开始吧！蒋先生，我先要冲湿您的头发，哦，水温刚好，您试试行吗？（边说边和护士长、床位护士共同给他用洗发香波揉搓他的头发）这样会不会太重？有什么不舒服请告诉我好吗？

Mr. Jiang：It's so comfortable and relaxing!（His wife used a towel to clean the lower part of his body. About ten minutes had passed and the room was filled with the fragrance of shampoo and body wash.）

蒋先生：太舒服了，觉得很轻松。（他的夫人用毛巾帮他搓着下身。约 10 分钟，屋里弥漫着洗发和沐浴露的芳香。）

Superintendent：（taking a look at the clock on the wall）Time is up. You cannot bathe any longer! Stop right now!

护理部主任：（看了眼墙上的时钟）时间到了。不能再洗了，马上停止吧！

Mr. Jiang：Let me shower for a little longer. It's extremely comfortable and I feel revived...

蒋先生：再让我冲一会儿吧，舒服极了，我好像感到自己又活回来了……

Superintendent：Mr. Jiang, your pulse is accelerating and you are sweating on the head. You can't shower any longer otherwise your blood vessels will dilate, which will lead to shock. You need to take a rest now. Come here, we are going to wrap you up with this large towel. Your head will also be wrapped up with a dry towel or else you would catch a cold.

护理部主任：蒋先生，您的脉搏在加速，头上在出汗，不能再冲了，否则血管继续扩张会休克的，现在需要休息。来，我们用大毛巾将您裹起来，头也要用干毛巾裹一下，否则会着凉感冒的。

Head Nurse：How are you feeling now? Are you very tired?

护士长：您现在感觉如何？是否很累？

Mr. Jiang：Very comfortable indeed. Being able to take a bath at this moment of my life, I will die without any regret!

蒋先生：真的很舒服，能够在这个时候洗上澡，我死而无憾了！

# Part Three

## Overseas Nursing Cases

## 海外护理集锦篇

# 1. A Job Interview 工作面试

Applicant: Good morning. Is this the Human Resources?
申请人：早上好。这是人力资源处吗？
Interviewer: Yes.Come in please.What can I do for you?
面试者：是的，请进。需要我帮忙吗？
Applicant: I'm here for an interview as requested.
申请人：我是应要求来面试的。
Interviewer: You are Miss Zhao Qi, aren't you?
面试者：你是赵祁小姐，对吗？
Applicant: That's right.
申请人：是的。
Interviewer: Have a seat, please.
面试者：请坐。
Applicant: Thank you.
申请人：谢谢。
Interviewer: I've read your resume. Have you brought your credentials?
面试者：我看过你的简历了。你带证件来了吗？
Applicant: Yes, here they are—my ID card, my diploma and my nursing license.
申请人：带了，在这—我的身份证、毕业证和护士执照。
Interviewer: You were a nursing major, weren't you?
面试者：你学的是护理专业，对吗？
Applicant: Yes, I was. I graduated from the Nursing Program of Tianjin Medical College.
申请人：是的，我毕业于天津医学高等专科学校护理专业
Interviewer: What nursing courses did you take at college?
面试者：你在学校上过什么护理课程？
Applicant: I had Basic Nursing Techniques, Adults'Nursing, Elderly Adults'Nursing, Mother and Infant's Nursing, Children's Nursing, Rehabilitation Nursing, Emergency Nursing, etc.
申请人：我学过护理学基本技能、成人护理、老年护理、母婴护理、儿童护理、康复护理、急救护理等。
Interviewer: How is your English proficiency?

面试者： 你的英语程度怎么样？

Applicant: Our program was designed to cultivate nurses whose English proficiency and professional skills are both excellent. I learned both general English and nursing English. And I've passed CET Band 6. This is my certificate.Besides，I've been taking oral English courses in an evening school for one year.

申请人： 我们专业的目标是培养既精通英语又有出色护理技能的护士。我既学过普通英语也学过护理英语，还通过了大学英语六级考试。这是我的证书。此外，一年来我一直在夜校上英语口语课程。

Interviewer: Could you tell me what kind of work experience you've had?

面试者： 你能跟我谈谈你有什么工作经历吗？

Applicant: I've worked in Tianjin Medical University General Hospital for more than two years.

申请人： 我在天津医科大学总医院工作两年多了。

Interviewer: What do you do exactly?

面试者： 你具体做什么工作呢？

Applicant: I'm in the Surgical Department. My work involves doing routine nursing care，giving preoperative and post operative cares，administering medications，and so on.

申请人： 我在外科。我的工作包括常规护理、术前和术后护理、给药等。

Interviewer: Have you ever worked in other sections?

面试者： 你在其他科室工作过吗？

Applicant: Yes. Before this I worked in the Medical Department for nearly one year. My responsibilities included taking nursing histories，keeping charts，giving injections，taking temperature and blood pressure，pre-paring patients for treatments，making bed，etc.

申请人： 是的。之前我在内科工作过将近一年。我的职责包括采集护理病历、填写各种记录表、打针、测体温和血压、为病人做治疗准备、铺床等。

Interviewer: Do you have any hobbies?

面试者： 你有什么业余爱好吗？

Applicant: Yes. I enjoy reading and listening to music，and I go jogging every day.

申请人： 我喜欢读书和听音乐，还天天去慢跑。

Interviewer: Do you think you have any advantages for the job?

面试者： 你认为自己做这份工作有什么优势吗？

Applicant: Well，I like helping people who are in trouble with health. I have some work experience. I'm a hard worker. I take work seriously. I'm caring and reliable. I'm good at communicating with people.

申请人： 嗯，我喜欢帮助有健康问题的人。我有一些工作经验。我工作努力认真。我有爱心，可信赖。我善于与人沟通。

Interviewer: Do you have any questions about the job?

面试者： 对这份工作你有什么要问的吗？

Applicant: Yes. I'd like to know if medical insurance is included in the payment for overseas nurses in your hospital.

申请人：有。我想知道你们医院给海外护士的工资中是否包含医疗保险。

Interviewer: Yes, we pay medical insurance for all staff.

面试者：包含，我们为所有的员工支付医疗保险费用。

Applicant: That's fine.

申请人：这很好。

Interviewer: Is there anything else you'd like to know?

面试者：还有别的什么想知道的吗？

Applicant: No, not at this time.

申请人：没有了，就现在这些。

Interviewer: Well, your qualifications for the job are excellent. But we have dozens of applicants to be interviewed. We cannot reach a final decision until we have talked to all of them.

面试者：好，你从事这份工作的资历条件很好。但是我们要面试几十个申请人。我们跟申请人全都谈过之后才能做最后决定。

Applicant: When can I know whether I'm accepted or not?

申请人：什么时候我能知道我是否被录用呢？

Interviewer: We'll call you next week. Thank you for coming, Miss Zhao.

面试者：下星期我们会给你打电话。谢谢你来面试，赵小姐。

Applicant: Thank you. I appreciate the time you've given me. I look forward to hearing from you.

申请人：谢谢。耽误您很多时间。期待您来电。

# 2. Introduction and Greetings

# 介绍和问候

Nurse Lana: Hello. My name is Lana.

拉娜护士：你好，我是拉娜。

Nurse Li Ping: Hi. I'm Li Ping. You may call me Ping.

李平护士：你好，我是李平，请称呼我平。

Nurse Lana: I haven't seen you before. You're new here, aren't you?

拉娜护士：我以前没见过你。你是新来的吗？

Nurse Li Ping: No. I came here one year ago.

李平护士：不，我来这里一年多了。

Nurse Lana: Where are you from?

拉娜护士：你来自哪里？

Nurse Li Ping: I'm from Xi'an. It is in China. What about you?

李平护士：我来自中国西安，你呢？

Nurse Lana: I'm from Jakarta in Indonesia. I'm a Registered Nurse, trained in critical care nursing. I'm now working as a staff nurse in the Intensive Care Unit (ICU). Most of my patients are being treated for respiratory problems. I've been working at A Hospital for two years. Which floor do you work in?

拉娜护士：我来自印度尼西亚雅加达。我是一名注册护士，曾在重症护理方面接受过培训，现在我在重症监护室工作，这里大部分的病人在治疗呼吸道疾患。我已经在A医院工作两年了，你在哪个科室？

Nurse Li Ping: I am working in third floor. It is a surgical unit. I take care of patients who are recovering from surgery.

李平护士：我在三病区工作，那是外科病区，护理术后恢复期的病人。

Nurse Lana: What's your responsibility?

拉娜护士：你的职责是什么？

Nurse Li Ping: Er...I have to set the trolley for sterile procedures such as surgical dressing and intravenous infusion, monitor patients vital signs regularly, do basic care such as bathing and feeding, etc.

李平护士：嗯……准备治疗车实施换药、静脉输液等无菌操作，常规监测病人生命体征，给病人喂饭、洗澡等基础护理。

Nurse Lana: Who is your supervisor?

拉娜护士： 谁是你的护士长？

Nurse Li Ping： Ms. Mary is our nurse manager. She supervises six staff nurses，four enrolled nurses and three health care assistants. We work on three rotating shifts. I prefer the morning shift which starts at 7 a.m. and finishes at 3 p.m. For the rest of the day，I will attend English classes. I don't like the late night shift. I feel very tired when I don't get enough sleep. Why did you come to work in America?

李平护士： 玛丽是我们的病房护士长，她管理 6 名注册护士，4 名助理护士和 3 名护理员。我们实行三班制，我喜欢早班，时间从早上 7 点至下午 3 点，因为我可以利用余下的时间参加英语课程班。我不喜欢晚班，因为得不到充足的睡眠时会感觉很累。你为什么来美国工作？

Nurse Lana： I have a few friends working in A Hospital，and they told me the hospital was hiring many foreign nurses. That's why I am here.

拉娜护士： 我有一些朋友在 A 医院工作，当时他们跟我说这所医院要招聘很多外国护士，因此我就来这里应聘。

Nurse Li Ping： Do you enjoy working here?

李平护士： 你喜欢这份工作吗？

Nurse Lana： It's quite all right. It has its ups and downs. Most of my patients are on the critical situation. They need a lot of care. It's really encouraging when a critical patient becomes stable and is moved to the general ward. Several of them returned to thank us. We also lost some patients. We feel sad for them，Anyway our care will go on...Oh，we've arrived. By the way，it's nice to talk with you.

拉娜护士： 非常喜欢。工作有快乐的时候，也有不快乐的时候，这里的病人大部分病情危重，他们需要精心照顾。当病人的病情从危重逐渐稳定到可以转到普通病房时的确很鼓舞人心，他们中有些人会回来感谢我们。当然，有时我们也会失去一些病人，会感到非常难过，不管怎样我们仍然得继续工作。哦！我们到了，顺便说一下，跟你聊天非常高兴。

Nurse Li Ping： It's been a pleasure talking with you，too.

李平护士： 我也是。

Nurse Lana： See you. Bye.

拉娜护士： 再见。

Nurse Li Ping： Bye.

李平护士： 再见

# 3. Orientating a New Nurse

# 为新护士介绍情况

Yanti：Good morning.I'm Yanti，the new nurse. I will work here from today.

燕蒂：早上好，我是新来的护士燕蒂，今天来报到。

Mary：Good morning，Yanti. I'm Mary，your nurse manager. Welcome to this ward.

玛丽：燕蒂，早上好，我是玛丽，你的护士长。欢迎来到我们病房。

Yanti：Glad to see you.

燕蒂：很高兴认识你。

Mary：I'll show you around. First let me introduce you to the doctor.

玛丽：我带你参观一下病房。首先，请允许我把你介绍给医生们。

（The nurse manager leads Yanti to the doctor's station.）

（护士长领燕蒂来到医生站。）

Mary：Good morning，Dr Li.

玛丽：李医生，早上好。

Dr Li：Morning，sister. I see you have a new staff with you.

李医生：护士长，早上好。我看到您跟一位新员工在一起。

Mary：Yes, Dr Li. I'd like you to meet Yanti，our new staff nurse. Yanti，this is Dr Li，our consultant physician.

玛丽：是的，李医生，这是燕蒂。燕蒂，这是我们的顾问医生——李医生。

Yanti：Good morning，Dr Li.

燕蒂：李医生，早上好。

Dr Li：Good morning，Yanti.

李医生：燕蒂护士，早上好 .

（The nurse manager then leads Yanti to the nurses'station.）

（护士长带领燕蒂来到护士站）

Staff nurse：Good morning，sister.

护士：护士长，早上好。

Mary：Good morning，staff nurse. This is Yanti，our new staff. She has become a member of our staff with effect from today.Yanti，meet Susie.

玛丽：早上好，这是新来的护士燕蒂，从今天开始她就是我们中的一员了。燕蒂，这是苏西。

Staff nurse：Hi，Yanti. Nice to be working with you.

护士： 燕蒂，你好，很高兴与你共事。

Yanti: Hello，Staff Nurse Susie. Glad to be working with you，too.

燕蒂： 苏西，你好，我也很高兴与你共事。

（In the office of the nurse manager）

（在护士长办公室）

Mary: Now let me give you some information about the ward.

玛丽： 现在请允许我向你介绍一下病房的基本情况。

Yanti: Yes，Sister.

燕蒂： 好的，护士长。

Mary: Ward 20 is a renal ward. We have 20 beds on this floor. Many of our patients are due to kidney problems. Most of them are diagnosed with acute nephritis. We've seen several cases of chronic renal failure. The patient in bed 3 is waiting for a kidney transplant. Our staff ratio is one nurse to five patients. The nurses work on two shifts. The duty roster is scheduled on a weekly basis. You get one day off every week.

玛丽： 20病房是肾病病房，本楼层我们有20张床位。这里的病人很多患有肾脏疾病，其中大部分是急性肾炎，也有一些慢性肾衰竭病人，3床的病人准备做肾移植手术。我们病房的护患之比是1∶5，按周排班，两天一换班，每周休息一天。

Yanti: I see. What about night shift?

燕蒂： 我明白了，夜班呢？

Mary: We've a pool of staff on permanent night shift. They work four nights and get three days off.

玛丽： 我们有一群护士专职上夜班，工作4晚，休息3天。

Yanti: How do I request for a specific day off?

燕蒂： 我怎么申请在特定的日期休息？.

Mary: You need to put in a request at least one week in advance. Alternatively，you can switch your schedule with another staff，but give me ample notice，at least two days before. Do you have any question about this？

玛丽： 你至少要提前一周提出请求，或者与其他护士换班，但是至少要提前两天告诉我。还有其他问题吗？

Yanti: Yes，what happens if I'm sick?

燕蒂： 是的。如果我生病了怎么办？

Mary: That's a good question. Call the ward manager at once when you're unwell. If she is not available，you can leave a message with the staff nurse on duty.

玛丽： 问得好。如果你感觉不舒服，立刻打电话给病房主管，如果她不在，你可以给当班护士留话。

Yanti: Okay，and what about breaks for lunch or dinner?

燕蒂： 好的，关于午餐或晚餐的休息时间呢？

Mary: The nurses are entitled to one hour of break for meals or dinner. You can help yourself to the drinks and beverages in the staff lounge. There is also a microwave oven for staff use. The hospital cafeteria is on level 3.

玛丽： 午餐休息时间为 1 小时，你可以随意喝员工食品柜中的饮料，还有一个微波炉可供使用。医院餐厅设在三楼。

Yanti： That sounds good.

燕蒂： 听起来不错。

Mary： I notice you have beautiful long hair and nicely polished nails. Here at hospital, we encourage our staff to keep their hair and nails short. The reasons are obvious. If staff prefer to keep their hair long, we require them to tie it up neatly. Is that all right with you?

玛丽： 你有漂亮的长发，指甲上涂有美丽的指甲油。在医院里，我们建议员工留短发、剪短指甲，原因显而易见。如果员工想留长发，我们要求挽发，你可以吗？

Yanti： Sure. That's not a problem at all.

燕蒂： 当然，没有问题。

Mary： One more thing, patients are our customers. Remember always show our respect, concerns and courteousness to our patients and their relatives.

玛丽： 另外一点，病人是我们的顾客，所以我们希望员工能尊重并有礼貌地对待病人和他们的探视者。

Yanti： Yes, of course. Is there anything else I need to know?

燕蒂： 当然，还有别的事情吗？

Mary： I think this is enough for today. Don't be afraid to contact any one of us whenever you need help. We're one big family here at our hospital.

玛丽： 今天就讲这些。当你需要帮助时，尽管联系我们。在玛丽医院我们是个大家庭。

Yanti： Thank you, Sister. I will do my best.

燕蒂： 护士长，谢谢您。我会尽力工作的。

# 4. Appointment

# 预约

## (1)

Nurse： Good morning，Dr. Smith's office. Can I help you?

护士： 早晨好，史密斯医生办公室。我能为你做什么吗？

Patient： Yes，it's Mrs. Bushman here. I would like to see the doctor as soon as I can. I am having trouble with my stomach again. It's terrible at this moment. I can hardly sleep during the night.

病人： 你好，我是布什曼太太。我要尽快看医生。我的胃病又犯了，现在疼得很厉害，晚上几乎不能入睡。

Nurse： Oh，I am sorry to hear that，Mrs. Bushman. Let me see if I can get you in this afternoon. No，I am sorry. It will have to be tomorrow morning，Friday，the eighteenth. I can give you an appointment with the doctor at 9：30 a.m. Will that be all right?

护士： 哦，听到这个我很抱歉，布什曼太太，我给你看看是不是能够预约在下午。不行，很抱歉，得要到明天早晨，也就是 18 号星期五。我可以给你安排早晨 9：30 与医生预约见面，这样可以吗？

Patient： Hmm，Friday the eighteenth? I have other plans tomorrow morning. But，I will have to go to the doctor instead. Health should always come first，right? I will be there at 9：30 tomorrow morning. Thank you.

病人： 嗯，18 号星期五？我还有其他的安排，但是我也只好去看病了。健康永远是第一位的，对不对？明天早晨 9：30 我会去医院。谢谢你。

## (2)

Patient： Hello. I'd like to make an appointment to see a dentist.

病人： 你好，我想预约一下看牙齿。

Doctor： Of course. Do you want to have an examination or do you have a particular problem.

医生： 好的，你想做一个检查还是有什么具体问题？

Patient： I'm having trouble with a tooth which is very painful to chew on.

病人： 我牙齿有问题，咀嚼东西非常疼。

Doctor： We'd better take a look at this tooth soon to find out what's wrong with it. If you are available, we have a vacant slot to see you tomorrow afternoon at 4 p.m.

医生：我们最好等一会儿检查一下牙齿，看看是什么问题。如果你方便的话，我们明天下午 4 点有个空位给你看看。

Patient: That's very thoughtful of you. I'll take that appointment.

病人：你对人真是细心周到。我接受这个预约。

Doctor: Can I have your name and contact number please?

医生：请问贵姓和联络电话。

Patient: My name is Mark Johnson and my phone number is 87697231. One more thing, what will you do tomorrow and how much is it likely to cost?

病人：我叫马克•约翰逊，我的电话号码是 87697231。还有一件事，明天你会怎么给我检查？费用大概是多少？

Doctor: I'll examine the tooth and probably need to take some radiographs. Once I know what's wrong with the tooth, I'll discuss the choice of treatment available with you. The initial consultation fee including the radiographs is about 160 dollars.

医生：我要检查你的牙齿，也许还需要拍一些射线照片。一旦知道了你牙齿的问题所在，我就会与你讨论一下可行的治疗方法。初诊费用包括拍射线照片，大概是 160 美元左右。

Patient: All right. Thank you very much. See you tomorrow.

病人：好的。非常感谢。明天见。

**(3)**

Nurse: Good morning. Dr. White's office.

护士：早上好，怀特医生办公室。

Patient: Good morning. This is Mary Smith. Can I speak to Dr. White?

病人：早上好。我是玛莉•史密斯。我能同怀特医生通话吗？

Nurse: I'm sorry he is talking with a patient right now. Can I help you? I'm Jane Franklin, a nurse at Dr. White's office.

护士：对不起，他现在正同病人谈话。我能帮你吗？我是怀特医生办公室的护士，名叫珍妮•弗兰克林。

Patient: Hello, Ms. Franklin. I have a son of three years old. His name is Robert Smith. Every month I take him to Dr. White for a health checkup.

病人：你好，弗兰克林女士。我有一个三岁的儿子，名叫罗伯特•史密斯。我每个月都领他去找怀特医生做健康检查。

Nurse: I've found the record of Robert's growth and development. Robert appears to have developed quite well.

护士：我找到了罗伯特成长发育的档案记录。他看起来一切都很正常。

Patient: I want to make an appointment. Is this afternoon OK for Dr. White?

病人：我想预约一下。今天下午怀特医生有空吗？

Nurse: I'm afraid Dr. White is occupied this afternoon. Would tomorrow morning be convenient for you, Mrs. Smith?

护士： 恐怕今天下午怀特医生没有空闲时间。史密斯太太，明天上午对你来说方便吗？

Patient： Tomorrow morning? Let me see. Tomorrow is Sunday. It's OK with me.

病人： 明天上午？让我想一想，明天是星期天，可以。

Nurse： Fine. How about 9：00?

护士： 那好，9 点怎么样？

Patient： Good. I'll be at Dr. White's office at 9：00 tomorrow morning with Robert. Thank you，Ms. Franklin.

病人： 行，明天上午 9 点我会带罗伯特到怀特医生办公室。谢谢你，弗兰克林女士。

Nurse： You are welcome. Goodbye，Mrs. Smith.

护士： 不客气。再见，史密斯太太。

## （4）

Mrs. Stan： Can I speak to Dr. Grant，please?

斯坦太太： 请问格兰特医生在吗？

Dr. Grant： Yes. This is Dr. Grant speaking. What can I do for you?

格兰特医生： 我就是，有什么需要帮忙的吗？

Mrs. Stan： Hello. This is Mrs. Stan，Dr. Grant.

斯坦太太： 格兰特医生，我是斯坦太太。

Dr. Grant： What's happening，Mrs. Stan?

格兰特医生： 你怎么不舒服了，斯坦太太？

Mrs. Stan： Oh，no，it's not me. My son Bill is sick.

斯坦太太： 哦，不，不是我。是我儿子比尔病了。

Dr. Grant： What's wrong with Bill?

格兰特医生： 比尔哪儿不舒服？

Mrs. Stan： He has red spots on his arms，on his shoulders...

斯坦太太： 他手臂上、肩膀上……长了红斑。

Dr. Grant： Does he have red spots all over his body?

格兰特医生： 他是不是全身都长了红斑？

Mrs. Stan： Yes，he does.

斯坦太太： 是。

Dr. Grant： Does he have a fever?

格兰特医生： 他有没有发热呢？

Mrs. Stan： Yes，he does. This morning his temperature was 39 degree centigrade.

斯坦太太： 哦，对了。今天早上他烧到了 39℃。

Dr. Grant： Well，that's too bad.

格兰特医生： 哎呀，那太糟了。

Mrs. Stan： What's the problem with Bill? He cried all day.

斯坦太太： 大夫，比尔究竟怎么了？他整天哭。

Dr. Grant： He has measles.

格兰特医生： 他出麻疹了。

Mrs. Stan：Measles? Oh，dear. Can you come and see him now?

斯坦太太：出麻疹？天啊！你现在可以来看他吗？

Dr. Grant：I'm going to have an operation this morning. But I can come this afternoon.

格兰特医生：今天上午我得给病人动手术。下午我可以来。

Mrs. Stan：Thank you，Dr. Grant.

斯坦太太：谢谢你，格兰特医生。

Dr. Grant：Please remember，do not scratch the red spots.

格兰特医生：记住，不能让他抓那些红斑。

Mrs. Stan：I won't let him do that. See you this afternoon，doctor.

斯坦太太：我不会让他抓的。下午见，医生。

Dr. Grant：Goodbye.

格兰特医生：再见。

## （5）

Nurse：Doctor's office. Jennifer speaking. How can I help you?

护士：医生办公室，我是詹尼佛。我能帮你什么忙吗？

Patient：I need to make an appointment with Dr. Harris.

病人：我需要与哈里斯医生预约看病。

Nurse：Do you know your chart number?

护士：知道你的病历簿编号吗？

Patient：No，sorry. It's at home and I'm at work right now.

病人：对不起，病历簿在家，我现在在上班。

Nurse：No problem. What's your name，please?

护士：没关系，请问贵姓？

Patient：William Henzell.

病人：威廉•亨泽尔。

Nurse：Okay. Mr. Henzell. Please hold one moment while I grab your chart，please.

护士：好的，亨泽尔先生。请稍等片刻，我拿一下你的病历资料。

Patient：Sure.

病人：好的。

Nurse：Thanks for waiting. Now，what do you need to see the doctor about?

护士：久等了，多谢。嗯，你需要让医生帮你看什么病呢？

Patient：Well，I have a rash all over my body. It itches badly.

病人：我浑身都起了红疹，痒得很厉害。

Nurse：Hmm. Dr. Harris is off tomorrow. Do you think it can wait until Wednesday.

护士：嗯，哈里斯医生明天休息。你能不能等到星期三再来看病？

Patient：Oh，I was really hoping to get in today or tomorrow. Maybe I'll have to go to the walk-in-clinic instead.

病人：噢，我真的希望能够预约到今天或者明天。也许我应该去随诊门诊部看病。

Nurse：Actually，we have had a cancellation for 2：00 p.m. today if you can get away from the office.

护士： 实际上有病人取消了今天下午 2 点的预约，我们有一个空缺，如果你能够从你的办公室赶过来的话。

Patient: Gee, it's almost 1: 00 p.m. already. I think I can make it if I leave right now.

病人： 哇，都快一点钟了。如果我现在马上赶过去的话，还能够来得及。

Nurse: We're running a bit behind schedule, so you can probably count on seeing the doctor around 2: 30.

护士： 我们比原定的时间安排晚了一点点，所以，你或许可以在 2: 30 左右找医生看病。

Patient: That's great. Thanks for fitting me in.

病人： 好极了。谢谢你给我安排了预约。

Nurse: No problem, Mr. Henzell. We'll see you in an hour or so.

护士： 不客气，亨泽尔先生。我们一个小时左右再见。

## (6)

Nurse: Hello, how can I help you?

护士： 你好，我能够帮你什么忙吗？

Patient: I've got an appointment with Dr. Adams.

病人： 我与亚当斯医生有个预约。

Nurse: Are you Ms. Moyers?

护士： 你是莫耶斯女士吗？

Patient: Yes, I am. I have an appointment at ten.

病人： 是的，没错。我预约在 10 点钟。

Nurse: We just need to fill in some information for our files. Could you fill out these forms?

护士： 我们只是要为档案材料补充一些信息。你可不可以填写一下这些表格呢？

Patient: Certainly (come back after filling out the forms). What is this form for?

病人： 当然了。(填完表格以后返回)这个表格是拿来干什么用的？

Nurse: It's just a privacy form informing you of our policies.

护士： 这是告诉你我们政策的个人资料表格。

Patient: Is that really necessary?

病人： 真的有必要吗？

Nurse: I'm afraid it is. Could you also sign that form?

护士： 恐怕有必要。在表格上也要签名，可以吗？

Patient: OK, there you go. Here's my insurance provider's card.

病人： 好了，可以啦。这是保险公司工作人员的名片。

Nurse: Thank you. OK, that'll be $20?

护士： 谢谢你。好了，请交 20 美元。

Patient: Why do I have to pay $20?

病人： 为什么要交 20 美元呢？

Nurse: It's the deductible for office visits required by your health care provider.

护士： 它是由健康医疗部门要求的可以扣除的门诊费。

Patient： But I'm insured, aren't I?

病人： 但是，我买了医疗保险，对不对？

Nurse： Yes, of course. Your health care provider asks for deductibles on office visits.

护士： 当然是的。健康医疗部门要求这个门诊扣除条款的设置。

Patient： Every time I turn around I've got some additional fee to pay. I don't know why I pay for insurance!

病人： 每次我来的时候都被要求支付额外的费用。我真的不知道我为什么还要买保险。

Nurse： I know it's frustrating. We also have a lot of paperwork. Every provider has different forms and requirements!

护士： 我知道这个会令人沮丧。我们还有许多书面工作要做。每个医疗部门都会有各种各样不同的表格和要求。

Patient： This can't continue on like this!

病人： 不能再继续这样了。

Nurse： I agree with that! Okay, you can go in now. Dr. Adams is waiting for you at his office.

护士： 我同意。好了，你可以进去了，亚当斯医生在办公室等你。

# 5. Receiving a New Patient

# 接收新病人

Nurse: Good afternoon. Are you Mr. John Lane?

护士：下午好。您是约翰•莱恩先生吗？

Patient: Yes, I am.

病人：是的，我是。

Nurse: I'm Li Lin, your nurse today. I'm going to take you to your room. Would you please follow me?

护士：我是李琳，今天我是您的护士。我马上带您到病室，请跟我来。

Patient: OK. Thank you.

病人：好的。谢谢。

Nurse: Here we are. Room 306 is for you, Your bed number is 28.

护士：到了。306是您的病室，您的床位号是28。

Patient: It looks very nice. Where should I put my personal articles?

病人：看起来很不错。我应该把私人物品放在哪里？

Nurse: You'd better only keep small everyday things in your bedside table, and here is a locker for you to put other things in. If you have any valuables, you can put them in the hospital safe, or you can ask your relatives to take them back home.

护士：您最好只把常用的小物品放在床头柜里，这里还有一个置物柜给您放其他东西。如果您有贵重物品，可以放在医院的保险柜里或者请家属带回家。

Patient: Thank you. What daily articles do I need to bring in?

病人：谢谢。我需要带什么日用品来？

Nurse: Toothbrush, toothpaste, slippers, towels, and so on.

护士：牙刷、牙膏、拖鞋、毛巾等。

Patient: Could I watch TV here?

病人：我能在这里看电视吗？

Nurse: You can watch TV in this single room. Here is the remote control. But you can't bring electrical appliances from home.

护士：您在这个单人病室可以看电视，这是遥控器。但您不能从家里带电器来。

Patient: What should I do if I want a nurse?

病人：如果我需要叫护士该怎样办？

Nurse: Here is the call button. If you press it, the staff at the Nurse's Station will be here as soon as possible. Besides, there is another call button in the bath room in case you need it.

护士： 这有呼叫按钮。您按了按钮，护士站的护士就会尽快过来。此外，卫生间里还有一个呼叫按钮，以防您需要。

Patient: When are the meal-times?

病人： 开饭是什么时间？

Nurse: 7: 30 a.m. for breakfast, 12 at noon for lunch, and 6 p.m. for dinner. You. can order meals and have them in the room, or you can go to the restaurant on the first floor. There are a variety of Chinese, Muslim and Western foods for your choice. When you need special diets, our clinical dietitian will approach you about it.

护士： 7 点半早餐，12 点午餐，下午 6 点晚餐。您可以订餐在病室吃，也可以到一楼的餐厅用餐。有各种各样的中餐、清真餐和西餐供您选择。您需要特殊饮食时，我们的临床营养师会来给您指导。

Patient: When are my relatives and friends allowed to visit me?

病人： 什么时间我的亲友可以来探视呢？

Nurse: The visiting hours are from 6 p.m. to 8 p.m. By the way, neither you nor your visitors can smoke inside the hospital.

护士： 探视时间是下午 6～8 点。顺便说一句，您和探视者都不能在医院里吸烟。

Patient: I see. Could you tell me when the doctor will come to see me?

病人： 我明白了。您能告诉我医生什么时候会来看我吗？

Nurse: Your doctor will come to see you soon. The ward rounds and treatment start at 8 a.m. every morning. Nurses on duty make two rounds of the wards during the night. Any more questions?

护士： 医生很快就会来看您的。每天早 8 点开始查房和治疗。夜班护士查两次病房。还有问题吗？

Patient: Not at the moment. Thank you very much.

病人： 暂时没有了。非常感谢。

Nurse: It's my pleasure. Would you mind changing into your pajamas? I'll be back in a few minutes to get information about your health history.

护士： 不客气。您换上病人服装好吗？过会儿我回来收集您的病史信息。

# 6. Introducing Environment

# 介绍病房环境

Nurse: Are you Mr. John?

护士：是约翰先生吗？

Patient: Yes.

病人：是的。

Nurse: I'm your nurse. This way, please. I'll take you to the ward.

护士：我是您的主管护士，请这边走，我带您去病房。

Patient: Thank you.

病人：谢谢。

Nurse: Here is your bed. The call button is here.You may push it if you need a nurse. This is your bedside table for such things as toiletries. If you have any valuable belongings, we'll keep them for you.

护士：这是您的病床。这是按钮，如果您要叫护士就请按它。这是床头柜，供您放洗漱用具等东西。如果您有贵重物品，我可以代您保管。

Patient: I see, thanks. Where is the restroom?

病人：谢谢。请问，卫生间在哪儿？

Nurse: On the left side of this door. And there is another one at the end of the corridor, in which you can take a bath.

护士：在这扇门的左边，在走廊的尽头还有一个，浴室也在那儿。

Patient: That's good.

病人：好的，我知道了。

Nurse: The sitting room is over there. You can have your meals, watch TV and have other recreational activities there. The ward is your home during your stay in hospital.

护士：休息室在那边，您可以在那里吃饭、看电视和进行娱乐活动。在您住院期间，病房就是您的家。

Patient: OK. I would like to know if my wife can visit me.

病人：请问，我的妻子可以来看我吗？

Nurse: Of course. She can visit you from 3 to 7 p.m. every day and from 8 to 11 a.m. on the weekend mornings.

护士：当然，她可以在每天下午3～7点及周末的上午8～11点来看您。

Patient: That's nice.

病人： 那太好了。

Nurse： By the way, please let me know if you leave the ward.

护士： 顺便说一下，如果您要离开病房，请通知我。

Patient： OK.

病人： 好的。

# 7. Introducing Regulations

# 介绍病房守则

Nurse: Hello, Mr. Johnson. I'm your nurse. Your doctor informed me of your admission.

护士：您好，约翰逊先生。我是您的护士，您的医生已经把您住院的事通知我了。

Patient: Hi.

病人：您好。

Nurse: This is your ward. You will be sharing it with another patient. There is a curtain between your beds for your privacy.

护士：这是您的病房，要与另一位病人合住。中间有帘子隔开，如果需要，可以把帘子拉上。

(The nurse leads Mr. Johnson into the ward.)

(护士带约翰逊生进入病房。)

Nurse: Good afternoon, Mr. Thomas. Here comes a new friend, Mr. Johnson.

护士：下午好，托马斯先生。来了位新朋友，约翰逊先生。

Patient (another one): Welcome, Mr. Johnson.I'm glad to have a roommate. I'm Paul Thomas.

病人(另一位)：欢迎您，约翰逊先生。很高兴有了一位室友。我是保罗•托马斯。

Patient: Thank you, Mr. Thomas. What toiletries should I bring in, nurse?

病人：谢谢，托马斯先生。护士，我应该带哪些日常用品？

Nurse: Toothbrush, toothpaste, comb, slippers, towels, soap and so on. You can put them in this drawer.

护士：牙刷、牙膏、梳子、拖鞋、毛巾、肥皂等。您可以把它们放在这个抽屉里。

Patient: Can I bring in a TV set or radio set?

病人：可不可以带电视或收音机？

Nurse: No, they are too noisy. But you may bring a walkman with head-phone.

护士：不可以，太吵了。不过可以带随身听，用耳机。

Patient: When can my relatives and friends come to see me?

病人：我的亲友什么时候可以来看我？

Nurse: Visiting hours are from 1 to 2 p.m. and 5 to 7 p.m. Each time only two visitors are allowed to enter the ward.

护士： 哦，探视时间是下午1～2点和5～7点，每次只允许两位探视者进入病房。

Patient: I see. How about the meals?

病人： 知道了。吃饭怎么办？

Nurse: Meal time is 8 a.m. for breakfast，12 noon for lunch，and 6 p.m. for dinner. We serve a variety of Chinese and Western food. Our clinical dietitian is available to help with special diet needs.

护士： 早上8点早餐，中午12点午餐，晚上6点晚餐。我们有丰富多样的中餐和西餐供应，还有临床营养师指导特殊饮食。

Patient: Thank you very much.

病人： 谢谢您的介绍。

Nurse: You are welcome.

护士： 别客气。

# 8. Discussing Meals and Food

# 与病人谈论饮食安排

Nurse: Welcome. I'm the nurse in charge of this ward. We hope you will feel at home here. This is Miss Rose Clinton.

护士: 您好。欢迎您。我是这个病房的护士。希望您能有家的感觉，这是护士罗丝•克林顿小姐。

Patient: Sorry to bother you all.

病人: 麻烦你们了。

Nurse: If you need anything, just press this button.

护士: 您若需要什么，就请按这个按钮。

Patient: Is it possible for my sister to stay here with me?

病人: 我姐姐可以在这里陪我吗？

Nurse: Yes, but she has to pay for her bed. Does she want have meals here too? We don t think it is necessary for her to stay. Your condition isn't so serious.

护士: 可以，但是得交陪住费。她也在这里吃饭吗？我认为她不需要陪住，您的病情不那么严重。

Patient: What are the hours here for meals?

病人: 这儿什么时候开饭？

Nurse: Patients usually get up at 7 a.m. Breakfast is at 8 a.m. The ward rounds and treatments start at 9 a.m. Lunch is at noon, after that it is nap time. Visiting hours are from 3 to 7 p.m. Dinner is at 6 p.m. Bed time is from 10p.m.

护士: 病人一般早 7 点起床，8 点吃早餐，9 点医生查房和做治疗，12 点午餐，饭后午睡，下午 3～7 点是探视时间，6 点晚餐，10 点熄灯。

Patient: Will you show me where the sitting-room, bathroom and telephone are?

病人: 请告诉我起居室、浴室和电话在哪儿好吗？

Nurse: Of course. Are you Muslim?

护士: 当然可以，您是伊斯兰教徒吗？

Patient: No, I am not.

病人: 不，我不是。

Nurse: Which kind of food do you prefer, Chinese or Western?

护士: 您喜欢吃中餐还是喜欢吃西餐？

Patient: I like Chinese food very much.

病人：我非常喜欢吃中餐。

Nurse：Have you eaten breakfast already?

护士：您吃早餐了吗？

Patient：Yes，I have.

病人：是，吃过了。

Nurse：How is your appetite?

护士：您的胃口怎样？

Patient：Not so good.

病人：不太好。

Nurse：What are your eating habits?

护士：您的饮食习惯怎么样？

Patient：I don't eat much. I would like to have a snack in the afternoon and before going to bed.

病人：我吃得不多。我希望在下午和睡前吃点东西。

Nurse：Are you allergic to any food?

护士：您对什么食物过敏吗？

Patient：I am allergic to sea food.

病人：我对海产品过敏。

Nurse：Do you like fruit?

护士：您喜欢水果吗？

Patient：Yes，Please give me some with each meal.

病人：是的，请每餐都给我些水果。

Nurse：Do you prefer a consomme or a cream soap?

护士：您喜欢清汤还是奶油汤？

Patient：I like rice porridge.

病人：我喜欢吃大米粥。

Nurse：Please try to eat a little more. It will help you recover more quickly.

护士：请多吃一些。这样可以帮助您早日康复。

# 9. Communications in the Ward

# 病房中的交流

Patient： It is too noisy.

病人： 太吵闹了。

Nurse： May I close the door?

护士： 我可以关上门吗？

Patient： OK. I am hungry.

病人： 好的。我饿了。

Nurse： I'll go and get you some cough drop.

护士： 我去给您拿点咳嗽药来。

Patient： May I have another pillow?

病人： 我可以再要一个枕头吗？

Nurse： Do you need some clean pajamas?

护士： 您要干净的睡衣裤吗？

Patient： Yes，thank you. Please bring me a dressing gown too.

病人： 是的，谢谢您。请再给我拿件晨衣来。

Nurse： Do you want to have a bed-bath?

护士： 给您擦个澡好吗？

Patient： I'd rather have a shower.

病人： 我想洗个淋浴。

Nurse： May I put these flowers away?

护士： 我把这些花收起来好吗？

Patient： Yes，please put these flowers in a vase.

病人： 可以，请将这些花放在花瓶里。

Nurse： Mr. Smith，there's a call for you.

护士： 史密斯太太，有您的电话。

Patient： Is it a long distance call?

病人： 是长途电话吗？

Nurse： No. It's from your embassy.

护士： 不是，是从你们大使馆打来的。

# 10. Caring for a Muslin Patient

# 护理穆斯林病人

Nurse：Hello，Mr Ali. Dr An has prescribed this medicine for you.

护士：你好，阿里先生，安医生已为你开了这种口服药。

Patient：I have my own medicine. It's in my bag.

病人：我自己有药，在包里。

Nurse：When did you take your medicine last time?

护士：你上次吃药是什么时间？

Patient：Last night.

病人：昨天晚上。

Nurse：What about this morning?

护士：今天早上吃药了吗？

Patient：Er...no...I've not taken my medicine this morning.

病人：嗯，没有……今天早晨我还没有吃药。

Nurse：No wonder. Mr Ali，how do you expect to control your epilepsy if you're not serious about taking your medicine. Now swallow these pills right away.

护士：难怪！阿里先生，如果你不认真吃药，如何控制癫痫。马上服下这些药片。

Patient：But nurse，I cannot. This is the fasting month. I'm not supposed to take anything including medicine in the daytime during this period.

病人：但是护士，我不能吃药。斋月期间，白天我不能吃任何东西，包括药物。

Nurse：Mr Ali，which is more important? Your life or your religion? I'm sure your Allah is understanding and not unreasonable? Now take this medicine Now.

护士：阿里先生，你的生命与你的信仰哪样更重要？我认为你的阿拉会明白的，他不会不讲道理的。请马上吃药。

Patient：Nurse. Don't you understand? I cannot take anything in the daytime. I'm not taking the medicine now.

病人：护士，难道你不明白吗？白天我不能吃任何东西，现在不能吃药。

Nurse：Now，Mr Ali，don't take it so serious. The doctors cannot help you if you're so stubborn.

护士：阿里先生，不要这样认为。这么固执，即使医生也帮不了你。

Patient：Hey，nurse. I don't like your manners. You're rude. I want to speak to the doctor.

病人：嘿，护士，我不喜欢你的服务态度，太粗鲁，我想跟医生说话。

Nurse: All right then.

护士： 那好吧。

(The doctor approaches the patient.)

(医生来到病人身边。)

Doctor: Hello, Mr Ali. I'm Dr An. How are you feeling? How may I help you?

医生： 你好，阿里先生，我是安医生，你现在感觉怎样？你有什么事吗？

Patient: Hello doctor. I'm really tired trying to explain to that nurse that I can't take my medicine now. She just doesn't understand. Doesn't she know the practices of Islam?

病人： 你好，医生，我很费力地跟护士解释说我现在不能吃药。她还是不明白，难道她不了解伊斯兰习俗？

Doctor: I see. Would you like to briefly tell me what happened?

医生： 我明白了，你能简单地告诉我刚才发生什么了吗？

Patient: Yes. I tried telling that nurse Li Ping that I'm observing the fasting month. During this period, we have to refrain from taking food or drinks, including medicine. Doctor, can you tell the nurse about this? She doesn't have any respect for me or my religion and she complains that I'm difficult and non-compliant.

病人： 好的，我费力地跟李平护士解释我遵守斋月禁食戒律，这期间我们必须禁饮食，包括药物。医生，你能把这些告诉护士吗？她不尊重我和我的信仰。并且说我难相处、不配合。

Doctor: Mr Ali. I understand how you feel. I do apologise for your unpleasant experience. The nurse is a new staff from China. She probably doesn't know much about your religion.

医生： 阿里先生，我很理解您的感受，向你道歉，给你带来的不愉快敬请谅解。护士是新来的，来自中国，她可能不了解你的宗教信仰。

Patient: Well then, she shouldn't be arguing with me.

病人： 那好吧，她不应该跟我吵架。

Doctor: Not to worry, Mr Ali. We'll sort this out later. We can work out an altrnative. Instead of taking your phenytoin 100 mg three times a day, we could change it to a single daily dose of 300 mg to be taken when you break fast, if that's all right with you.

医生： 不要担心，阿里先生，一会我们会处理此事的。我们可以做个选择，服用苯妥英钠 100 毫克 / 次，3 次 / 日；如果你觉得合适的话，也可 300 毫克 / 次，1 次 / 日，开斋时服用。

Patient: Yes, doctor. Thank you very much, Dr An. I feel so much better now.

病人： 好的，安医生，谢谢你。我现在感觉好多了。

Doctor: Good. I'll inform the nurse about this.

医生： 很好，关于这些我会通知护士的。

(Nurse Li Ping returns to check on the patient.)

(李平护士来为病人做检查)

Nurse: Mr Ali. I'm sorry about what happened just now. It's my mistake. I should have been more sensitive.

护士： 阿里先生，对于刚才发生的事情我向你道歉，是我的不对，我应该更体谅你一些。

Patient: It's okay. I didn't know you're new.

病人： 好了，我不知道你是新来的。

Nurse: Thank you for your understanding. I'll be careful in future. Let me know if you need anything.

护士： 谢谢你的理解，以后我会注意的。如果你有需要请及时告诉我。

# 11. Nursing Assessment

# 护理评估

## （1）

Nurse： Mr. Lane，in order to make nursing records for you，I need to get some information about your health history. Would you mind if I ask you a few questions?

护士： 莱恩先生，为了给您建立护理病历，我可以问您一些问题吗？我需要收集一些您的健康情况资料。

Patient： Of course not.

病人： 当然可以。

Nurse： What brought you to hospital today?

护士： 今天您为什么来医院？

Patient： I began to have bad abdominal pains and severe diarrheas last night. I've been to the washroom for nearly ten times since midnight. Now my belly is still hurting but when I go to the washroom，nothing comes out. I feel awful.

病人： 昨天夜里我开始腹痛得要命，腹泻得厉害。从午夜到现在我去过差不多十次洗手间了。现在我的肚子还很疼，但去洗手间却什么都拉不出来。我感觉很难受。

Nurse： What did you have for dinner yesterday evening?

护士： 昨天晚饭吃的什么？

Patient： I had spicy hot pot with some friends，I might have eaten too much.

病人： 我和朋友吃的辣火锅，可能吃得太多了。

Nurse： Have you got stomachache，nausea or vomiting?

护士： 您有胃疼、恶心或呕吐吗？

Patient： My stomach aches a little but I've got neither nausea nor vomiting.

病人： 胃有点疼，但没有恶心和呕吐。

Nurse： Have you ever been hospitalized before?

护士： 您以前住过院吗？

Patient： No，this is the first time. Before this I always thought I had been in good health. I haven't got any diseases except for common colds.

病人： 没住过，这是第一次。这之前我一直觉得自己身体健康。除了普通感冒我从来没得过其他病。

Nurse： Could you tell me something about your parents' health conditions?

护士： 您能告诉我您父母的健康状况吗？

Patient: My mother passed away.

病人： 我母亲去世了。

Nurse: I'm sorry to hear it. Do you know what caused her death?

护士： 真遗憾。您知道她去世的原因吗？

Patient: She died of a heart attack.

病人： 她是心脏病突发去世的。

Nurse: What about your father?

护士： 那么您的父亲呢？

Patient: He has high blood pressure.

病人： 他患有高血压。

Nurse: Are you allergic to any food or medicine?

护士： 您对什么食物或药物过敏吗？

Patient: When I eat crab, I will develop rashes.

病人： 我吃螃蟹会起皮疹。

Nurse: Do you have any food restriction except seafood?

护士： 除海鲜外，您有什么食物不能吃吗？

Patient: No.

病人： 没有了。

Nurse: Do you smoke?

护士： 您抽烟吗？

Patient: One or two when I am tired or anxious.

病人： 在疲劳或焦虑时会抽一两根。

Nurse: Do you drink alcohol?

护士： 您喝酒吗？

Patient: I have a little red wine or beer sometimes.

病人： 有时喝点红酒或啤酒。

Nurse: How is your bowel movement usually? Do you have it everyday?

护士： 您通常大便怎么样？天天有大便吗？

Patient: I usually pass stool once a day, but sometimes I have constipation.

病人： 我通常每天大便一次，但有时会有便秘。

Nurse: Are you on any medication?

护士： 您在服用什么药吗？

Patient: No.

病人： 没有。

Nurse: That's all for now. Thank you for your cooperation. If you have any questions, please feel free to ask me. Next I'm going to take your temperature, pulse and blood pressure.

护士： 就这些问题了。谢谢您的合作。如果您有任何问题，请随时问我。接下来我要测您的体温、脉搏和血压。

## (2)

Nurse: Thank you for giving me so much information about your health history. Now I need to take your temperature. Would you please put the thermometer under your armpit for five minutes?

护士：谢谢您给我这么多您的健康情况信息。现在我需要测量您的体温。请把体温计夹在腋下5分钟。

Patient: OK. How many times should I have my temperature taken everyday?

病人：好的。我每天应该测几次体温？

Nurse: Usually your temperature must be taken twice a day. If you have a fever, it will be every four hours.

护士：通常必须每天测两次。如果发烧，每4小时测一次。

(5 minutes later...)

(5分钟后……)

Nurse: Can I have the thermometer please?

护士：请把温度计给我好吗？

Patient: Here you are. Do I have a fever?

病人：给您。我发烧吗？

Nurse: A little. It's 37.8℃. It will go down soon with the treatment going on, Don't worry. Now let me count your pulse rate.

护士：有一点发烧，37.8℃。随着治疗的进行，体温会很快降下去。别担心。现在让我数数您的脉搏。

Patient: How is it?

病人：怎么样？

Nurse: 84 per minute. It's quite normal. I also have to take your blood pressure. I need your assistance.

护士：每分钟84次，很正常。我还得测您的血压。我需要您的配合。

Patient: All right. I will do whatever you ask me to do.

病人：好的。我听您的。

Nurse: Would you please roll up the sleeve of your left arm? I'm going to wind this cuff round your upper arm.

护士：请卷起左臂袖子好吗？我要把袖带绑在您的上臂上。

Patient: OK, no problem.

病人：行，没问题。

Nurse: Your blood pressure is one hundred and twenty over eighty mmHg.

护士：您的血压是120/80mmHg。

Patient: Is it normal?

病人：正常吗？

Nurse: Yes, it is.

护士：是的，正常。

Patient: Oh, I'm relieved. I've always been worried about it because both my father and grandfather are suffering from hypertension.

病人：哦，我放心了。我一直担心我的血压，因为我父亲和爷爷都患有高血压。

Nurse: Then you have to keep monitoring your BP. Hypertension has a very obvious hereditary tendency. From now on, you'd better not do the jobs that are too tiring and stressful. You should eat little meat and salt, but have lots of vegetables and fruits. And what's more, stay away from alcohol and give up smoking.

护士：那么您应该经常监测血压。高血压有非常明显的遗传倾向。从现在起，最好不要做太辛苦紧张的工作。您应该少吃盐，少吃肉，多吃蔬菜水果。此外，忌烟，禁酒。

Patient: I will try to follow your cooperation advice in life. Thank you very much.

病人：我会尽力照您的建议安排我的生活。非常感谢您。

Nurse: It's my pleasure.

护士：这是我的荣幸。

**(3)**

Nurse: Good morning, Mr. Lane. I'm Yan Fei, the nurse on duty. Did you eat or drink anything this morning?

护士：早上好，莱恩先生。我是值班护士闫菲。您今天早上吃东西喝水了吗？

Patient: No, I didn't. I was told to fast after midnight for the blood test this morning.

病人：没有。我接到通知说，午夜后不能进食喝水，今天早晨验血。

Nurse: Great. Thanks for your cooperation.

护士：很好。谢谢您的合作。

Patient: I'm very thirsty. I usually drink some water as soon as I wake up.

病人：我很渴。我通常一醒来就喝点水的。

Nurse: It will be very soon. Then you can have something to drink, Can I have your arm please?

护士：抽血会很快的。然后您就可以喝水了。您把手臂伸出来好吗？

Patient: This one. My veins don't stand out clearly.

病人：这只手臂吧。我的静脉不明显。

Nurse: I'll try to do it with great care, Mr. Lane. Relax, please.

护士：我会非常仔细地寻找，莱恩先生。请放松。

Patient: I will try.

病人：我尽量。

Nurse: Now make a fist, and don't look at it if you feel nervous. Here, the needle is in.

护士：现在握拳。如果您紧张，就不要看这里。好，针进去了。

Patient: How much blood do you need?

病人：需要抽多少血？

Nurse: I will just draw 8 ml. That's enough blood, and you can release your fist now. All right, it's done. You must press this area with the cotton wool for a while to stop bleeding.

护士：只抽8毫升。血够了，您可以松拳了。好，结束了。您必须用药棉在这里按一会儿以便止血。

Patient: Is that all?

病人：这就结束了吗？

Nurse: Yes, Mr. Lane. Don't be too nervous next time. The doctor has also ordered to collect your urine and stool specimens. Here are two containers with your name labels on them.

护士：是的，莱恩先生。下次不要太紧张了。医生还吩咐采尿和便标本。这是两个贴了您名字标签的标本盒。

Patient: How can I collect urine sample?

病人：我怎么采尿标本呢？

Nurse: Put on this pair of disposable gloves and hold this little cup. First pass some urine out and then pass urine into the cup till it's 1/3 full.

护士：带上这副一次性手套，捏住尿杯。先排出一点尿，然后把尿排到尿杯中，1/3杯就够。

Patient: What about stool specimen?

病人：便标本呢？

Nurse: Take a clean bedpan to the washroom. Pass your stool in the bedpan and don't throw the toilet paper into it. Then collect a little lump of stool with this stick and put it in this small paper box.

护士：带一个干净的便盆到洗手间。把大便排在便盆里，别把卫生纸扔进去。然后用这支小棒采集一小块便标本放在这个小纸盒里。

Patient: Where should I put the containers with specimens?

病人：我应该把采集完的标本盒放在哪里呢？

Nurse: On the table just outside the washroom please.

护士：放在一处洗手间的桌子上。

Patient: I've got it. Thank you.

病人：我明白了。谢谢。

Nurse: You're welcome.

护士：不客气。

# 12. Morning Care

# 晨间护理

Nurse： Good morning，Mr. Tailor. I'm Liu Qian，your nurse today. Did you sleep well last night?

护士： 早上好，泰勒先生。我是刘倩，您今天的护士。昨晚睡得好吗？

Patient： Not very well. I woke up at 3 a.m.this morning.

病人： 睡得不太好。我凌晨三点就醒了。

Nurse： You should tell your doctor about it.

护士： 您应该跟您的医生说说。

Patient： I think so.

病人： 我是这样想的。

Nurse： Let me help you to clean up.

护士： 让我来帮您梳洗。

Patient： All right.

病人： 好的。

Nurse： Would you like to brush your teeth first?

护士： 您想先刷牙吗？

Patient： Yes，I would.

病人： 好的。

Nurse： Are the ulcers in your mouth still hurting?

护士： 您嘴里的溃疡还疼吗？

Patient： They've got much better since you gave me the solution to rinse my mouth. My pajamas are all wet from sweating during the night. Can I have them changed?

病人： 您给我药水漱口后好多了。我夜里出汗，衣服都湿了。我可以换换衣服吗？

Nurse： Of course. I've already brought some clean ones for you. I'II give you a bed-bath and then I'II help you to change.

护士： 当然可以。我已经为您带来了干净衣服。我先给您做个床上擦浴，然后帮您换衣服。

Patient： That's great.

病人： 太好了。

Nurse： Would you please turn over to the other side? l'II rub your back with a hot towel and then massage it with alcohol and talcum powder.

护士：　请您翻过身去好吗？我用热毛巾给您擦擦背，然后用酒精和滑石粉按摩。

Patient:　What for?

病人：　这有什么作用呢？

Nurse:　It can stimulate your blood circulation to prevent pressure ulcers.

护士：　主要是为了促进血液循环，预防压迫性溃疡。

Patient:　What are pressure ulcers?

病人：　什么是压迫性溃疡？

Nurse:　They are usually called bedsores. They generally result from persistent pressure on the back.

护士：　就是人们通常说的褥疮。褥疮一般是背部持续受压引起的。

Patient:　I see.

病人：　我明白了。

Nurse:　You've got clean clothes now. I'm going to change the bed sheets, quilt cover and pillow case.

护士：　您换好干净衣服了。我准备换床单、被罩和枕套。

Patient:　Do I have to get up?

病人：　我需要起来吗？

Nurse:　No, you don't. I can do the change without your getting out of bed.

护士：　不必。您不用下床我就能换。

Patient:　All right.

病人：　好的。

Nurse:　We're done. You look much more comfortable now.

护士：　我们都弄好了。您看上去舒服多了。

Patient:　Yes, I am very comfortable. Thank you very much.

病人：　是的，我很舒服。非常感谢。

Nurse:　Would you mind if open the windows to air the room?

护士：　我开窗给房间通通风，您不介意吧？

Patient:　Of course not.

病人：　当然不。

Nurse:　I'll be back to close them after a little while.

护士：　过一会儿我会回来关窗的。

Patient:　Thank you.

病人：　谢谢。

Nurse:　My pleasure.

护士：　不客气。

# 13. Helping a Patient

# 帮助病人

## (1)

Nurse： Good morning, Mr. Adams. How are you doing today?

护士： 早晨好，亚当斯先生。今天你还好吗？

Patient： Horrible! I can't eat anything! I just feel sick to my stomach. Take the tray away.

病人： 糟糕透了，我吃不了东西，我胃里感到恶心。把盘子拿走。

Nurse： That's too bad. I'll just put this over here for now. Have you felt queasy for very long?

护士： 太遗憾啦。我暂时把它放一边儿。你感到恶心有很久了吗？

Patient： I woke up during the middle of the night. I couldn't get back to sleep, and now I feel terrible.

病人： 我半夜醒来后就再也睡不着了。现在我感到糟糕透了。

Nurse： Have you been to the toilet? Any diarrhea or vomiting?

护士： 你去过卫生间吗？有没有任何腹泻或者呕吐？

Patient： I've been to the toilet twice, but no diarrhea or vomiting. Perhaps, I should drink something. Can I have a cup of tea?

病人： 卫生间我去过两次。但是我没有腹泻或者呕吐。也许我应该喝点什么。我能喝杯茶吗？

Nurse： Certainly, I'll get you a cup immediately. Would you like black tea or peppermint tea?

护士： 当然可以，我马上给你倒一杯。你是要红茶还是薄荷茶？

Patient： Peppermint, please. Do you think I could have another blanket? I'm so cold. I think I'm getting the chills.

病人： 请给我薄荷茶。能不能再给我一床毯子？我感觉非常冷。

Nurse： Here's an extra blanket. Let me tuck you in.

护士： 再给你一床毯子。让我帮你盖好。

Patient： You're so sweet. What is your name?

病人： 你真好。你叫什么名字？

Nurse： My name is Alice. I'll be on shift during the day for the next few days.

护士： 我叫爱丽丝。以后这几天我都值白班。

Patient： Hello, Alice. My name is Jack. Nice to meet you.

病人： 你好，爱丽丝。我叫杰克。见到你真高兴。

Nurse： Let's get you feeling better, Jack! Is there anything else I can get for you?
护士： 让我们帮助你感觉舒服点，杰克。我还可以帮你做什么别的事情吗？
Patient： That's alright. I think a cup of tea and a warm blanket should help.
病人： 可以啦。我想一杯茶和一床毛毯应该可以了。
Nurse： OK. I'll be back as soon as the tea is ready.
护士： 好的，茶准备好我就回来。
Patient： Thank you.
病人： 谢谢你。

**(2)**

Patient： Nurse, I think I might have a fever. It's so cold in here!
病人： 护士，我想也许我发烧了。这里好冷啊！
Nurse： Here, let me check your forehead.
护士： 来吧，让我摸一下你的额头。
Patient： What do you think?
病人： 你认为怎么样？
Nurse： Your temperature seems raised. Let me get a thermometer to check.
护士： 你的体温好像是升高了。我拿个温度计给你量一下。
Patient： How do I raise my bed? I can't find the controls.
病人： 怎么样才能够把我的床摇高？我找不到控制把手。
Nurse： Here you are. Is that better?
护士： 在这里，好点了吗？
Patient： Could I have another pillow?
病人： 能不能再给我一个枕头？
Nurse： Certainly, Here you are. Is there anything else I can do for you?
护士： 当然可以，给你。还有别的其他事情要我帮你做吗？
Patient： No, thank you.
病人： 不用了，谢谢。
Nurse： OK, I'll be right back with the thermometer.
护士： 好的，我去拿温度计，马上就回来。
Patient： Oh, just a moment. Can you bring me another bottle of water, too?
病人： 哦，稍等一下，能不能再给我拿瓶水来？
Nurse： Certainly, I'll be back in a moment.
护士： 当然可以，我一会就回来。

**(3)**

Relative： Excuse me, nurse.
探视者： 打扰一下，护士。
Nurse： yes?
护士： 什么事？

Relative：Can you tell me the way to the pharmacy，please?

探视者：你能告诉去药房的路吗？

Nurse：Yes，sure. But it's quite a long walk from here.

护士：当然了，但是离这里很远。

Relative：It's all right.

探视者：没关系。

Nurse：Well，take the lift down to Level 1. When you go out of the lift，turn right and walk all the way down the corridor. You will pass the Radiology Department on your left. Keep walking till you get to the Urology Centre.

护士：好，乘电梯到一楼，出电梯向右转，一直沿着走廊走，你将会看到放射科在你的左手边，继续向前走直到泌尿外科中心。

Relative：I see.

探视者：我明白。

Nurse：Turn right and go straight to the end of the annex building. Look for the signage that says"East Wing". Follow the arrow sign. Further down you will see Gynaecology Clinic. You can't miss it because of its distinctive design and the mural painting.

护士：向右转，继续走直到裙楼的尽头，留心"东翼"指示牌，顺着箭头标志走，你会看到妇科门诊，那里有独具特色的设计和壁画，你一定能找到。

Relative：Hmmm...Okay.

探视者：嗯，好的。

Nurse：Go past the Gynaecology Clinic，and then you'll find the atrium of the main building. Look out for the taxi stand. The pharmacy is next to it. Ask the customer service staffs at the information counter if you get lost.

护士：走过妇科门诊，你会来到主楼的大厅。留心的士站点，药房就在它旁边。如果你迷路了，可以到咨询台询问客服主管。

Relative：How long does it take to get there?

探视者：到那里大约需要多长时间？

Nurse：It will take you about ten minutes.

护士：大约需要10分钟。

Relative：Thank you very much.

探视者：非常感谢你。

Nurse：You're welcome.

护士：你太客气了。

# 14. An Intromuscular Injection and a Skin Test

# 肌内注射和皮试

## (1)

Nurse： Good morning. Are you Mr. Addison，Bed 48?

护士： 早上好，您是48床的艾迪森先生吗？

Patient： Yes，I am.

病人： 是的，我是。

Nurse： The doctor has ordered to give you an injection of penicillin. Do you know if you are allergic to it?

护士： 医生下医嘱给您注射青霉素，您知道自己是否对青霉素过敏吗？

Patient： I have no idea. I've never had this shot.

病人： 不知道。我从来没打过这种针。

Nurse： I'm going to do a skin test first to see if you have any sensitivity. Now，please roll up your sleeve and rest your forearm on the table and relax.

护士： 我会先做皮试，看看您是否过敏。现在请卷起袖子，前臂放在桌子上，放松。

Patient： OK.

病人： 好的。

Nurse： It's done. I'll be back in 20 minutes to look at your reaction. If you feel any discomfort，such as dizziness，sweating or chest pain，please press the call button.

护士： 做完了。我会在20分钟之后回来看皮试反应。如果您感到任何不适，如头晕、出汗或胸痛，请按呼叫按钮。

Patient： OK.

病人： 好的。

(20 minutes later)

(20分钟后)

Nurse： Time is up.

护士： 时间到。

Patient： How is my skin test result?

病人： 我的皮试结果怎样？

Nurse： There's no redness or swelling. You're not allergic to penicillin. I'm going to give you the injection. Please wait. I'll be in a moment.

护士：没有红肿。您对青霉素不过敏。我马上给您注射。请稍等，我很快就回来。

（A moment later）

（几分钟后）

Patient: Where do you give it?

病人：在哪注射？

Nurse: In the buttocks.

护士：在臀部。

Patient: There's a lump on my left buttock from the last week's injection. What shall I do?

病人：因为上星期打的那些针，我的左臀有个硬块。我该怎么办？

Nurse: Let me have a look. You can put hot towels on it for fifteen minutes three times a day. If it doesn't get better，we'll try physiotherapy.

护士：让我看看。您最好用毛巾热敷 15 分钟，每天敷 3 次。如果没有好转，我们再试试理疗。

Patient: Thank you for your advice.

病人：谢谢你的建议。

Nurse: I'll give the injection in your right buttock today. Would you please unite your belt and pull your trousers lower?

护士：今天我会在您的右臀上注射。请您解开腰带，把裤子拉下来一些，好吗？

Patient: Please be gentle.

病人：请轻点。

Nurse: I will. I'll sterilizing the skin...and it's done. Did it hurt?

护士：好的。我在给皮肤消毒……注射完了。疼吗？

Patient: No，never felt a thing.

病人：一点也不疼。

Nurse: If you feel uncomfortable，please call me right away.

护士：如果您感到不舒服，请立刻按铃叫我。

Patient: OK. Thank you.

病人：好的，谢谢。

Nurse: You're welcome.

护士：不客气。

**（2）**

Nurse: Mr. Bush，you have pneumonia and will need to give you some penicillin injection. First，I'll give you a penicillin skin test. Have you used penicillin before?

护士：布什先生，您患的是肺炎，需要注射青霉素。首先要给您做个青霉素过敏试验。您以前用过青霉素吗？

Patient: Yes，I have.

病人：用过。

Nurse: Are you allergic to it?

护士：那您对青霉素过敏吗？

Patient： No，never.

病人： 不，从来不过敏。

Nurse： Are you allergic to any other medicine?

护士： 您对其他药物过敏吗？

Patient： No.

病人： 没有。

Nurse： OK. Please give me your right hand.

护士： 那好，请伸出右手。

Patient： All right.

病人： 好的。

Nurse： If you feel any discomfort，such as dizziness，sweating or chest pain，please tell me.

护士： 如果您感到头晕、出汗、胸痛，或者有任何不舒服的地方请告诉我。

Patient： I will. May I ask some questions?

病人： 好的。我能问几个问题吗？

Nurse： Yes，certainly.

护士： 当然可以。

Patient： I don't understand why you take my temperature and feel pulse several times a day.

病人： 我不明白为什么您每天给我测好几次血压和脉搏。

Nurse： An individual's temperature，pulse，respiratory and blood pressure are called vital signs. They are measured to detect any changes in normal function. They are also used to determine a patient's response to treatments. A change in condition can be recognized from the vital signs.

护士： 一个人的体温、脉搏、呼吸和血压叫做生命体征。通过测量生命体征，我们可以监测人体正常功能的变化，判断病人对治疗的反应。病情变化也可以从生命体征上表现出来。

Patient： I didn't know they were so useful.

病人： 真没想到有这么大用途。

（20 minutes later）

（20 分钟后）

Nurse： There is no red or swelling. You are not allergic to penicillin. Please untie your belt and pull your trousers lower. I'll give you a penicillin injection.

护士： 没有红肿，您不过敏。请解开腰带，把裤子拉下来一些。我要给您打一针青霉素。

Patient： Please do it gently.

病人： 请轻一点。

Nurse： I will. Do you feel a sting where I press? Bend your left leg and relax your muscles...

护士： 我会的。觉着我压着的地方刺痛吗？把左腿弯起来，肌肉放松……

# 15. An Introvenous Infusion

# 静脉输液

**（1）**

Nurse： Good morning，Mr. Bryant. It’s time to start your IV.

护士： 布莱恩特先生，上午好。该给您输液了。

Patient： Could you tell me about how the IV fluid helps me?

病人： 对不起，您能告诉我输这些液体的作用吗？

Nurse： Of course.The fluids will provide energy for you and prevent electrolytic imbalances after operation.

护士： 当然可以。输入的液体能为您提供能量，还可预防术后电解质失衡。

Patient： Would you please let the fluid drop more quickly?

病人： 请您把液体滴速调快点儿好吗？

Nurse： No.Your IV fluids must be given slowly so as not to overburden your heart.

护士： 不可以的。您的静脉输液必须慢速，不然会增加心脏负荷。

**（2）**

Nurse： Good morning. Are you Mr. Lane. Bed 28?

护士： 早上好。您是28床莱恩先生吗？

Patient： Yes. I am.

病人： 我是。

Nurse： It’s time to give you today’s IV treatment. It’ll take a couple of hours. Do you need to go to the washroom or something before that?

护士： 到给您做今天的静脉输液治疗的时间了。输液需要几小时。您需要先上洗手间或做什么准备吗？

Patient： I don’t. I’m ready.

病人： 不需要，我已经准备好了。

Nurse： Good.

护士： 很好。

Patient： What is in the bottle?

病人： 瓶子里是什么药？

Nurse： It is a glucose and NS solution with some medicines in it. Now I’m going to wind a tourniquet round your arm to look for a good vein. Please make a fist.

护士：是加了药的葡萄糖和生理盐水溶液。现在我要用止血带扎住您的手臂找个明显的静脉。请握拳。

Patient：Please be gentle.

病人：请轻点。

Nurse：I will. I'm sterilizing. Please don't move until I tell you. The needle is in. Please release your fist. I'm turning on the IV.

护士：好的，我在消毒。我不叫您动时请不要动。针进去了。请松拳。我要打开调节器了。

Patient：Can I move now?

病人：我能动了吗？

Nurse：No，you can't move until I tape it up. All right. It's all set.

护士：等我把它粘牢您才能动。好，都弄妥了。

Patient：Can you make fluid run faster? I don't want to be confined in bed for a long time.

病人：能让液体流快点吗？我不想好长时间下不了床。

Nurse：I'm afraid not. The IV should drip at the speed as you can see in the drip chamber now.

护士：恐怕不行。输液就应该是现在您看到的滴管里的速度。

Patient：Why?

病人：为什么？

Nurse：If your IV fluid runs too fast，It will overload your heart. You can sit up if you fell tired.You may stand up if you like. Whatever you do，you should keep your IV site lower than your heart.

护士：如果您的静脉液体流得太快，会使您的心脏超负荷。您感觉累了可以坐起来。如果您愿意，站起来都行。无论您做什么，必须保持输液部位低于心脏。

Patient：I see.

病人：我明白。

Nurse：If you feel any pain or see any swelling，please press your call button at once. Don't worry.I'll be back from time to check it.

护士：如果您感觉这里疼或看到肿起来，请立即按呼叫按钮。别担心。我会随时回来查看的。

Patient：Thank you.

病人：谢谢。

Nurse：My pleasure.

护士：不客气。

# 16. Talking with a Patient about His Surgery

# 与病人谈论手术

## (1)

Nurse: I saw that the surgeon and anesthesiologist talked with you. Do you have any questions about what they said?

护士：我看到外科医生和麻醉师跟您谈话了，对他们说的您还有什么问题吗？

Patient: Well, Dr.Clinton said to me, 'You will be NPO tonight.' And he mentioned an IV.What does that mean?

病人：哦，克林顿医生对我说："您今晚是 NPO。"他还提到Ⅳ，这些是什么意思？

Nurse: Well, as preparation for the surgery you have been on a liquid diet today. After midnight you cannot eat or drink anything. That is called NPO. An Ⅳ is a needle that is inserted into a vein in your arm. We'll start one tonight to give you fluids and any necessary medicine.

护士：好，作为手术前的准备，您今晚要实行流质饮食。午夜后您就不能吃喝任何东西了，这就叫 NPO。Ⅳ是一根扎入您手臂静脉的针头，我们今晚开始通过Ⅳ给您输液体和必要的药。

Patient: When will I go to surgery?

病人：我什么时候做手术？

Nurse: You'll leave here at about 7 a.m. Early in the morning the nurse will shave your abdomen, and then give you a premedication that will make you very sleepy. You won't be able to get out of bed after you get the shot.

护士：您早上 7 点离开这儿。明早会有护士为您清洁腹部，然后给您术前用药，这将使您昏昏欲睡。吃了药后您就起不来床了。

Patient: When will I come back?

病人：我什么时候回来呢？

Nurse: Well, your surgery is at 8 a.m. After surgery you will spend a few hours in the Recovery Room. After your condition is stable, you will come back here, probably not before 2 p.m. When you come back, you will still be very sleepy.

护士：您的手术在 8 点开始。手术后您要在恢复室休息几个小时。您的情况稳定后，就会回到这里，大概不会在下午 2 点以前吧。回来的时候，您还会在睡。

Patient: Will it be painful?

病人：我会很痛吗？

Nurse：Abdominal surgery may be painful，be sure to tell the nurse if you have pain and she will give you a pain shot for it. We want you to be comfortable，and we will be asking you to cough，breath deeply，and do leg exercises. These are important to prevent postoperative complications.

护士：腹部手术一般会很痛。如果痛就叫护士，她会给您止痛药。我们希望在要求您咳嗽、深呼吸和做腿部练习的时候您能感觉舒服。这对避免术后并发症状很重要。

Patient：What kind of complications?

病人：什么并发症？

Nurse：Well，anesthesia and bed rest can cause some problems with your lungs and legs circulation. As soon as you are awake，we will be saying"take a deep breath，cough."This is to help prevent pneumonia. We will be getting you out of bed the morning after surgery to help the blood circulation in your lower body.

护士：麻醉与卧床可能引发肺部问题和腿部血流不畅。你一醒过来，我们会让你深吸气、咳嗽以避免肺炎。明天早上我们还会帮您下床，促进您下肢的血液循环。

Patient：What is this machine?

病人：这是什么机器？

Nurse：That is an incentive spirometer. It is to help you breath deeply. This also helps to prevent pneumonia. Why don't you try it now? The indicator goes up when you inhale deeply.

护士：这是一台诱发型肺量计。它能帮助您深呼吸，还能帮助避免肺炎。为什么不试试？当您深吸气时，这指针就会浮上来。

Patient：Like this?

病人：就这样？

Nurse：Yes，good. If you have any questions，please let me know.

护士：对，很好。如您有任何问题，请告诉我。

Patient：I will. Thank.

病人：我会的，谢谢。

## （2）

Nurse：Good morning，Mr. Smith. I'm Wang Hua，your nurse today. Has Dr. Davis told you that you are going to be operated on tomorrow morning?

护士：早上好，史密斯先生。我是王华，今天我是您的护士。达维斯大夫通知您明天上午做手术了吗？

Patient：Yes，I was told yesterday.

病人：是的，昨天告诉我的

Nurse：Have you signed the surgical consent form yet?

护士：您签手术同意书了吗？

Patient：Yes，I have. What time will the operation start?

病人：是的，签了。手术什么时候开始？

Nurse: At 9: 00. But you'll have to get pre-medication and leave for the Operating Room at least half an hour before that. If your wife and other relatives come to see you, they must be here by 8: 00.

护士：上午9点钟。但是您得接受术前药物，要提前至少半小时离开病房去手术室。如果您的妻子和其他亲属来见您，必须8点前到这里。

Patient: How long am I going to stay in the operating room?

病人：我会在手术室待多长时间？

Nurse: It is hard to say. It will depend on the operation procedures and your recovery from the anesthesia. And after the surgery, you'll stay in the Recovery Room for some time until your condition is stabilized.

护士：很难说。这取决于手术过程和麻醉恢复的情况。手术后，您会在恢复室待一段时间，直到您的状况稳定。

Patient: I see. This is the first time I'm in hospital for surgery. I'm really scared.

病人：我明白了。这是我第一次住院做手术。我真的很害怕。

Nurse: Take it easy, Mr. Smith. The surgeon who is going to give you the operation is very experienced and considerate. Everything will work out fine. Don't worry.

护士：别紧张，史密斯先生。给您做手术的外科医生经验非常丰富，考虑也很周到。一切都会顺利的。不要担心。

Patient: Well, I'll try not to. Will I feel pain during the operation?

病人：好吧，我会尽量不担心。手术中我会感觉疼吗？

Nurse: As you're going to have a general anesthesia, you won't have any feel.

护士：由于您将进行全身麻醉，您不会有任何感觉。

Patient: Thanks. Now I don't feel as nervous as before.

病人：谢谢。现在我不像先前那么紧张了。

Nurse: As part of the preparation for the surgery, you have to have a liquid supper this evening, and absolutely nothing by mouth after midnight.

护士：作为手术准备工作的一部分，您今天晚饭只能吃流食，而且午夜之后绝对不能吃或喝任何东西。

Patient: I see.

病人：我明白。

Nurse: The nurse on the evening shift is going to give you a skin preparation and an enema.

护士：晚班护士会给您备皮和灌肠。

Patient: I've got it. Thank you for telling me so much.

病人：我知道了。感谢您告诉我这么多。

Nurse: You're welcome.

护士：不客气。

**（3）**

Nurse: We are going to do the operation on you tomorrow. I hope you won't be nervous.

护士：明天我们就要给您做手术了，希望您不要紧张。

Patient: I will try not to, but will it hurt?

病人：我尽量，但手术会不会很痛？

Nurse: You will be anesthetized, so you won't feel pain until it off. Have you signed your consent yet?

护士：您将被麻醉，所以手术期间您不会觉得痛。您在手术同意书上签字了吗？

Patient: How should I write it?

病人：该怎么写呢？

Nurse: "I (name) the undersigned have requested and consented to a certain operation." That's all. We need the seal of your embassy and the signature of your Ambassador on the consent form.

护士："我（名字）签名人申请并同意做某种手术。"然后签上名字就行了。我们需要在这张同意书上盖上你们大使馆的印鉴，还需要你们大使的签字。

Nurse: I will have to shave around the area of operation.

护士：我要把手术区周围的毛剃一下。

Patient: I have never been in a hospital before. I'm very scared.

病人：我从来没住过医院，我害怕极了。

Nurse: There is nothing to worry about. The doctor who will operate on you is very experienced and considerate. If you have any discomfort during the operation, please don't hesitate to tell him. I'll give you an enema tonight. After that, please don't take any food or water before the operation.

护士：不必担心，给您做手术的医生富有经验而且细致耐心。手术当中您有什么不舒服，尽管向他提出来。我今天晚上要给您灌一次肠。这以后直到手术前请不要再吃东西或喝水了。

Patient: How do you do it? Does it hurt?

病人：您怎么做呢，痛吗？

Nurse: I'II insert a rubber tube into your anus and let the soapsuds solution flow into your rectum. Please let me know if you feel a distension. I'II stop the flow. Try to hold it in for a few minutes before you expel it. That will produce a better result.

护士：我先给您肛门里插根橡皮管，再往（直肠）里送些肥皂水。您觉着肚子胀，就说话，我就不灌了。您先尽量憋几分钟再排便，这样效果就会好些。

# 17. Preparing an Operation

# 手术准备

## (1)

Nurse： Good afternoon，Mrs. Brown. Do you know you're scheduled to have an operation tomorrow?

护士： 下午好，布朗夫人。您知道您明天要做手术了吗？

Patient： Yeah，but what time am I going to have it?

病人： 是的，可具体是什么时间呢？

Nurse： The operation starts at nine o'clock in the morning. But you will have to get injections about 30 to 45 minutes before you leave for the surgery. If your family comes to see you before the operation，they should be here by 7：30 a.m.

护士： 手术上午 9 点开始，但您要在离开病房去做手术前 30～45 分钟打针。如果您的家人要在手术前看您，应该在早上 7：30 前到这儿。

Patient： I see.

病人： 我知道。

Nurse： Did your doctor tell what kind of operation you're going to have?

护士： 您的医生告诉您要做什么手术了吗？

Patient： Yeah，I'm going to have cystectomy.

病人： 是的，我要做膀胱切除手术。

Nurse： All right. Have you signed the consent?

护士： 好的，您在手术同意书上签字了吗？

Patient： Yes，here it is.

病人： 是的，在这儿。

Nurse： I would like to explain the preparation for the operation. If you have any question，please stop me.

护士： 我要为您说明手术准备工作，您如有问题，请打断我。

Patient： OK.

病人： 好。

Nurse： First of all，we'll prepare you by shaving and cleaning your abdomen. After shaving，we would like you to take a bath or shower.

护士： 首先，我们要为您刮除手术区的体毛并清洁腹部，之后您要洗个澡或冲个淋浴。

Patient: I see.

病人：明白。

Nurse: You're going to have a liquid meal for dinner and you'll get sleeping pills at nine. You should take in absolutely nothing by mouth after midnight. In the early morning you'll have an enema.

护士：今晚您要吃流食，晚 9 点服安眠药。午夜后不能进食任何东西。明天一早要进行灌肠。

Patient: How long am I going to stay in the operating room?

病人：我要在手术室待多长时间？

Nurse: It's hard to tell. It will depend on operating procedure and your recovery from the anesthesia. You'll probably return to this room in the afternoon.

护士：很难说，这取决于手术的进程和您从麻醉苏醒的时间。您可能要在明天下午回到病房。

Patient: I see.

病人：明白了。

Nures: You look worried. Do you have any concerns?

护士：您有点儿焦虑，有什么问题吗？

Patient: Nurse, will this operation hurt a lot?

病人：护士，这个手术很痛吗？

Nurse: No. You're going to have general anesthesia. So during the operation you'll not feel anything. You'll find yourself back in your room after the operation.

护士：不会。您将处于全身麻醉，手术期间您不会有任何感觉。手术后您将发现您已经回到您的病房中。

Patient: OK. Thank you, nurse.

病人：好，谢谢你，护士。

## (2)

Nurse: Good evening, Mr. Smith. I'm Gu Fang, the nurse on evening shift. You are going to have a subtotal gastrectomy tomorrow morning, aren't you?

护士：晚上好，史密斯先生。我是顾方，夜班护士。您明天早上做胃次全切手术，对吗？

Patient: Yes, I am.

病人：是的。

Nurse: As part of the preparation for the surgery, I have to shave off the hair around the operation area. Are you ready?

护士：作为手术准备的一部分，我得剃去手术区周围的毛发。您准备好了吗？

Patient: Yes, but...

病人：准备好了，不过……

Nurse: Don't be shy. You see. I've drawn on the curtain between your bed and the other one. Nobody can see you except me. You have to stay still until I finish it lest the razor should hurt you.

护士： 不用害羞。您看。我已经把您的床和另一张床之间的帘子拉上了。除了我没有人能看到您。您必须保持不动，直到我做完，以免剃刀伤到您。

Patient： I will.

病人：好的。

（Shaving）

（备皮进行中）

Nurse： OK. It's finished. And I also have to give you an enema.

护士： 好了。备皮做完了。我还得给您灌肠。

Patient： Why do I need it? I'm not constipated.

病人： 为什么要灌肠？我不便秘。

Nurse： It is necessary to flush out your intestine in order to keep your bowel clean for the operation.

护士： 为了保持手术时肠道清洁，必须冲洗您的肠道。

Patient： I see.

病人： 我懂了。

Nurse： Please stay in bed. I'll be back with the enema appliances.

护士： 请躺在床上，我马上取灌肠用具来。

（A moment later...）

（片刻之后……）

Patient： How do you do it? Does it hurt?

病人： 怎么灌肠呢？会不会痛呀？

Nurse： I'll insert this rubber tube into your anus and let the soap suds solution flow into your rectum. It won't hurt at all.

护士： 我会把这个橡皮管插入肛门，让肥皂水流进直肠。一点也不疼。

Patient： I see.

病人： 我明白了。

Nurse： While I'm doing it, you may feel a little distension. So please take a deep breath with your mouth open. After it's finished, you'd better hold it for ten minutes before you expel it. That may produce a better result.

护士： 我做灌肠时，您可能会觉得有点腹胀。请张开嘴深呼吸。灌肠完毕后，您最好憋10分钟再排便。这样效果更好。

Patient： I've got it.

病人： 我知道了。

Nurse： Let's begin. Would you please lie on your left side? If you feel distension, please let me know. I'll slow the flowing down.

护士： 开始吧。请您朝左侧躺好吗？如果您觉得腹胀，请告诉我。我会放慢液体流的速度。

（The enema is going on）

（灌肠进行中）

Patient： How much solution is there left in the bottle? I can't hardly hold much longer.

病人：瓶子里还剩多少液体？我憋不住了。

Nurse：It will be finished soon. Take a deep breath...Good. Now we are through. Try to lie on your back or on the right side for a few minutes. Then I'II help you to the toilet.

护士：快完了。深呼吸……好。现在我们完成了。试着平躺或朝右侧躺几分钟。然后我扶您上厕所。

Patient：Oh，I don't feel so uncomfortable now. I think I can manage by myself.

病人：哦，现在我不觉得那么不舒服了。我想我自己可以应付。

Nurse：Please feel free to call me if you need me. Do you remember you can't have any food or water after midnight?

护士：如果您需要我，请随时按铃叫我。还记得午夜后不能吃东西或喝水吗？

Patient：Yes，I do.

病人：是的，我记得。

Nurse：Then try to have a good sleep.

护士：那么尽可能睡个好觉。

Patient：I'll try. Thank you.

病人：我尽量。谢谢。

Nurse：My pleasure.

护士：很高兴为您服务。

# 18. Post-operative Care

# 术后护理

## (1)

Nurse： Mr. Jones，how are you feeling?

护士： 琼斯先生，您感觉怎么样？

Patient： Terrible. Why did you get me out of bed today? I just had surgery yesterday.

病人： 糟透了。为什么您今天就要我起床？我昨天刚做完手术。

Nurse： It can prevent complications.

护士： 早点儿起床能避免手术并发症。

Patient： I've never heard of that. When my dad had surgery，he was in bed for a week.

病人： 我从来没听说过。我爸爸做手术的时候，他在床上躺了一周。

Nurse： They used to do that. Now we know that getting up early is better.

护士： 那过时了。现在我们知道，早些起床更好。

Patient： But it hurts. And I feel dizzy.

病人： 但我很痛，痛死了。我还感觉晕。

Nurse： You were given a pain shot an hour before you got up. You should get up slowly. Look ahead and don't look down; you will feel less dizzy.

护士： 您起床前一小时已经用过止痛药。您应该慢慢起来。向前看，别向下看，您就觉得不那么晕了。

Patient： What is that machine? What is it for?

病人： 这个机器是什么？干什么用的？

Nurse： This is an incentive spirometer. It is to help you to breathe more deeply. Patients can get pneumonia after surgery because they are in pain and don't breathe deeply. This machine helps prevent pneumonia.

护士： 这是诱发型肺量计，它能帮助您深呼吸。病人手术后因为疼痛不愿做深呼吸可能会发生肺炎，这台机器能帮病人避免肺炎。

Patient： Why did the doctor listen to my stomach?

病人： 医生为什么要听我的肚子？

Nurse： He was listening for bowel sounds. As soon as your bowels are moving again，you can start to eat again.

护士： 他在听肠鸣音。一旦您的肠管开始恢复蠕动，您就可以吃东西了。

Patient： All I want to do is sleep. Why are you keeping me up?

病人：我现在就想睡觉，您干嘛总是打搅我？

Nurse：It is my job to make sure you don't have any complications. If you do the deep breathing and get out of bed often，you will be able to go home quicker.

护士：使您避免任何并发症是我的工作。如果您坚持深呼吸和多起床，您就能早点儿回家。

Patient：I'll try to do as you say.

病人：我会试着按您说的做。

**（2）**

Nurse：Good morning，doctor.

护士：医生，早晨好。

Doctor：Good morning. How is the patient after surgery?

医生：早晨好，病人手术后情况如何？

Nurse：The patient has a slight pain in the wound. Some blood has been oozing from the draining wound; the dressing has been changed once.

护士：伤口有点痛。伤口引流有些渗血，换过一次敷料。

Doctor：That's good.

医生：那很好。

Nurse：Does he still need the Ⅳ and penicillin?

护士：静脉输液和青霉素是否继续给？

Doctor：Yes.

医生：继续。

Nurse：（To the patient）You look a little better today.

护士：今天看来您精神好一些。

Patient：Yes，but lying in bed all day，I feel uncomfortable all over.

病人：是的，不过整天躺着我觉得全身不舒服。

Nurse：You can get out of bed today. Sit on the edge of the bed，and if you don't feel dizzy you can get out of bed.

护士：您今天可以下床，先在床边坐坐，没有头晕就可以下床了。

Patient：But my abdomen feels stuffed.

病人：不过我感到腹胀得很。

Nurse：Did you pass any wind?

护士：您排气了没有？

Patient：No.

病人：没有。

Nurse：You can lie on your side more often. If the wound does not hurt，you can get out of bed and walk around. That will help peristalsis of the intestine，which means you will pass gas a bit more easily and the distension will go away.

护士：可以多侧卧，如果伤口不痛可下床活动，那样有助于恢复肠蠕动，使气体排出减轻腹胀。

Patient：The wound is painful and it is hard to cough up the sputum.

病人：伤口痛，而且有痰又难咳出来。

Nurse：You should sit up. That will help you breath deeper and cough out sputum more smoothing, and prevent pneumonia.

护士：您应该坐起来，那样可以帮助您深呼吸，使痰较容易咳出，并防止肺炎。

Patient：All right.

病人：好的。

Nurse：Did you drink any water?

护士：您喝过水了吗？

Patient：Yes.

病人：喝过。

Nurse：Does you stomach feel stuffed or do you feel nauseated?

护士：您感觉胃胀和恶心吗？

Patient：No

病人：没有。

Nurse：That's good. You can start on a fluid diet now and probably porridge in two days.

护士：那很好，您可以开始吃流质，过两天吃稀饭。

Patient：Thank you. How much longer do I have to stay in hospital?

病人：谢谢。我还要住院多久？

Nurse：You can go home in about a week

护士：一个星期左右便可出院了。

**（3）**

Nurse：Good morning，Mr. Hill. I'm Zhang Fan，your nurse today. How are you feeling now?

护士：早上好，希尔先生。我叫张帆，今天是您的护士。您现在感觉怎样？

Patient：Much better.

病人：好多了。

Nurse：Have you passed the gas yet?

护士：您排气了吗？

Patient：Yes，I did it last night.

病人：是的，昨晚排气了。

Nurse：Good.

护士：很好。

Patient：Can I move in bed?

病人：我能在床上活动吗？

Nurse：Yes，of course. Actually you should get out of bed as soon as possible.

护士：当然能。其实您应该尽快下床活动。

Patient：My wound is still hurting.

病人：我的伤口还疼呢。

Nurse：You must have some movement in order to prevent intestinal adhesion. Let me help you to get up. Put your hand on your wound，and walk around the room slowly. Yes， that's right.

护士： 您必须活动活动，为的是预防肠粘连。我来帮您起床。把手按在伤口上，在屋子里慢慢走走。对，就这样。

(Talking while walking...)

（边走边聊……）

Patient: Can I eat something today?

病人： 今天我能吃点东西吗？

Nurse: Since you have passed the gas，you can start to have some liquid diet today.

护士： 既然您已经排气了，今天您可以开始吃流质饮食。

Patient: Great. When will I be able to leave the hospital?

病人： 太好了。我什么时候能出院？

Nurse: Your sutures will be removed seven days after the operation. You can go home after that if everything works out well.

护士： 术后七天拆线。如果一切顺利，拆线之后您就可以回家了。

Patient: I'd like to hear that.

病人： 我就想听到这个。

Nurse: Please go back to bed to take a rest. You can get up again to have a walk later.

护士： 请先回床上休息一会儿。过会儿再下床走动。

Patient: Ow，my wound is really hurting. It's over 3 hours since I had the last pain shot. I need medicine to stop the pain.

病人： 哎哟！我的伤口真疼呀。上次打止疼针到现在已经三个多小时了，我需要止疼药。

Nurse: It seems to be a little early to give you another pain shot，This medicine has a very strong effect and the doctor has ordered medication at four hours interval. Can you stand it for a while?

护士： 现在打下一次止疼针似乎有点早。这药效力很强，医生下医嘱要求间隔四小时用药。您能忍一会儿吗？

Patient: Oh，no，I can't stand it any longer.

病人： 不行，我忍受不住了。

Nurse: I see. Then I will call the doctor to see if I can give you a pain killer. Please relax and don't worry.

护士： 我明白了。那么我打电话给医生看看是否可以给您止痛药。请放松，别担心。

Patient: Thanks a lot.

病人： 多谢。

Nurse: You're welcome.

护士： 不客气。

# 19. Physical Assessment

# 身体检查

Nurse： Mr. James，I now need to do a physical assessment. Would you please change into this patient gown and lie down on the bed?

护士： 詹姆斯先生，我要为您做一个身体检查，请您换上这个病号服并躺在床上。

Patient： Certainly.

病人： 没问题。

（While Mr. James is changing，the nurse washes her hands.）

（在詹姆斯先生换衣服的时候，护士在洗手。）

Nurse： Please lie on your back. Let me put your head up a little. Is that more comfortable?

护士： 请仰卧。让我把您的头抬高些，这样舒服吗？

Patient： Yes. It is also less painful if I bend my knee a little.

病人： 是的。如果我将膝盖弯一点，疼痛也会轻一点。

Nurse： First I am going to listen to your abdomen. Do you feel any pain when I push on your abdomen?

护士： 我先听听您的肚子。我按您的肚子时您感觉痛吗？

Patient： Yes.

病人： 是的

Nurse： Take a deep breath in through your nose and let it out through your mouth. This will help you relax.

护士： 通过鼻子深深吸气，并通过嘴呼气。这有助于您放松。

Patient： Yes，it does.

病人： 是，确实管用。

Nurse： Do you have any trouble with constipation or diarrhea?

护士： 您有便秘或腹泻的毛病吗？

Patient： Usually，it is quite regular. But I haven't had a bowel movement for three days.

病人： 通常很正常，但我有三天没解大便了。

Nurse： Now I will check your feet. Please push against my hands.

护士： 现在我来检查您的脚。请蹬我的手。

（As the nurse checks the symmetrical strength of the.feet，she checks the skin color and temperature and the pulse.）

（在护士检查双脚力量对称的时候，她还检查了他的皮肤颜色以及体温和脉搏）

Patient: Is everything okay?

病人：都正常吗？

Nurse: Yes. Now I need to listen to your heart. Please don't talk. (The nurse assesses the heart sounds.) Now I am going to listen your lungs. Please sit up. Please take a deep breath in, hold it, and let it out. Again, again. Now breath normally. Thank you.

护士：是的。现在我要听听您的心脏，请别说话（护士仔细听心脏的声音）。我现在要听一下您的肺部。请坐起来，深吸一口气，憋住，呼出。再来一次，再来一次。现在请正常呼吸。谢谢。

Patient: What is going to happen?

病人：下面做什么？

Nurse: I am going to start an Ⅳ to give you fluids. You are NPO that means you cannot eat or drink anything. I'll be taking your temperature every four hours. In the morning you will have more blood tests and x-rays. Since we don't know the cause of the pain, we cannot give you any pain medicine. It might hide your symptoms.

护士：我要给您做静脉输液。您是NPO，就是说您不能吃喝任何东西。我每四小时为您测量一次体温。上午您还要做更多的检查和X线检查。由于不知道您疼痛的起因，我们不能给您服用止痛药。那会掩盖您的症状。

Patient: What if it becomes worse?

病人：如果更痛怎么办？

Nurse: Whenever you feel pain, you can do deep breathing. It will help you to relax. I need to prepare the IV now. I'll be back soon.

护士：感觉痛的时候，您可以做深呼吸。这会帮助您放松。我要去准备静脉输液了，马上就回来。

Nurse: Mr. Black, I am going to take your vital signs.

护士：布莱克先生，我要测量您的生命体征。

Patient: What are vital signs?

病人：什么是生命体征？

Nurse: Your temperature, heart rate, respiration rate and blood pressure. Please open your mouth. Thanks. Now keep it close.

护士：您的体温、心率、呼吸频率和血压。请您张开嘴。谢谢，请闭上。

(The nurse put the thermometer into Mr.Black's mouth, and checks his blood pressure. Then, takes the thermometer out.)

（护士将体温表放入布莱克先生的口中，并测量血压，然后将体温表取出。）

Patient: What was my temperature?

病人：我的体温是多少？

Nurse: Thirty-seven degrees.

护士：37℃。

Patient: And my blood pressure?

病人：血压呢？

Nurse: One hundred and twenty over eighty mmHg.

护士： 120/80 mmHg。

Patient： Is that normal?

病人： 正常吗？

Nurse： Yes. Now I need to listen to your heart and lungs. Take a deep breath in. Again.

护士： 是的。现在我要听听您的心肺。深吸一口气。再来一次。

Patient： Okay, Thank you.

病人： 好，谢谢。

# 20. Gathering Information about a Sick Child

## 询问患儿病史

Nurse: Are you Susan Johnson's mother?

护士：您是苏珊•约翰逊的母亲吗？

Mother: Yes, I am.

母亲：是的。

Nurse: How old is she?

护士：她多大了？

Mother: Almost ten months.

母亲：快10个月了。

Nurse: What brought her to hospital today?

护士：今天为什么来医院？

Mother: She has got diarrheas for one day and they have been getting worse since last night.

母亲：她腹泻一天，昨天夜里加重了。

Nurse: About how many times so far?

护士：到现在为止大约多少次？

Mother: More than ten times. The stool is watery and in large quantities and it looks like egg soup.

母亲：10多次了。大便是稀水而且量很多，像蛋花汤一样。

Nurse: Is there any pus or blood in it?

护士：大便里有脓或血吗？

Mother: I can see some pus in it.

母亲：有，我看到一些脓。

Nurse: How are her usual bowel movements?

护士：她平常大便怎样？

Mother: They were quite regular and normal, once or twice a day.

母亲：以前她大便很规律很正常，每天一两次。

Nurse: How about her appetite? Do you breast-feed her?

护士：她的胃口怎么样？您给她哺乳吗？

Mother: Yes, I have breast-fed her since she was born, and she was gaining weight nicely. But she has lost her appetite for one day.

母亲：是的。从她出生就是我给她哺乳，她长得很快。但她已经一天没胃口了。

Nurse： Have you given her any complementary foods?

护士： 您给她添加辅食了吗？

Mother： Yes，I have. She began to have complementary foods when she was three months. At first she only had juices and yolk，and then vegetable puree，and lately meat puree.

母亲： 是的，我加了。她从三个月开始加辅食。最初只加果汁和蛋黄，然后加菜泥，最近加了肉泥。

Nurse： What did she eat yesterday and the day before? Has she ever vomited?

护士： 她昨天和前天吃了什么？她有没有呕吐？

Mother： She had nothing special the day before yesterday—just my milk and some meat puree. But she started vomiting milk yesterday afternoon，just after I nursed her.

母亲： 前天她没吃什么特别的东西——就是我的奶和一些肉泥。昨天早晨我喂奶之后她就开始吐奶。

Nurse： Can she drink any water?

护士： 她能喝水吗？

Mother： At first she drank quite a lot. She seemed rather thirsty. But now when she drinks some in，she will throw it out.

母亲： 刚开始喝得很多，她似乎很渴。但现在喝进去就会吐出来。

Nurse： Let me have a check-up. Well，her skin is not very elastic and her eye sockets have sunken in.

护士： 我来给她检查一下。嗯，皮肤弹性不太好，眼眶也凹下去了。

Mother： I think she has lost some weight. She used to be quite plump，but now she looks pine and she feels lighter in my arms. I'm so worried.

母亲： 我觉得她体重都减轻了。以前她胖嘟嘟的，但现在看上去瘦了，抱在我怀里也轻了。真担心啊。

Nurse： She's got signs of dehydration and acidosis. We must have her stool tested at once. Would you please help me to get a specimen?

护士： 她有脱水和酸中毒的体征。我们必须立刻给她化验大便。您能帮我弄一点她的大便标本吗？

Mother： Here is her diaper I had just changed for her before you came in. You can get some from it.

母亲： 这是您进来之前我给她换的尿垫。您可以从这上面取点。

Nurse： OK. I'll ask the doctor if we can give her an intravenous infusion immediately. Hopefully she will be better soon.

护士： 好的。我问问大夫是否可以立刻给她静脉输液。希望她很快好起来。

Mother： Thank you very much.

母亲： 非常感谢。

Nurse： It's my pleasure，

护士： 乐意为您服务。

# 21. Collecting a Blood Sample from a Sick Child

# 采集患儿血样

Nurse A： Do you have a minute，Mary？

护士甲： 玛丽，你有时间吗？

Nurse B： Yes，I do. Why?

护士乙： 是的，我有。什么事？

Nurse A： Can you help me to take a blood sample?

护士甲： 你能帮我采个血样吗？

Nurse B： Of course. Let's go.

护士乙： 当然可以。走吧。

（Two nurses come into the ward.）

（两个护士来到病室。）

Nurse A： Excuse me，Mr. Wood. I'm Yang Liu，your son's nurse. The doctor has ordered a blood test for your son. Would you please wait outside the room for a moment?

护士甲： 打扰了，伍德先生，我是杨柳，您儿子的护士。医生下医嘱为您儿子验血。请您在病室外等一会儿好吗？

Father： I'm afraid he will cry.

父亲： 我怕他会哭闹。

Nurse A： Please do not worry. I'll just draw a little blood from him. My colleague will help me to comfort him.

护士甲： 别担心。我就抽他一点点血。我的同事会帮我哄他。

Father： OK. I will stay outside of the room to wait. Be good，Tim.

父亲： 好吧。我会在病室外等。乖乖的，蒂姆。

Nurse A： Hello，Tim. I'm Yang Liu. How are you today?

护士甲： 你好，蒂姆，我是杨柳。今天你感觉怎样？

Child： Much better.

患儿： 好多了。

Nurse A： I'm going to take some blood from you. She is Li Xin. She is going to help me to hold you. Don't move while I do this. I won't hurt you much.

护士甲： 我要给你抽点血。她是李欣。她会帮我扶住你。我抽血时，你不要动。我不会弄疼你的。

Child： I'm scared of needles! I don't want to have my blood taken!

患儿： 我怕针！我不要抽血！

Nurse A： Do you want to be a brave boy，Tim?

护士甲： 蒂姆，你想当个勇敢的小伙子吗？

Child： Yes，I do.

患儿： 是的，我想。

Nurse A： Brave boys aren't afraid of needles.

护士甲： 勇敢的小伙子是不怕针的。

Child： But...

患儿： 可是……

Nurse A： It will be just like a little ant bite，I promise. Will you help us?

护士甲： 抽血就像蚂蚁轻轻咬一下，我保证。你愿意帮我们吗？

Child： All right. If you promise me it won't hurt，I will be good.

患儿： 好吧。如果你保证我不会疼，我会乖乖的。

Nurse A： That's fine，Tim. I'm going to clean the area first. You will feel a bit cold. Hold Li Xin's hand if you are nervous. It will only take a few seconds.

护士甲： 很好，蒂姆。首先，我要清洁抽血的地方。你会感觉有点凉。如果你紧张，就抓住李欣的手。只需要几秒钟就好。

Child： Be gentle，please.

患儿： 轻点，求你了。

Nurse A： I will.

护士甲： 我会的。

Nurse B： Now look at me，Tim. How old are you?

护士乙： 现在看我这儿，蒂姆。你几岁了？

Child： I'm six.

患儿： 我6岁了。

Nurse B： Do you go to kindergarten or stay with your grandma and grandpa while your mother and father are at work?

护士乙： 你爸爸妈妈上班时你去幼儿园还是跟爷爷奶奶在一起？

Child： I go to pre-school classes and I'm the monitor.

患儿： 我去学前班，我是班长。

Nurse B： How great you are! What do you want to do in future?

护士乙： 你真棒！你将来想做什么呢？

Child： I want to be a pilot.

患儿： 我想当飞行员。

Nurse A： It's done，Tim. You are such a good boy. Your dream will come true.

护士甲： 抽完了，蒂姆。你真是个好孩子。你的梦想会实现的。

Nurse B： Tim，you are so brave. Now you can let go of my hand and relax. I will press the spot for a little while until the bleeding stops.

护士乙： 蒂姆，真勇敢。现在你可以放开我的手，放松。我按一会儿抽血的地方止住出血。

Nurse A： Mr. Wood，you may come in now. Your son is so cute.

护士甲： 伍德先生，现在您可以进来了。您的儿子真可爱。

Father： Thank you. When can I get the result of the test?

父亲： 谢谢。什么时候能知道验血结果？

Nurse A： You can call Tim’s doctor for it in the afternoon.

护士甲： 下午您可以打电话问蒂姆的医生。

Father： I see. Thank you very much.

父亲： 我明白了。非常感谢。

Nurse A： You’re welcome.

护士甲： 不客气。

# 22. A Survey for Health Records

# 健康档案调查

Nurse: Good morning, Mrs. Woods. Thank you for coming to the Community Health Center. I got the information for the health of you and your husband last time. In order to set up the health records for your family, I also need to help you to out the form for Basic Indicators of Urban Household. Could I ask you some questions?

护士：上午好，伍兹太太。首先感谢您光临社区保健中心。上次我采集了您和您丈夫的健康档案信息。为了建立您家庭的健康档案，我还需要帮您填写《城镇居民家庭基本状况表》。我能问您几个问题吗？

Resident: Of course, no problem.

居民：当然可以。没问题。

Nurse: How far is your home to the nearest clinic, the highway, the shop and the police station, respectively?

护士：您家离最近的诊所、公路、商店和派出所分别有多远？

Resident: Let me see. About 800 m to the nearest clinic, 500 m to the highway, 300 m to the shop and 1000 m to the Police Station.

居民：让我想想。离得最近的诊所约 800 米，到公路 500 米，到商店 300 米，到派出所 1000 米。

Nurse: Do you live in a house or apartment?

护士：您住独栋房还是公寓？

Resident: I live in an apartment.

居民：我们住在公寓。

Nurse: Which floor do you live on?

护士：您住在几楼？

Resident: It's on the first floor.

居民：住一楼。

Nurse: How big is it in area and how many bedrooms are there in it?

护士：您的公寓多大面积，有几间卧室？

Resident: It's $160m^2$ with 3 bedrooms in it.

居民：160 平方米，有 3 间卧室。

Nurse: Does it have good lighting all year around?

护士：您家全年采光都好吗？

Resident: It is quite bright all year around except in winter when the daylight is short.

居民：除了冬季白天很短的日子，其他时间都很明亮。

Nurse: So the lighting is average. Is the airing very good?

护士：采光算中等。通风好吗？

Resident: Yes, it is.

居民：是的，通风很好。

Nurse: How many people are living in your apartment now?

护士：目前有几个人住在您家？

Resident: Only my husband and I.

居民：只有我和我丈夫。

Nurse: So the average area per person is 80 $m^2$. Do you have own privacy space?

护士：那么人均面积是 80 平方米。您有自己的隐私空间吗？

Resident: One of our bedrooms is used as a study. That is where my husband usually stays. I usually stay in the living room or in the kitchen.

居民：我们把一个房间当作书房。那是我丈夫常待的地方。我通常待在客厅或厨房。

Nurse: How big is the study?

护士：书房多大？

Resident: 12$m^2$

居民：12 平方米 .

Nurse: So you have 12 $m^2$ privacy housing area. Can your apartment keep you warm when it is cold?

护士：那么您家有 12 平方米的个人隐私房面积。天冷时您家暖和吗？

Resident: It used to be very cold in winter. Since the new heating system was built and the double-glazing windows replaced single glazing ones a few years ago, it has been very warm and comfortable.

居民：过去我家在冬天非常冷。自从几年前建了新的供暖系统并把单层玻璃窗换成双层玻璃窗，我家就非常温暖舒适了。

Nurse: Do you feel the air dry or humid in your home?

护士：您感觉家里的空气干燥还是湿润？

Resident: It is dry in winter but humid in summer. We sometimes use airconditioning to dehumidify it in summer.

居民：家里空气冬天干燥，夏天湿润。夏天我们有时会用空调除湿。

Nurse: Is there fume in your kitchen when you cook?

护士：您做饭时厨房里有烟吗？

Resident: No, our kitchen has very good ventilation.

居民：没有，我家厨房排风非常好。

Nurse: Do you put raw and cooked foods in separated containers and cut them with different knives and on different chopping boards?

护士：您把生熟食品分开用不同的容器装、并用不同的刀和砧板切吗？

Resident: Yes, I do.I pay great attention to food hygiene.

居民：是的，我把生熟食品分开切，我非常注意饮食卫生。

Nurse: Do you have the gas pipeline?

护士：您用管道煤气吗？

Resident: Yes，we do.

居民：是的，我们用。

Nurse: Do you use sitting toilet or squatting one?

护士：您用坐厕还是蹲厕呢？

Resident: Sitting one.

居民：坐厕。

Nurse: Would you mind telling me the total annual income of your family in the past three years?

护士：您介意告诉我您家过去三年每年的收入吗？

Resident: Well，my husband gets a fairly good salary. I also had a salary two years ago，so we had $45，000 in 2007. I've got retirement pension since 2008. Now our total income is $35，000 every year.

居民：嗯，我的丈夫有相当不错的薪水。我两年前也有工资，所以我家 2007 年总收入时 45，000 美元。2008 年以来我拿退休金了。现在我家每年总收入是 35，000 美元。

Nurse: How much do you spend each year in the past three years?

护士：您家过去三年总花费是多少？

Resident: We paid the last mortgage for our apartment in 2007. It was $6，000 a year. Our living expenditures plus travel expenses were about $12，000 each year.

居民：2007 年我们付完了公寓的贷款，这笔钱是每年 6000 美元。我们家的生活支出加上旅游费用约是每年 12 000 美元。

Nurse: When did you and your husband get married?

护士：您和您丈夫是哪年结婚的？

Resident: In 1978.

居民：1978 年。

Nurse: When did you get your first kid? How many children have you got?

护士：您什么时候生的第一个孩子？您有几个孩子？

Resident: My son was born in 1979. He is our only child.

居民：我儿子是 1979 年出生的。他是我们的独子。

Nurse: When did he start school?

护士：他是哪年开始上学的？

Resident: In 1986.

居民：1986 年。

Nurse: Did the family have any problems during these times?

护士：在这期间家里出过什么问题吗？

Resident: Our son is a good boy. The only problem was that he ran away from home once when he was 16 because there was an argument between him and us about his future.

居民： 我儿子是个好孩子。唯一的问题是，他 16 岁时离家出走一次，因为我们和他之间为他的前途起了争执。

Nurse： When did he leave home?

护士： 他什么时候离开家的？

Resident： He left home to go to college in another city in 1998.

居民： 他在 1998 年离开家去了另外一个城市上大学。

Nurse： Has he ever come back to live with you since then?

护士： 那之后他回来跟你们一起住过吗？

Resident： No. He has his own family now. He comes to see us once a week.

居民： 没有。现在他有自己的家庭。他每周回来看望我们一次。

Nurse： Has your life been changes a lot since he moved out?

护士： 他搬出去后你们的生活变化大吗？

Resident： Well，we felt quite lonely for almost five years，but now we get used to it.

居民： 嗯，开始有将近五年我们感到很寂寞，但现在已经习惯了。

Nurse： Have you been feeling bored since you retired?

护士： 您退休后有没有感觉无聊？

Resident： Yes，a little. I have to kill time by watching TV or playing net games.

居民： 是啊，有点。我靠看电视或玩网络游戏打发时间。

Nurse： There are quite a few activity groups in our community. You may find something interesting to do if you join one of them.

护士： 我们社区有不少活动小组。如果您参加一个小组，可能会找到些有趣的事情做做。

Resident： I'll go there to have a try.

居民： 我会去那里试试。

Nurse： Thank you for your time and cooperation.

护士： 谢谢您花这么多时间跟我们合作。

Resident： Thank you for doing so much for us.

居民： 谢谢您为我们做这么多。

# 23. Dyspnoea

# 呼吸困难

Nurse: Mrs. Ryan, have you noticed a change in your husband's mental state recently, does he get confused?

护士：赖安太太，近来您注意到您丈夫精神状态有什么变化吗？他是不是变得意识不清楚了？

Mrs. R: Now you come to mention it he does seem a bit dotty sometimes. You know, not always knowing where he is.

赖安太太：正如你所说的，有时他似乎有些古怪，他常常不知道他在哪儿。

Nurse: Hello Mr. Ryan, tell me about the problems you have with your breathing.

护士：您好赖安先生，请告诉我您的呼吸有什么问题。

Mr. R: I'm breathless most of the time but the infection made it much worse—I was really frightened and felt that I was fighting for breath until the treatment started to work.

赖安先生：以前大多数时间我都是喘不上气，但是这次感染让呼吸情况更糟了—我真的很恐惧，并且感到我正在挣扎着呼吸，这种感觉一直持续到治疗开始生效。

Nurse: Before the infection how was your breathing? Were you breathless sitting still?

护士：感染以前您的呼吸情况怎么样？您坐着仍然喘不上气吗？

Mr. R: Oh no, only when I tried to walk about.

赖安先生：哦，不是，只有走动时才那样。

Nurse: Can you normally get upstairs in one go ?

护士：您通常一口气能走上楼来吗？

Mr. R: Only if I rest on the landing and get my breath back.

赖安先生：我一次只能上到楼梯平台，必须在那里休息一会，使我的呼吸平稳下来。

Nurse: How far can you walk on the level without getting breathless?

护士：您在平地上能走多远而不气喘？

Mr. R: I can get as far as the back garden but I'm fair jiggered after.

赖安先生：我最远能够走到后花园，但是走到那里后我就喘不上气了。

Nurse: Is there anything else about your breathing? Do you wheeze?

护士：关于您的呼吸还有其他情况吗？您喘息吗？

Mr. R: Yes, I do wheeze and my chest often fells tight, but Dr Singh is going to put me on something new, so hopefully that will do the trick.

赖安先生：是的，我喘起气来呼哧呼哧的，并且我的胸口常有种紧缩感。不过辛大夫打算给我点新的药，希望那种药会有效。

Nurse： Hope so. What medicine were you taking at home before you came into the ward?

护士： 但愿如此。您来住院前在家里服用什么药？

Mr. R： The blue inhaler，and the antibiotics from the GP for the infection.

赖安先生： 为了治疗感染，全科医生给我用了蓝色的雾化吸入和抗生素抗感染。

Nurse： Are you using oxygen at home?

护士： 您在家里吸氧吗？

Mr. R： Yes，for up to 15 hours a day. It's OK，we have a machine that takes some gases out of the air and leaves the oxygen for me，so the missus doesn't need to keep changing cylinders and I can get around in the house and out as far as the back garden.

赖安先生： 是的，一天持续吸氧 15 小时。它是非常有效的，我们有台机器它能从空气中吸取一些气体并把氧气提供给我。所以我的太太不需要不断为我更换氧气罐，我能够在屋里到处溜达，还能够出去到后花园。

Nurse： What else helps your breathing?

护士： 在您的呼吸上还需要其他帮助吗？

Mr. R： Well-sitting up and leaning on the table help，but when I'm very chesty it's better to sleep downstairs in an armchair. At lest the wife gets some sleep even if I don't. A while ago I started doing relaxation exercises and that helps when I feel panicky，but they didn't work last night—worse luck.

赖安先生： 需要扶我坐起来并靠在桌子旁边，当我严重咳嗽时，我最好睡在楼下带扶手的椅子上。即使我不能睡觉，至少我妻子可以睡一会。刚才我在做放松训练，在我恐慌时很有帮助，但是昨天晚上没起作用——命苦啊！

Nurse： Do you still smoke?

护士： 您还抽烟吗？

Mr. R： No，not for years.

赖安先生： 不，我已经好几年没抽了。

Nurse： When did you stop smoking?

护士： 您是什么时候戒烟的？

Mr. R： I used to smoke roll-ups and I cut myself down to ten a day，and then I said'that's it. No more'and I haven't smoked for five years. It was hard but I was determined to stick to no smoking.

赖安先生： 我以前常吸烟卷，然后每天限制在 10 支，然后我说，"就抽这些了，不能再抽了"。我已经有 5 年没吸烟了。这很难，但是我决定坚持不再吸了。

Nurse： That's good，but do you still cough?

护士： 这很好，您还咳嗽吗？

Mr. R： Yes，cough and bring up stuff. I had a smokers' cough，when I was in the Army，but now I cough any time of the day or night.

赖安先生： 是的，咳嗽并且有痰。我在部队的时候有吸烟咳嗽，但是现在无论是白天还是晚上我都不停的咳嗽。

Nurse: What colour is the sputum you cough up? Has the amount increased?

护士：您咳出的痰液是什么颜色的？痰量增加了吗？

Mr. R: Really green because of the infection, and much more, and my mouth tastes foul.

赖安先生：由于感染，痰液是绿色的，量非常多，还有点臭。

Nurse: We sent a specimen to the laboratory earlier, so I'II get you some sputum pots and tissues and some mouthwash. The physiotherapist is on his way up to see you, so he will help you to cough and clear your chest. Do you have any pain with the cough?

护士：我们已经送了一个痰标本到化验室，我将给您痰盂和一些纸巾还有一些漱口水。理疗师正在来看您的路上，他将协助您咳嗽并且清理您的胸部。您咳嗽时胸部疼痛吗？

Mr. R: Not at the moment.

赖安先生：现在还没有出现这种情况。

Nurse: What about washing and dressing? Are you able to manage or do you need some help.

护士：洗澡穿衣怎么样？您能够自己完成还是需要一些帮助？

Mr. R: Just need some help to wash my back and feet. She does it at home.

赖安先生：仅需要别人帮我洗后背和脚，她在家里帮我洗。

Nurse: How is your appetite? What about eating and drinking?

护士：您的胃口怎么样？吃喝怎么样？

Mr. R: I'm trying to have a drink every hour like you said, but I can't face a big meal.

赖安先生：我按您所说的尽量每小时都喝水，但是我不能一顿吃太多。

Nurse: I will ask the dietician to visit and discuss it with you, but for today I can give you some nourishing drinks and order snacks or light meals for you.

护士：我将请膳食专家来会诊并和您谈论这个问题，但是今天，我可以给您提供一些营养饮料并为您订一些小吃或便餐。

Mr. R: Thanks, that sounds spot on.

赖安先生：谢谢你，这听起来挺好的。

Nurse: Your bed is close to the bathroom and lavatory. Will you be able to walk or will a wheelchair be easier?

护士：您的床靠近浴室和厕所。您是自己走着去还是有一辆轮椅容易些？

Mr. R.: It's not far I can get there, but after washing I might need some help back.

赖安先生：到那里不太远，我能够走到那里，但是洗完澡之后，我需要有人帮助我回来。

Nurse: How are you sleeping?

护士：您的睡眠情况怎么样？

Mr. R.: Don't worry I'll sleep OK tonight—after today with having to call the ambulance and everything I'm knackered.

赖安先生：不用担心，今晚我会睡得很好——今天由于不得不叫救护车和一些事，我觉得很疲劳。

Nurse: Is there anything you would like to ask me.

护士：您还有其他的事情要问我吗？

Mr. R：No，thanks. You and the doctor explained what was going on earlier and I do understand about COPD. An 'expert patient' you might say.

赖安先生：没有了，谢谢你！你和医生提前解释了还要做什么，并且我也确实了解了慢性阻塞性肺病。你可以说我是个“专家病人”了。

Nurse：Just ring the bell if you need me. I think Mrs Ryan went to phone your son and have a cup of tea while we did the paperwork. I'II bring her in to you when she gets back.

护士：如果您需要我帮忙时，请您按铃叫我。当我们在做这个文书工作时，我想您的太太去给您的儿子打电话了，并且顺便喝点茶。等她一回来我就带她来见您。

# 24. Migraine

# 偏头痛

Miss. C： My heads are getting worse. I wish I knew what brings it on.

卡特女士： 我的头痛越来越严重，我想知道这是什么造成的。

Nurse： When did you start having migraine?

护士： 您什么时候出现周期性偏头痛的？

Miss. C： Oh，years ago when I was still at school，but now they're coming every couple of weeks.

卡特女士： 啊，几年前我还在上学的时候出现的，但是现在它还每几周就发作一次。

Nurse： How does that differ from before?

护士： 现在发作与以前发作什么不同了呢？

Miss. C： I only had them once in a blue moon，but always when I was planning to do something special.

卡特女士： 过去只是偶尔才发作，而且通常是在我计划做一些特殊事情的时候。

Nurse： Can you think of any reasons why they're coming more often?

护士： 您能想出目前发作更频繁的一些原因吗？

Miss. C： Well，I've got a new job and it's more stressful.

卡特女士： 哦，我刚找到一份新的工作，压力很大。

Nurse： Can you do anything about that?

护士： 针对压力，您有什么办法吗？

Miss. C： No chance at the moment.

卡特女士： 还没有。

Nurse： What about things likes certain foods，or drinks. Have you noticed any link?

护士： 像某些食品或饮料等一些东西，与您的偏头痛有什么联系吗？

Miss. C： I know to lay off chocolate. But now it's really spooky. Sometimes I have a sip of wine and my head feels tight and I just know that a migraine is on its way，and other times I have two or three glasses and get away with it.

卡特女士： 我知道要戒掉甜食，但现在的确有些见鬼了。有时候我喝一小口葡萄酒，我的头就紧绷绷的，我就知道偏头痛又要发作了，有时候我喝两三杯却没事。

Nurse： Is it a particular type of wine?

护士： 都是一种葡萄酒吗？

Miss. C： No，sometimes red and sometimes white wine.

卡特女士： 不，有时候是红葡萄酒有时候是白葡萄酒。

Nurse： Does anything special make it worse once you've got the pain?

护士： 当您头痛时，有什么特别的事情会使它加剧吗？

Miss. C： Yes, any bright light. You know like sunlight on water. It's no problem because I always have my dark glasses with me until I can get into bed.

卡特女士： 是的，任何强烈的光线都会，比如说，水面上的阳光。这倒不成问题，因为我常常戴墨镜，直到上床睡觉。

Nurse： What about the migraine attacks? Have they changed?

护士： 头痛发作呢，有什么变化呢？

Miss. C： The throbbing is much worse. It's so bad I have to lie on the bed and try to sleep.

卡特女士： 它跳动得更厉害了。痛得很剧烈以致于我不得不躺在床上设法睡觉。

Nurse： Do you take anything for the pain?

护士： 为此您吃什么药？

Miss. C： I always used to take a pain killer and the pain would soon go off, but no joy now. Nothing seems to shift the pain.

卡特女士： 过去我常常吃止痛药，头痛很快就消失了。但是现在不行，吃什么也缓解不了。

Nurse： Which painkillers?

护士： 什么止痛药？

Miss. C： Mostly Paracetamol but sometimes Ibuprofen. It depends on what I have with me.

卡特女士： 大多数时候是扑热息痛，有时候是布洛芬，要看我随身带的什么药。

Nurse： Over the last few years much better drugs have become available for migraine.

护士： 近几年又出现了一些治疗偏头痛更好的药。

Miss. C： Yes, I knew that, but it didn't matter while the Paracetamol still worked OK.

卡特女士： 是的，我知道。不过没关系，扑热息痛对我还有效。

# 25. Confusion

# 神志混乱

Mrs. G： Hello Nurse. My husband seems quite settled now. Would you like me to answer those questions?

乔治夫人： 护士，您好！我丈夫现在看起来平静多了。您愿意我来回答那些问题吗？

Nurse： Hello. Yes，now's a good time. Tea will be here half an hour or so. Will you be staying to have tea with Mr George?

护士： 你好！可以，现在时间正好。这里大约每半个小时就会提供一次茶点，您要待下来和乔治先生一起来点茶点吗？

Mrs. G： Yes，that would be nice. It's a real treat to sit down and have a meal that someone else has got ready.

乔治夫人： 是的，那很好。这真是一个款待，可以坐下来享用别人已经准备好的东西。

Nurse： Being the only carer is such hard work.

护士： 要做一个照顾者是很艰难的工作。

Mrs. G： At home he wouldn't let me out of his sight for a minute. You can imagine how hard it is to get a meal.

乔治夫人： 在家里他一分钟也不愿意我离开他的视线。您可以想象我要吃上这样一顿饭有多难了。

Nurse： Yes，how are you feeling now that Mr George is here with us?

护士： 是啊。现在您觉得乔治先生和我们待在一起怎么样啊？

Mrs. G： I know it was the right decision and had it all out with the people from the Social，but I'll miss him not being at home. It had to happen. I'm completely done in.

乔治夫人： 我知道这是个正确的决定，并且已经和社工们都说明白了，但是他不在家我会想念他。肯定会。我感到累坏了。

Nurse： Tell me about Mr George.

护士： 和我说说乔治先生吧。

Mrs. G： I wish you could have seen him before all this happened. He was so on the ball and always helping people. He was in the merchant navy and spent months away，so I was used to being on my own before he retired.

乔治夫人： 我多么希望在这一切发生之前你就见过他。他以前是那么有活力，总是帮助别人。他在商船队时一外出就是几个月，所以他退休之前我常常是自己待在家。

Nurse: Have you got family nearby?

护士: 您家人离得近吗?

Mrs. G: I won't be lonely. Our lad lives just around the corner. I really lost my Bob when his mind started to go.

乔治夫人: 我并不孤独,我们的儿子就住在附近。当鲍勃精神开始出现问题时,我真正地失去了他。

Nurse: When did you first notice?

护士: 您什么时候开始注意到这一点的?

Mrs. G: Hard to say, I suppose you expect your memory to get worse, so you put the little lapses down to him getting older.

乔治夫人: 不好说。我想你知道记忆力都会逐渐下降的,于是我就把他的衰退归结于他正在变老。

Nurse: Well we all lose our glasses and forgot names.

护士: 哦,我们都会忘记拿眼镜和想不起来一些名字。

Mrs. G: Yes, but it was more than that. He seemed muddled by everyday things like making a pot of tea. He would put the tea bags in the kettle or make the tea with cold water.

乔治夫人: 是。但是不仅仅是这些,他看起来会被泡茶这样的日常事情弄糊涂。他会把茶叶袋放到水壶里或者用冷水泡茶。

Nurse: How was he in himself?

护士: 他自己有什么感觉呢。

Mrs. G: At first he knew something was wrong. He was frustrated and would fly off the handle with me and I would snap back. I didn't realise he couldn't help it.

乔治夫人: 开始他还知道有些事不对劲。他心情沮丧,容易对我冒火,我会迅速反驳。我没有意识到他不能做这些。

Nurse: How do you feel about it now?

护士: 现在您觉得怎么样了?

Mrs. G: Real bad. I feel weepy just talking about it. Silly isn't it?

乔治夫人: 很糟糕。一说起来我就想哭。很可笑是吧?

Nurse: No it's not silly, not at all.

护士: 不,那不可笑,一点也不。

Mrs. G: After forty years married we knew what the other was thinking most of the time and now we're not even on the same wavelength.

乔治夫人: 结婚 40 年了。我们大多数时间都知道彼此在想什么。而现在我们却无法理解对方的意思。

Nurse: What other things have been happening?

护士: 还发生什么事情了?

Mrs. G: He would witter on and on about the same thing and asking me the same question. I'd say to him'Bob you're driving me up the wall', he'd smile and next minute do it again. But he hardly says a word now.

乔治夫人: 他总是不停地唠叨同一件事,问我同一个问题,我对他说"鲍勃,你简直快让我发疯了！"他笑笑，下一分钟却还会这样。可是他现在一句话也说不了了。

Nurse： What about washing and dressing?

护士： 他洗澡和穿衣服怎么样？

Mrs. G： Gets in a right pickle with dressing. I have to help him. It's as if he can't remember what to do. Getting him to shave is a right carry-on, he just won't do it and pushes me away if I try to help. I hate to see him so scruffy. He was always so particular with his turn out. I don't know whether you'll have better luck with him.

乔治夫人： 他穿衣服有些困难，我不得不帮他，他好像记不得要做什么。给他刮胡子就是很好的例子，他就是不刮，如果我帮他，他还把我推到一边。我不愿意看到他这样邋遢，原来他对衣着外貌总是十分讲究的。我不知道您在照顾他时运气是否会比我好些。

Nurse： The care assistants have special training sessions and they're all used to looking after people who have problems like Mr George's.

护士： 护理助理们有专业的培训课程，并且他们都习惯照顾存在像乔治先生这样问题的人。

Mrs. G： But they won't know how to stop him getting in a lather.

乔治夫人： 但他们不知道如何使他停止焦躁。

Nurse： Would you like to meet the team who will caring for Mr George, so you can tell them about the best way to do things? Most relatives say it's reassuring.

护士： 那您愿意见见将要照顾乔治先生的成员吗？这样可以告诉他们照顾的最好方式。大多数家属觉得这样能够放心。

Mrs. G： That would put my mind at rest about leaving him here. I will just say that he seems to like sitting in front of the box. He can't know what's on but he does seem calmer. Before he got this bad he was forever changing channels and I never got to see the end of anything.

乔治夫人： 那我会放心地把他留在这里。我只能告诉他们，他看起来像是愿意坐在电视机前。他不知道在演些什么，但是他看起来更平静些。在他发脾气之前他一直更换频道，我从来没能看到过任何节目的结尾。

Nurse： How frustrating for you. Does Mr George wander about?

护士： 对您来说这多沮丧啊。乔治先生有徘徊行为吗？

Mrs. G： In the last few months it started. He kept wandering off during the day. He was off like a shot and he'd be in the road before I got out the house. I was sure he'd be under a car at any moment. And then he stopped knowing day and night and would get up at all hours of the night. That really scared me. What if he'd turned on the gas? He was always fiddling with it during the day.

乔治夫人： 最近几个月开始出现。他整天走来走去。他动作很快，没等我走出房子，他已经到马路上了，我相信他随时都会被车压了。后来他分不清白天黑夜了，总是整晚不睡觉。这真让我感到害怕，如果他打开了煤气，该怎么办啊？他白天的时候总是摆弄它。

Nurse： That must have been a real worry.

护士： 那的确让人担心。

Mrs. G： I'd lay there in the dark listening for him getting up，and when I dropped off any little noise would wake me. That's what really decided me about him coming here.

乔治夫人： 黑暗中我躺在那里，就听见他起床的声音。当我睡着时，任何细小的声音都会把我吵醒的。这才让我真正决定让他到这来。

Nurse： I just heard the tea trolley go by. We can finish this later if you like.

护士： 我刚刚听到餐车经过。如果您愿意，我们先结束这次谈话吧。

Mrs. G： I could do with a cuppa，I'm parched.

乔治夫人： 我想要杯茶，我有点口渴。

# 26. Stroke

# 卒中

Nurse：Mrs. Egbewole，do you have any problems with your speech?

护士：艾格贝沃尔太太，您说话有困难吗？

Mrs. E.：It is slurred sometimes，but that's because my mouth doesn't work properly.

艾格贝沃尔太太：有时模糊不清，但那是因为我的嘴不能好好地说话。

Nurse：How does that make you feel?

护士：那会让您有什么感觉？

Mrs. E.：I feel really embarrassed，especially if I'm talking to someone new.

艾格贝沃尔太太：我觉得很不安，尤其是与陌生人谈话时。

Nurse：Haw can we help?

护士：我们能为您做什么？

Mrs. E.：I'll be all right as long a people give me enough time to get the words out. It gets me flustered if people are impatient.

艾格贝沃尔太太：如果给我足够时间让我把话说出来，我会感到好些。如果和我交谈的人不耐烦，我就慌乱了。

Nurse：I'll make sure that is recorded in your care plan and that all members of staff know to give you plenty of time to tell us things. Did you see the speech and language therapist after the stroke?

护士：我保证这些情况都会被记录到您的护理计划中，并且所有工作人员都会给您足够时间去告诉我们一些事情的。您卒中之后看过语言治疗专家吗？

Mrs. E：Yes，but I couldn't handle it so soon after losing my husband.

艾格贝沃尔太太：看过，但是我失去我的丈夫（我的丈夫死了）之后我就不能去看了。

Nurse：How would you feel about trying again with speech and language therapy?

护士：您认为再尝试做语言治疗怎么样？

Mrs. E：If you think it might help I'm willing to give it another go.

艾格贝沃尔太太：如果你觉得有帮助，我可以再试试。

Nurse：Fine. I'll organise a referral. Is there anything else that's troubling you?

护士：好的。我会提出一个转诊介绍。您还有其他让您烦恼的事情吗？

Mrs. E：Well，yes，there is，and it's all down to the muscles in my face not working properly. I can't help dribbling.

艾格贝沃尔太太：是的，还有，是因为我的脸部肌肉不能正常活动(引起)。我不自觉就流口水了。

Nurse：You obviously know about keeping the skin round your mouth clean and dry because there is no sign of soreness.

护士：您的口周没有发炎的迹象，说明您显然知道保持嘴周围的清洁和干燥。

Mrs. E：Yes. The nurses on the stroke unit really stressed good skin care. But another thing that worries me is the look of my face—it's really lopsided and when I try to smile I must look dreadful.

艾格贝沃尔太太：是的，在卒中病房时，护士经常强调良好的皮肤护理。让我担忧的另一件事是我脸的样子，它总是倾向一方，当我试着笑时看起来一定可怕极了。

Nurse：Maybe the speech and language therapist can suggest something to help, but you could mention it to Dr Newell. She will be in this afternoon.

护士：语言治疗专家可能给您一些有帮助的建议，但您应该向纽维尔医生提起这件事，今天下午她会来这里。

Mrs. E：That's a good idea.I will add it to my list of questions I have for her.

艾格贝沃尔太太：好主意，我会把这个加到要问她的问题当中。

Nurse：How is your sight? I see you have spectacles/glasses on at the moment.

护士：您的视力怎么样？现在我看您戴了眼镜。

Mrs. E：Yes, I'm blind as a bat without them and have needed help for years. I used to have contact lenses, but after my stroke I found it too difficult to take them out, so I got some specs.

艾格贝沃尔太太：是的，没有眼镜我像蝙蝠一样瞎，几年来一直都需要别人帮助。我过去常戴隐形眼镜，但卒中之后我发现把它们取出来很难，于是我就戴眼镜了。

Nurse：Do you have a second pair for reading or does the one pair do for everything?

护士：您看书时有另外一副眼镜还是做什么事情都用一副眼镜？

Mrs. E：They are bifocals and I am supposed to look through a different bit for reading. But if the print is very small, such as on food labels, I use a magnifying glass instead.

艾格贝沃尔太太：我的眼镜是双焦点的眼镜，看书时必须用不同的部分来看。但是如果印刷的字体很小，比如食品商标，我就用放大镜来代替眼镜。

Nurse：Did you bring the magnifying glass in with you?

护士：您随身带着您的放大镜吗？

Mrs. E：Oh yes, my carer packed everything but the kitchen sink.

艾格贝沃尔太太：是的，我的家庭护士给我带全了除厨房用的以外所有东西。

Nurse：Who normally cleans your spectacles?

护士：通常由谁为您清洗眼镜呢？

Mrs. E：My lovely carers do that, I can't with only one good hand.

艾格贝沃尔太太：常常是我可爱的(是指喜欢的)家庭护士清洗，靠一只手我可没法弄。

Nurse: Would you like me to give them a clean now?

护士：现在我来帮您清洗好吗？

Mrs. E: Thanks. they're not very clean and it makes things look blurred.

艾格贝沃尔太太：谢谢你，它们是不太干净，戴着看东西模模糊糊。

Nurse: Do you have any other problems with your eyes? Sometimes a stroke can affect vision. such as seeing things double.

护士：您的眼睛还有其他问题吗？有时卒中能影响人的视力，像看东西双重影。

Mrs. E: Oh no，I was lucky. When I was younger I suffered terribly with migraine and then I used to see flashing lights with a zigzag pattern before the headache came on. If I'm out in a cold wind my eyes start running but that's normal.

艾格贝沃尔太太：哦，没有了。我还幸运。年轻时我患有严重的偏头痛，在头痛开始前我常常看到一些弯曲的闪烁亮光的东西。遇到冷风我的眼睛会流泪，但那是正常的。

Nurse: Definitely normal，it certainly happens to me.

护士：确实正常，我也这样。

# 27. Hearing Impairment

# 听力损伤

Nurse: Hello Mr. Sandford, I'm Nurse MacGregor. I understand that you have come to see us about your hearing.

护士：你好，桑德福特先生，我是护士麦格里戈。我知道您是来看你的听力的。

Mr. S: Hello, everyone calls me Nick. My hearing is no good I can't hear them on the telly or the boss at the shop.

桑德福特先生：您好，人人都喊我尼克。我的听力不太好。我听不到电视上或商店老板说什么。

Nurse: Can you hear me all right?

护士：您能听到我说话么？

Mr. S: Yes.

桑德福特先生：能。

Nurse: What would you like me to call you?

护士：您愿意我称呼您什么？

Mr. S: You can call me Nick if you like.

桑德福特先生：如果你愿意叫我尼克好了。

Nurse: OK. Has your hearing always been bad Nick?

护士：好的。尼克，您的听力一直这么差吗？

Mr. S: Not as bad—it's really bad now and I can't hear the telly

桑德福特先生：以前没有这样，现在是很糟糕了，我听不到电视上说什么。

Nurse: What do you like on the telly?

护士：您喜欢看什么电视节目？

Mr. S: I watch Eastenders and Coronation Street, they're the best and I like the football as well.

桑德福特先生：我看 Eastenders 和 Coronation Street，它们是最好的节目，我还喜欢看足球赛。

Nurse: What helps you to hear?

护士：什么对您的听力有所帮助呢？

Mr. S: Like now when I can see you and nobody else is talking. When I'm calm.

桑德福特先生：像现在这样我能看到你，又没有其他人说话的时候。还有当我安静的时候。

Nurse： Anything else?

护士： 还有什么时候？

Mr. S： The ear wash but it feels funny.

桑德福特先生： 洗耳时，不过感觉奇怪。

Nurse： We can have a look inside your ears with the special light to check for wax, you might need another ear wash to help you hear.

护士： 我们可以用一种专门的灯来检查您耳朵里的蜡状物，您可能还需要一次冲洗来帮您听东西。

Mr. S： OK.

桑德福特先生： 好吧。

Nurse： Have you got a hearing aid?

护士： 您有助听器吗？

Mr. S： Don't like it.

桑德福特先生： 我不喜欢它。

Nurse： What don't you like?

护士： 您为什么不喜欢它？

Mr. S： It's broken.

桑德福特先生： 它坏了。

Nurse： Have you got it with you? Perhaps the technician can mend it.

护士： 您带在身上了吗？或许技师可以修一下。

Mr. S： Here it is, but it's no good.

桑德福特先生： 在这儿呢，不过那没用。

Nurse： I'll take it to the technician in a bit. Does anything else happen as well as not being able to hear?

护士： 过一会儿我把它拿给技师。除了听不到，您还有什么问题吗？

Mr. S： Roaring and buzzing in my ears.

桑德福特先生： 我耳朵里有轰鸣声和嗡嗡声。

Nurse： Anything else?

护士： 还有呢？

Mr. S： My ears feel stuffed up and I get giddy and stagger.

桑德福特先生： 我的耳朵感觉被塞紧了，觉得眩晕还摇摇晃晃的。

Nurse： Do you fall over?

护士： 您摔倒了吗？

Mr. S： I know it's coming, so I sit down.

桑德福特先生： 我知道会摔倒，就坐下来。

# 28. Anxiety

# 焦虑

Nurse: Hello Mr. Reeves. I'm Nurse Owen. is it all right if I ask you some questions?
护士：你好，瑞威先生。我是欧文护士，能问您几个问题吗？
Mr. R: Yes.
瑞威先生：可以
Nurse: I understand that you have had some panic attacks.
护士：我知道您有过恐慌发作。
Mr. R: Yes. when I had to go back to work after the weekend。
瑞威先生：是的，在我过完周末回去工作时。
Nurse: Tell me what happened
护士：能告诉我是怎么回事吗？
Mr. R: It came out of the blue. I felt uneasy and came over all sweaty. My heart was pounding and my chest felt like it would burst. I thought I was about to snuff it.
瑞威先生：突然出现的。我感觉不舒服，出汗、心跳加速、胸像要炸开一样，我觉得我快死了。
Nurse: What did you do?
护士：您是怎么处理的呢？
Mr. R: I tried to calm down and take some big breaths，but it didn't work and I had to get off the bus in a hurry and pushed my way off. People must have thought I was round the bend.
瑞威先生：我试着镇静下来，做深呼吸，但是没用。我只能下车，走路。人们一定认为我有精神病。
Nurse: Did you get to work in the end?
护士：最后您上班了吗？
Mr. R: No，I needed to get home.
瑞威先生：没有，我需要回家。
Nurse: Were things any better once you got home?
护士：您回家后感觉是否好些了？
Mr. R: The panic had gone. hut I felt edgy.
瑞威先生：恐慌没有了，但是觉得不安。
Nurse: How do you mean?

护士： 什么意思？

Mr. R： I couldn't settle to anything and was fidgety all day.

瑞威先生： 我不能平静地做任何事，而且整天坐立不安。

Nurse： Tell me about your job.

护士： 说一些关于您工作的事情吧。

Mr. R： I work for an insurance company in the claims department.

瑞威先生： 我在一家保险公司的索赔部工作。

Nurse： What does that involve?

护士： 工作内容包括什么呢？

Mr. R： I deal with claims from clients. It's mainly people damaging things at home or perhaps they have had a break-in. It must be dreadful and I worry about getting the claims agreed quickly if someone has had a break-in.

瑞威先生： 我处理顾客的索赔案，主要是一些家里有物品损坏或是遭到盗窃的顾客。如果有人遭到盗窃，那真是让人不快，而且我急于尽快令人满意地处理完。

Nurse： Do your managers put pressure on you to complete claims within a set time?

护士： 你们部门经理会施加压力让您在固定时间内完成这些案件吗？

Mr. R： Yes, it's all about targets and outcomes, but you must know. It's like that in the NHS these days.

瑞威先生： 是的。但你必须知道，这都是与目标与成果有关的，正像这些日子在国家医疗卫生服务部门中的事情。

Nurse： Yes, most people seemed to have pressures at work.

护士： 是啊，大多数人在工作当中看起来都有压力。

Mr. R： It started when I wanted be the quickest to get claims sorted out.

瑞威先生： 每当我想最快地澄清这些案件事实的时候，我就感到压力了。

Nurse： What happened?

护士： 会发生什么状况呢？

Mr. R： I was working against the clock and I managed for a while, but then I felt that I must complete everything the same day.

瑞威先生： 我争分夺秒地工作，但这样不多久，我就会感觉我必须在同一天内完成所有事。

Nurse： Was that realistic?

护士： 这样现实吗？

Mr. R： No, but I couldn't see that. I stayed most evenings, but seemed to get less and less done.

瑞威先生： 不现实。但是我察觉不到这一点。我几乎总是熬夜，但完成的工作看起来却越来越少。

Nurse： Why do you think that happened!

护士： 您觉得为什么会这样呢？

Mr. R： I couldn't concentrate and went from job to job without finishing it. I couldn't deal with claims that were anything out of the ordinary.

瑞威先生： 我不能集中精力，总是还没完成一项工作就转向了另一项工作。我不能处理那些不太平常的案件。

Nurse: How did you cope?

护士：那您如何应付呢？

Mr. R: Well I didn't cope. I just put them to the bottom of my pile of work.

瑞威先生：我应付不了。我只是把它们放在一大堆工作的最后面。

Nurse: How has the work situation affected your daily life?

护士：这种工作状态给您的日常生活带来什么影响了呢？

Mr. R: I'm finding it hard to get out of the house for work in the mornings.

瑞威先生：我发现自己早晨很难离开家门去上班。

Nurse: Anything else?

护士：还有呢？

Mr. R: Same sort of problems as the ones at work. I can't concentrate on one thing and keep starting things and then leaving it to start something else. Doing the shopping is a nightmare. I just wander from aisle to aisle picking items up and putting them down. It takes me over an hour and then I forget lots of items.

瑞威先生：还有就像工作时遇到的同样问题。我没办法专心于做某一件事，总是不停地开始一件事又扔下它去开始其他事。购物对我而言就像噩梦一样让人痛苦。我只是在货架之间不断徘徊，把商品拿起来又放下，这样会花去我一个多小时，而我还是忘了很多东西。

Nurse: Do you feel under stress?

护士：您感受到压力了吗？

Mr. R: Most of the time.

瑞威先生：大部分时间都会这样。

Nurse: What sort of things make you feel stress?

护士：什么事情让您感到有压力？

Mr. R: Work obviously, but things at home can hassle me as well.

瑞威先生：很显然是工作，但家里的事情也会让我紧张。

Nurse: At home?

护士：家里的？

Mr. R: Yes, paying bills on time and the state of the garden, it's like a jungle. When I feel uptight I get really fussy about piddling things that don't matter.

瑞威先生：是。准时付账单和整理花园，都像团乱麻。当我感到心情焦躁，就会为一些无关紧要的琐事而发脾气。

Nurse: What do you normally do to relieve the stress?

护士：通常您会怎样缓解压力呢？

Mr. R: Listening to music helps and I've started doing yoga again.

瑞威先生：听音乐会有帮助，而且我已开始练习瑜伽。

Nurse: Your GP thought that our team might be able to offer you some help.

护士：您的全科医生认为我们能够为您提供些帮助。

Mr. R: Yes, we discussed some of the options, but I need more details.

瑞威先生：是的，我们讨论了一些可供选择的方案，但是我们还需要更多细节。

# 29. Depression

# 抑郁

Nurse: Hello, I'm Nurse Sanchez. May I call you Mel?
护士：你好，我是山迟子护士。可以称呼你迈尔吗？
Mel: If you like.
迈尔：如果你想，可以。
Nurse: What would you like to talk to me about?
护士：你愿意和我谈点什么？
Mel: You know, I moved here last term when my mum and dad split up.
迈尔：你知道，上学期我爸爸妈妈离了婚我就来到这里。
Nurse: Yes, you came from St. Mary's didn't you?
护士：你来自圣玛丽市，是吧？
Mel: Yeah, it was cool there.
迈尔：是的。那里很好。
Nurse: How are you settling in here?
护士：在这儿住着怎么样？
Mel: Don't know really.
迈尔：真的不知道。
Nurse: What about the people in your class? Have you made any friends?
护士：班上同学怎么样？你已经交到朋友了吗？
Mel: They've all known each other since year 7. They don't want me—they think I'm stupid.
迈尔：他们从七年级就很彼此熟悉了。他们不需要我，他们认为我很笨。
Nurse: Is that what you think?
护士：你觉得是这样么？
Mel: Yeah, because of the row I had with that girl who's always talking.
迈尔：是的。因为我和一个总是讲话的女生吵过架。
Nurse: How do you feel about the quarrel?
护士：你对那次吵架有什么想法？
Mel: It's getting me down.
迈尔：它让我情绪很低落。
Nurse: Have you felt like crying at all?

护士：你想过大哭一场么？

Mel: I'm usually OK, as long as they don't keep picking on me. During PE I burst into tears when they made a thing about not picking me for their team. They said I was naff at sport.

迈尔：如果他们不总捉弄我，我一般会好点。在体育课上，他们故意要花招不让我成为他们的队员，我就突然大哭起来。他们说我在体育方面是个笨蛋。

Nurse: Do feel like breaking down at other times?

护士：你其他时候会突然烦躁吗？

Mel: Yeah, sometimes at home for no reason, but my mum says I should try not to take things to heart.

迈尔：是的。在家里有时会不明原因的就这样。但我妈妈说我应该别把事情都放在心上。

Nurse: Did you tell your mum that you just felt like crying.

护士：你告诉过你妈妈你想哭吗？

Mel: I don't want to worry her. She's having a bad time.

迈尔：我不想让她担心。她现在也不是很好。

Nurse: Because of the divorce?

护士：因为离婚么？

Mel: Yeah, she was gutted.

迈尔：是的，她非常难过。

Nurse: How have you been feeling generally?

护士：你平常感觉怎么样？

Mel: Sort of sad and fed up.

迈尔：感到有点悲伤和厌烦。

Nurse: Are you able to enjoy the things you used to do?

护士：你能在过去经常做的事情中享受到乐趣吗？

Mel: I can't be bothered to get dolled up.You can't go out on your own.

迈尔：我再怎么打扮得漂亮也还是厌烦。依靠自己没有办法好起来的。

Nurse: What about hobbies?

护士：爱好怎么样？

Mel: I used to help out at the local riding stables.

迈尔：以前在当地骑马的马棚里会对我有些帮助。

Nurse: Yes?

护士：是吗？

Mel: I gave it up when we moved to this place. I can't get interested in anything now.

迈尔：当我搬到这地方我就再没去。我现在对什么也不感兴趣。

Nurse: Apart from what you have told me, is there anything else you are particularly worried about?

护士：除了你已经告诉我的，你还有什么特别担心的么？

Mel: Yeah, I'm frantic about my exams.

迈尔： 是的，对于我的考试我急得发狂。

Nurse： What are you planning to do?

护士： 你有什么打算么？

Mel： Yeah，I really want to go to university to do law，so I need good grades.

迈尔： 有，我很想上大学学法律，这样我需要好成绩才行。

Nurse： It's difficult changing schools just before exams.

护士： 在考试之前转校比较难。

Mel： Tell me about it.

迈尔： 是的。

Nurse： How is your studying going?

护士： 你的学习情况怎么样？

Mel： I should do a plan，but I keep putting it off，It's easier to watch TV.

迈尔： 我愿意做一个计划，但总是拖延，很容易去看电视。

Nurse： How are you sleeping?

护士： 睡眠怎么样？

Mel： It's difficult to drop off worrying about my revision.

迈尔： 担心复习，所以很难睡着。

Nurse： What about your appetite?

护士： 胃口还好吧？

Mel： OK，if you count junk food. If my mum is out I just have chips.

迈尔： 不错，如果你是指吃零食。如果我妈妈不在家，我就吃些薯片。

Nurse： When you feel sad do you ever feel like harming yourself?

护士： 当你伤心时曾经想过要伤害自己吗？

Mel： No，not really. I know my mum needs me and I'm set on being a lawyer.

迈尔： 没有，真的没有。我知道我妈妈需要我，并且我还决心要当律师。

Nurse： Do you think you could talk to your mum about how you're feeling?

护士： 你觉得你能够告诉你妈妈这些想法吗？

Mel： I suppose it would be best.

迈尔： 我想那会很好。

Nurse： The doctor might be able to help as well.

护士： 医生可能还会帮你。

Mel： Yeah，thanks.

迈尔： 是的。谢谢你！

# 30. Scald

# 烫伤

Nurse： Hello again Mrs. Kaur. Have the painkillers worked?

护士： 考尔太太您好！吃了止痛药已经起作用了吗？

Mrs. K： Hello Nurse. Yes，the pain is much less. My arm just feels sore.

考尔太太： 您好，护士！是的，疼痛减轻多了，就是手臂还有些痛。

Nurse： The plan is to keep the scald dry and warm and let it heal. I've come to put a dressing on your arm.

护士： 医嘱要保持烫伤处温暖干燥，促进愈合。我来给你的手臂缠上绷带。

Mrs. K： I don't want anything that will stick.

考尔太太： 我不要那些东西，会粘住的。

Nurse： The dressings we use don't stick anymore，they are made to be nonadherent.

护士： 我们用的绷带不会粘住的，它们被制成无黏性的了。

Mrs. K： I remember the pain years ago when dressings did stick.

考尔太太： 我还记得几年前被绷带粘住的痛苦。

Nurse： The dressing only needs to be on for a few days and the scald will heal. It was a good thing that you knew the first aid for scalds，cooling the skin down certainly stopped it getting any worse.

护士： 绷带只需要用几天，伤口就会愈合的。您知道烫伤的首要处理措施，冷敷伤口可防止恶化。

Mrs. K： I saw a thing on the telly about what to do with burns. But what about some burn ointment? It must need something.

考尔太太： 我在电视上看到过如何处理烧伤，不过那种烧伤软膏怎么样？我的伤口一定需要些软膏什么的。

Nurse： If you leave the dressing on for two or three days the scald will heal without any other treatment.You can take mild painkillers such as paracetamol if your arm is sore.

护士： 如果您缠上绷带 2～3 天，伤口会愈合的，不需要其他任何措施。如果手臂疼痛您可以吃点扑热息痛这样的止痛药。

Mrs. K： I don't like the idea of taking it off myself.

考尔太太： 我可不喜欢自己动手拆绷带。

Nurse： Well today is Saturday，so it should all be healed by Monday. You can get an appointment with the practice nurse for Tuesday and she can take off the dressing and check your arm.

护士：哦，今天是星期六，这样到下周一应该会完全愈合。您可以和开业护士约好，周二她会为您拆下绷带并检查一下手臂。

Mrs. K：Sounds sensible，I will do that. I really feel such a fool—how could I pour boiling water over myself. I am doing all the silly things my granny did when she was 80.

考尔太太：听起来不错，我一定会的。我觉得自己真可笑——怎么会把开水倒到自己身上呢？我正在做一些我祖母80岁才做的愚蠢事情。

Nurse：How do you think it happened?

护士：您觉得是怎么回事？

Mrs. K：I can't seem to judge where the cup is. It's the same when I pour orange juice into a glass. And the kettle is so heavy.

考尔太太：我似乎不能判断茶杯的位置。当我把橘子汁倒进杯子时也会这样，而且这水壶太重了。

Nurse：Have you had your eyes checked recently?

护士：最近您检查过眼睛吗？

Mrs. K：My routine test must be due very soon—I will phone on Monday.

考尔太太：很快就到我的常规体检了。我星期一会打电话的。

Nurse：Could you talk to the practice nurse about the trouble you have when pouring fluids?

护士：您愿意告诉开业护士您倒水时的烦恼吗？

Mrs. K：Yes，do you think I should tell her about how things are blurred and sometimes lines look very odd and wavy?

考尔太太：可以。你觉得我应该告诉她看东西是怎样的模糊，有时水流的线看起来非常不固定还摇摆吗？

Nurse：That sounds like a good idea. But what can you do to make the kettle easier to use?

护士：听起来是个好主意。但是你怎么做才能使你的水壶好用一点？

Mrs. K：I forget it's only me having a drink and usually fill it too full.

考尔太太：我忘了就只有我喝茶，我把它装得太满了。

Nurse：Yes，I just fill mine without thinking. I have seen smaller kettles. Perhaps you would find that easier.

护士：的确，我也会无意地就把水壶灌满水。我见过小的水壶，可能对你会好用一点。

Mrs. K：My daughter can get me one when she goes to the big shops.

考尔太太：我女儿去大商店能帮我买一个。

# 31. Taking Medicine

# 服药

Nurse：The antibiotics for you to take home have come up from the pharmacy and l would like to go over what you need to do.There are instructions on the labels. but it helps if we talk it through as well.

护士：您的抗生素已经从药房里取来了。我再重复一遍您该如何服用。药物标签上有说明，但是如果我们再共同从头到尾再说一下是有好处的。

Mr. A：Yeah，OK then. I want to get it right. It was a bit of a fright ending up in here just for a cat bite gone septic.

安德森先生：是的，那样很好。我也想弄明白，仅仅因为猫咬后就引起脓毒导致住院，真让人感到恐怖。

Nurse：What seems like such a minor thing can quickly get really bad. There are three separate antibiotics to take—here look. There are two penicillins：flucloxacillin and phenoxymethylpenicillin.You need to take these every six hours and an hour before food or on an empty stomach. These are the best ones for your infection and you have already told us that you are not allergic to penicillin.The other antibiotic is metronidazole，which you need to take every eight hours，but this time with or after food.

护士：有些看起来无关紧要的事情就有可能突然变得很糟糕。看这里有三种抗生素要吃，两种青霉素类：苯氧甲苯西林和氟氯西林，要每 6 小时吃一次，在饭前一小时或空腹服用。您已经告诉我们你对青霉素不过敏，这些药对你的感染而言是最好不过的。第三种是甲硝唑，每 8 小时服用一次，饭中或饭后服。

Mr. A：Yeah，no problems with penicillin and I'm used to taking tablets—with the Epilim twice a day and the Torem first thing.

安德森先生：是的，我吃青霉素没问题的。我已经习惯吃药片——常常每天吃两次德巴金并且早晨就吃拓赛 TM。

Nurse：Will there be any problem with having to take two before food and one with or after food?

护士：您对饭前吃两种药，另一种药饭中或饭后吃还有什么问题吗？

Mr. A：No，I already need to remember to take the Epilim after food.

安德森先生：没有。我早已经记住饭后吃德巴金了。

Nurse：What about writing out a chart? That would help，especially if you cross off doses as you take them.

护士： 做个计划表怎么样？那会有所帮助的，尤其是您可以吃了药就把它划掉。

Mr. A： I don't write so well，but one of our kids can do it.

安德森先生： 我写不好，但我们的一个小孩会来做的。

Nurse： It is important to take the antibiotics at regular times and to finish the seven-day course even if your hand seems better.

护士： 重要的一点是，即使您的手看起来有所好转，您也要按时吃药坚持到七天的疗程。

Mr. A.： Why can't I stop once it looks better?

安德森先生： 看起来好转了为什么我还不能停止吃药呢？

Nurse： Finishing the course means that the treatment will kill off all the bugs the infection is cured，and it is very important the bugs don't become immune to the antibiotics.

护士： 完成疗程意味着治疗会杀死所有病菌，感染被治愈，而且非常重要的是病菌目前还没有对抗生素产生耐药性。

Mr. A： What like that MRSA has? OK. I'll carry on to the end.

安德森先生： 就像MRSA？好吧，我会坚持到底的。

Nurse： Yes，just like MRSA，but you haven't got that.There are a few other things I need to tell you about the metronidazole. It is important to swallow the tablets whole with plenty of water. And you shouldn't drink alcohol while you are taking them and for two days after you stop—it can cause a nasty reaction with nausea and sickness. You might have a furred tongue and your urine can be dark.

护士： 是的，就像MRSA，但您不会出现那种情况。还有甲硝唑的一些其他事情我要告诉您。吞服药片时要喝足够的水，这点很重要。你吃药时以及停药后两天之内都不要饮酒，那会引起恶心和呕吐。您的舌头可能会生苔，尿的颜色可能会变深。

Mr. A： That's a blow. I could really do with a couple of pints. Thanks for the warning about my pee. That would have really put the wind up me.

安德森先生： 真是个打击。我能喝好几个品脱的啤酒。谢谢您提醒服药后我小便的颜色，否则那真会让我紧张的。

Nurse： Have you got plenty of Epilim and Torem at home?

护士： 您家里还有德巴金和拓赛TM这些药吗？

Mr. A： Yeah—I never run out of tablets. I dread having another fit now that they have settled down.

安德森先生： 是的，我从来都不用完药。虽然现在它平静下来了，但我就害怕痉挛再次突然发作。

Nurse： Have you any questions or bits you don't quite understand?

护士： 您还有什么问题或是不太明白的地方吗？

Mr. A： It's a lot to take in. Can you go through it all again please?

安德森先生：要记的东西太多了，请您再说一遍好吗？

Nurse: You're right it is a lot of information. Let's start with the three antibiotics and when to take them...

护士：您说得对，的确有很多信息。让我们从这三种抗生素药物及何时服用开始……

# 32. Joint Stiffness and Pain

# 关节僵硬和疼痛

Ms. W：Hello Nurse. Have you sorted out my physiotherapy appointment yet?

韦恩女士：您好，护士。你安排好我的物理治疗了吗？

Nurse：Yes，the physiotherapist is coming to treat you here.What do they usually do?

护士：是的。物理治疗师将会来这儿为您治疗。他们通常做什么呢？

Ms. W：In the past I had heat treatment，but now they concentrate on gentle exercise and making sure that my hand splints are still helping and not making my skin sore.

韦恩女士：过去我做过热疗。但现在他们着重于温和疗法，确保我手上夹板仍能起作用，而且不会使皮肤疼痛。

Nurse：Tell me how your mobility is affected by the arthritis.

护士：说说关节炎怎样影响到您的活动。

Ms. W：I have trouble getting in and out of bed，or the bath，and I need help to get out of a low chair.

韦恩女士：我上下床或洗澡都有麻烦，而且从矮的椅子上站起来也需要帮助。

Nurse：What about walking?

护士：走路怎么样？

Ms. W：Getting about is hard. I get around the house with the walking aid and tend to use a wheelchair when I go out. The car has been modified so at least I'm independent. I can go shopping and out with my pals.

韦恩女士：四处走动有些困难，我用步行辅助设备绕着房子走动，当出去时就要用轮椅了。汽车都已经做过修改，这样至少我可以不依赖别人。我可以和朋友们一起购物或出去。

Nurse：Yes，that is important.

护士：是的，这很重要。

Ms. W：I'm not going to be an invalid，always needing help and griping about the unfairness of it all.

韦恩女士：我可不想成为残疾人，总是需要帮助而且抱怨什么都不公平。

Nurse：How do you stay so positive?

护士：您怎么会这样自信呢？

Ms. W：After my joints，especially my hands，got really bad and I had to give up work I thought 'I'm only forty and can't just do nothing'. So I looked at ways I could be busy and useful.

韦恩女士： 在我的关节，尤其是手病情严重，不得不放弃工作后，我想我才 40 岁，可不能就这样无所事事。于是我就找各种办法忙碌起来并且成为有用之人。

Nurse： What do you do?

护士： 您做什么呢？

Ms. W： I go into the local primary school three mornings a week and listen to the children read. It's a great feeling when you hear them improve and become more confident. Just lately I started helping on a telephone helpline for people with disabilities—there are special hands-free phones so I don't need to use my hands much.

韦恩女士： 我每周到当地小学三次，去听孩子们读书。当你听到他们读书有进步变得更加自信时，那种感觉真的不错。后来我开始为一家残疾人求助热线帮忙。那里有专门的不需用手操作的电话，这样我就不用多动手了。

Nurse： We can sort out your care plan now and make sure that we include the help you need.You must tell me your usual routine for the hand splints as you're the expert. Can you arrange for your own wheelchair to be brought in?

护士： 现在我们可以制订出你的护理方案，以便确保把您需要的帮助都包括进去，您必须告诉我手指打夹板后能做的日常事务，因为您已经成内行了。您能把您的轮椅带进来吗？

Ms. W： My brother can fetch it at lunchtime if i give him a ring.

韦恩女士： 如果我给我兄弟打个电话，他会在午饭时间把它带来。

Nurse： What about other activities. Do you have difficulty using your hands?

护士： 其他活动怎么样？动手时您有困难吗？

Ms. W： Yes，the pain and stiffness in my hands and wrists really hold me back. My hands look so awful with the finger joints all puffed up and it's so frustrating and it really riles me when I can't do something simple like doing up buttons. It's always worse in the morning when you need to wash and dress，which is a real pain when I'm due at school.

韦恩女士： 是的。我的手和腕关节疼痛僵硬确实让我不能动。我的手看起来真是糟糕，关节都肿了，当我连系扣子这样简单的事情都做不了时，真感到失望和恼怒烦躁。通常在早晨要洗漱或穿衣时更为糟糕，在学校里做这些事真是麻烦。

Nurse： Are there any other movements that you find difficult?

护士： 您还发现其他方面的活动有困难吗？

Ms. W： Anything where I have to grip and move my wrist like holding the kettle and pouring.

韦恩女士： 凡是需要紧握和活动手腕，像提茶壶倒水这样的时候都有困难。

Nurse： Again we can plan what help you will need from us while you're here. Do you see the OT for help with this?

护士： 我们再来计划一下您在这儿需要我们为您提供什么帮助。您见过治疗师并寻求帮助吗？

Ms. W： Yes，she has been so helpful—lots of gadgets to help me do things，like dressing and cooking, for myself, and so many ideas about how to do things without getting tired or making the pain worse.

韦恩女士：是的。她的确可以提供帮助——有许多小器具可以用来帮我自己做像穿衣和烹调这样的事情。也有许多要领是关于做事怎样减少疲劳或不导致疼痛加剧的。

Nurse: Perhaps your brother can bring in the gadgets you need in here when he comes with the wheelchair. What do you think?

护士：当您兄弟来送轮椅时或许能带过来您在这里需要的小器具，您说呢？

Ms. W: OK. I hadn't thought of that.

韦恩女士：对呀！我怎么没想到呢？

Nurse: The rheumatology nurse specialist will be up later to review your drugs with Dr Wong, and co-ordinate all the other practitioners—I expect you know them both quite well by now.

护士：风湿病护理专家会来与王医生再讨论一下您的用药，并且与其他人员共同协商。我想到现在为止，您已经很熟悉他们两人了吧。

Ms. W: Yes, I certainly do.

韦恩女士：那是当然。

Nurse: Do you need anything for pain?

护士：您还需要止痛药吗？

Ms. W: No, not at the moment, thanks. I took all my morning drugs at home and I'd rather wait to see what happens after the drug review.

韦恩女士：不，现在不需要，谢谢。在家里我已经吃了早晨的药了。我更想等着看药物讨论之后的情况。

# 33. Ataxia

# 共济失调

Nurse: Hello Mr Lajosiki. I understand that you have come in today to have a fatty lump removed from your back and the plan is to send you home later this afternoon.

护士：您好，拉乔斯奇先生。据我了解您今天来这儿切除您背上的一个脂肪肿块，按计划下午就可以送您回家了。

Mr. L: Yes, that's right. The lump needs to come off—it gets in the way of the waistband of my trousers. I shall be glad to see the back of it. Did they tell you that I have Parkinson's disease?

拉乔斯奇先生：是的，是这样。这个肿块应该去除——它正好在我扎腰带的地方，我很高兴把它切除了。他们告诉你我有帕金森病了吗？

Nurse: Yes, it's in your notes from the assessment clinic. How does it affect you?

护士：是的，在您的门诊评估记录上有，它对您产生了什么影响呢？

Mr. L: The walking is the worst. It's difficult to start moving and I'm so slow. All I can do is shuffle to start with and then my steps get shorter and I get faster and faster, can't stop, and like as not over I go. I've really lost my nerve. If you saw me you would think I was the worse for drink.

拉乔斯奇先生：行走最差。开始迈步时有困难，走起来又非常缓慢。我只能拖着脚迈步，接着我的步子越来越小，走得越来越快而停不下来，似乎自己不能控制要摔倒。我已经丧失勇气了。如果你见了我，一定会把我当做醉汉。

Nurse: Do you have any other movement problems?

护士：您还有其他活动的问题吗？

Mr. L: I get that freezing where I'm rooted to the spot. It mostly comes on out of the blue, but I worked it out that trying to do more than one thing at once will bring it on. The shaking in my hands is bad and it's hard to do some things because my arms are so stiff.

拉乔斯奇先生：我会站在那儿没法儿动，像生了根似地站在那儿。这经常来得突然，但是我找到答案了，即当我试图同时做多件事的时候就会引起。我手抖得厉害，由于我的手臂太僵硬，有些事情无法做。

Nurse: What things are particularly difficult for you?

护士：什么事情对您来说特别困难？

Mr. L: It sounds daft，but it's mainly things like turning over in bed，reaching out for a cup，getting up out of a chair and turning round once I'm up.

拉乔斯奇先生：听起来有些荒唐，主要是像在床上翻身、伸手拿杯子、从椅子站起来和站着转身这样的事情。

Nurse: Are there things that help?

护士：有什么事情是可以有帮助的吗？

Mr. L: I've learnt a few tricks such as having a good firm mattress and a high-backed chair with arms. The others things are really simple，like other people waiting until I'm ready to move and giving me time to do things for myself. When I freeze，the physio told me to try stepping over an imaginary line，or to count 'one—two'out loud with each step and that does help.

拉乔斯奇先生：我知道了些小技巧，像有一个稳固的好床垫和高椅背带有扶手的椅子。其他事情也很简单，像让其他人等着我到我自己能动，并且给我时间来自己做事。当我动不了时，理疗师告诉我试着踏过一条想象当中的线或每迈一步大声数着"一、二"，这样的确很有帮助。

Nurse: What about other activities，such as those needing fine movements?

护士：其他活动怎么样？比如那些需要精细动作的？

Mr. L: Doing up shoelaces or buttons is impossible，so that material that sticks to itself is very handy. What's it called?

拉乔斯奇先生：系鞋带和纽扣是不可能的，因此那种可以自己粘在一起的东西非常便利，它叫什么来着？

Nurse: Oh，you mean Velcro. It's very useful，we use it a lot in the rehab unit.

护士：噢，您说的是维可牢尼龙搭扣吧，它很管用。我们在康复科用得很多。

Mr. L: I get loads of cramp attacks at night，so I'm awake half the night. Before the Parkinson's I could just pop out of bed and it would go.

拉乔斯奇先生：我在晚上总是抽筋，所以半夜我会醒来，在得帕金森病之前我还可以起床而且很顺利。

Nurse: Not so easy now.

护士：现在不那么容易了。

Mr. L: How right you are. I wish it would settle down.

拉乔斯奇先生：您说得很对，我多希望这种病能停止下来。

Nurse: I gather that your medication has just been changed.

护士：我知道最近您的口服药有所变化。

Mr. L: Yes，I said to the Doc that the cramp had gone on too long and he said I could try some different tablets.

拉乔斯奇先生：是的。我告诉医生我抽筋持续的时间变长，他说我可以试试其他的药。

Nurse: Any luck with the new tablets?

护士：新药管用吗？

Mr. L: Early days，but I think the cramps have eased off.

拉乔斯奇先生：现在说还早，但我觉得抽筋已经减轻了。

# 34. Anorexia

# 食欲减退

Nurse: Hello Miss Hyde-Whyte，I'm Nurse Mosquera. I would like to ask you some questions. Will that be all right？

护士：您好，海德•怀特女士。我是穆斯库拉护士。我想问您一些问题，现在可以吗？

Miss. H: Hello—please call me Maggie. The rest is such a mouthful.

海德•怀特女士：您好！请叫我玛吉。其余的字叫起来太长。

Nurse: I will need to weigh you and measure your height，but first a few questions.

护士：我要为您称体重、量身高。不过先回答几个问题吧。

Miss. H: I'm sure that I have lost weight—all my clothes hang on me.

海德•怀特女士：我确实体重已经下降——我的衣服穿上都宽宽松松的。

Nurse: How often do you eat and drink?

护士：您的饮食是怎么安排的？

Miss. H: Well I used to have breakfast，a proper cooked lunch and something on toast or a sandwich in the evening.

海德•怀特女士：哦。我习惯吃早餐，中午烹调一顿很好的午餐，晚上吃吐司蘸点东西或者一份三明治。

Nurse: Has something changed?

护士：现在变了吗？

Miss. H: I used to really enjoy cooking，have a G&T and then sit at the table with a nice meal，but now I've got no appetite and I just pick at it. My dad would have said you don't eat enough to keep a bird alive.

海德•怀特女士：我过去非常喜欢做饭，喝点 G&T，然后坐在桌旁享受一顿美餐。而现在我没有胃口，只是吃一点点东西。我爸爸说我吃的东西还不够喂鸟。

Nurse: Why do you think your appetite has decreased?

护士：您觉得您的食欲为什么会下降呢？

Miss. H: Two reasons I think. I've had mouth ulcers for ages. Probably my false teeth don't fit anymore; and I have been sick a few times after meals.

海德•怀特女士：我想有两个原因。我得口腔溃疡有年头了。可能我的假牙不太合适了，并且有几次吃完饭就恶心、吐。

Nurse: I'll look at your mouth in a moment and see if any treatment would help. It might be a good idea to see your dentist about the poorly fitting dentures. Tell me about the vomiting.

护士： 我会立刻检查您的口腔，看是否有什么治疗措施能管用。让您的牙医看一下您那副不太合适的假牙，可能会是个好主意。说一下呕吐的情况。

Miss. H： If I eat a proper meal I soon feel sick and then I'm sick. The food just comes back.

海德•怀特女士： 如果我吃了一顿饭，很快就会觉得恶心然后就呕吐。吃的东西又出来了。

Nurse： Are you sick at any other time?

护士： 其他时间您恶心吗？

Miss. H： No，only after food.

海德•怀特女士： 不，只是在饭后。

Nurse： What colour is the vomit？Is there any blood or bile?

护士： 呕吐物是什么颜色的？有血液或者胆汁吗？

Miss. H： No blood and it's not green or yellow like bile. The colour varies it depends on what I've eaten.

海德•怀特女士： 没有血，也不像胆汁那样发绿或者发黄。颜色都不一样，要看我吃的什么东西了。

Nurse： Sometimes blood can look like coffee grounds—anything like that?

护士： 有时血液可能呈咖啡渣样——有像那样的东西吗？

Miss. H： No，nothing like that.

海德•怀特女士： 不，一点儿也不像。

Nurse： How do you feel afterwards?

护士： 然后有什么感觉呢？

Miss. H： That's the strange thing. Once I've been sick I feel fine. My stomach feels uncomfortable before I'm sick，but that feeling soon goes afterwards.

海德•怀特女士： 真是奇怪，一旦我吐了，感觉就会好点。呕吐之前我的胃很不舒服，吐后这种感觉就不见了。

Nurse： When you were eating normally what sort of food did you cook?

护士： 您胃口正常时，一般都做什么食物？

Miss. H： Proper meals—meat or fish and lots of veg. and I always had dessert or some cheese. No point doing all that if I'm going to be sick.

海德•怀特女士： 平常的饭菜——鱼或肉和很多蔬菜，然后总是吃些甜点或干酪。如果感到恶心那就什么也不能吃了。

Nurse： How often do you usually shop for food?

护士： 您多长时间买一次东西来做饭？

Miss. H： Most days. It's nice to get out and have a chat with people.

海德•怀特女士： 大多每天都去。出去并与人们聊天是很愉快的。

Nurse： What do you eat and drink now?

护士： 现在吃的喝的都有什么呢？

Miss. H： I know that I must eat something，so I have things like scrambled egg on toast，soup and milky drinks. It's not unpleasant but I know it's not enough.

海德•怀特女士： 我知道我必须吃点东西，所以我有煎鸡蛋土司面包、汤和乳制品饮料。它不是不好，但我知道这不够。

Nurse： Let's see how much you weigh.What's your normal weight?

护士： 我们来看看您多重，您的正常体重是多少？

Miss. H： Before the vomiting started I had been about 10 stone for as long as I can remember.

海德•怀特女士： 在开始呕吐之前，在我的记忆中一直都是10英听。

Nurse： We use the kilogram for weight，but I can tell what it is in stones and pounds.

护士： 我们常用公斤来表示体重。不过我可以告诉您用英听和磅表示是多少。

Miss. H： What's the verdict then. Have I lost much?

海德•怀特女士： 那么测量结果是多少，我轻了许多吗？

Nurse： I'm afraid you have lost about 11 kilograms.You weigh 52 kilograms; that's 8 stone 2 pounds，so that's nearly 2 stone less than usual. We will have to keep an eye on your weight.

护士： 很抱歉，您已经轻了差不多11公斤。您的体重是52公斤，也就是8英听2磅，这样比正常轻了大约2英听。我们会关注您的体重的。

Miss. H： Well，it's no surprise my clothes are much too big.

海德•怀特女士： 哦，怪不得我的衣服都这么大呢。

Nurse： I'm going to refer you to the dietician and ask her to come and do a full nutritional assessment and see how we can provide you with enough nutrients and fluid while we wait for all the tests to be done. Meanwhile，we can order things like scrambled eggs，and give you soup and drinks with added nutrients if you're sure that won't make you sick.

护士： 我建议您去求助一下膳食专家，请她过来做一个完整的营养评估，我们等着做完所有的检验之后，看看怎样为您提供足够的营养和水分。同时，我们可以预定一些食物，像煎鸡蛋、有更多营养的汤和饮料，如果您确保不会引起恶心的话。

Miss. H： I'm sure that will be fine，thank you.

海德•怀特女士： 我想那不错，谢谢你！

# 35. Excessive Drinking

# 饮酒过多

Nurse：Hello Mr. Wakefield. How are you today?

护士：您好！威克菲尔德先生。今天感觉怎么样？

Mr. W：Not up to much.You know—it's hard to feel interested in anything these days.

威克菲尔德先生：不怎么样。你知道吗？这些日子我很难对什么提起兴趣来。

Nurse：Yes，it must be about six months since your wife died.

护士：是的，我知道。您妻子离开应该有6个月了吧。

Mr. W：It will be exactly six months on Wednesday. Her dying like that really hit me for six. Tom does his best，but I miss her so much. I can't keep on like this.

威克菲尔德先生：到星期三就整整6个月了。她的去世简直把我分成了六块。汤姆已经尽力了，但我还是如此地怀念她。我不能总是这样下去。

Nurse：What do you mean?

护士：您的意思是？

Mr. W：I can't leave Tom to run everything，but I feel dreadful.

威克菲尔德先生：我不能让汤姆来应付一切，但是我感觉糟透了。

Nurse：In what way do you feel unwell?

护士：您哪些方面感觉不好呢？

Mr. W：Most of it's my own fault. I know it's bad for me.

威克菲尔德先生：大多是我自己的事，我知道这样对自己也不好。

Nurse：Bad for you?

护士：对您不好？

Mr. W：The evenings are so long without her and at first I thought a couple of drinks would help me unwind and get through until bedtime.

威克菲尔德先生：没有她，夜晚是如此漫长。起初我以为喝两杯会让我放松，直至睡觉。

Nurse：Did it help?

护士：有帮助吗？

Mr. W：Not really and I ended up having more than a couple of drinks.

威克菲尔德先生：实在不管什么用。最终我喝了两杯还要多。

Nurse：Many more?

护士：那么多？

Mr. W： Oh yes，most evenings I manage a bottle of wine and some whisky，and then regret it in the morning.

威克菲尔德先生： 是的。大多晚上我喝一瓶葡萄酒和一些威士忌，而早晨起来我又后悔。

Nurse： How do you feel in the morning.

护士： 早晨您感觉怎么样？

Mr. W： Headache and generally lousy. I can't face breakfast and I'm often sick.

威克菲尔德先生： 头痛而且难受。我不能看到早餐，经常恶心。

Nurse： Do you take anything for the headache?

护士： 您吃什么来止痛呢？

Mr. W： A couple of aspirin，but they give me terrible indigestion.

威克菲尔德先生： 两片阿司匹林，但它们给我带来可怕的消化不良。

Nurse： You have obviously been thinking about the amount of alcohol you drink.

护士： 您显然已经注意到您饮酒的量了吧。

Mr. W： Yes，it's worrying me. What if I can't stop and become an alcoholic or something?

威克菲尔德先生： 是的，这让我担忧。我若是不停止，不就会成酒鬼之类的人了？

Nurse： How much do you think you're having in a week?

护士： 您觉得您每周喝了多少？

Mr. W： I know that there are sensible limits in units，but I don't know what they are.

威克菲尔德先生： 我知道要有一个较合理的限度标准，但我不知道是什么。

Nurse： Most men can safely drink 3-4 units a day without a significant Risk. A unit is 10 grams of alcohol and this is half a pint of standard strength beer or one glass of wine or one pub measure of spirits. Some stronger wines have more than 1 unit. The recommended level is 21-28 units for a man spread over 1 week. It's best to avoid binge drinking and keep 1 or 2 days when you don't drink.

护士： 大多男性每天喝 3～4 单位没什么大碍。1 单位等于 10 克酒精，即半品脱标准度数的啤酒、一杯葡萄酒或 1 酒吧单位的烈性酒。一些烈性酒要多于 1 单位。男性推荐标准为每周 21～28 单位。在您喝酒时最好避免狂饮（无控制地饮酒）或持续一两天不喝酒。

Mr. W： My intake is well over the sensible limit. Most nights I probably have over 10 units. I need to do something about it.

威克菲尔德先生： 我的摄入量远远高于合理限度。大多数晚上我喝的很可能都要多于 10 单位。我需要怎么做呢？

Nurse： You seem to have made up your mind to reduce your intake of alcohol. Have you thought about how you might do this?

护士： 看起来您已经下决心减少饮酒量了。您想过怎么做吗？

Mr. W： I don't want to give up drinking completely. In the past I enjoyed a drink in moderation and that's what I want to aim for. Some people say that they never touch a drop，but that's not for me.

威克菲尔德先生：我不想完全戒酒。过去我喜欢适量地饮酒，这就是我的目标。有些人说他们滴酒不沾，但那不适合于我。

Nurse：It's good to have a realistic goal，and drinking in moderation may have health benefits，such as reducing heart disease.

护士：有一个现实的目标很好，并且适量饮酒还有助于健康，比如能减少心脏病的发生。

Mr. W：All this booze has made me put on weight，so it will be healthier if I cut down on drinking and lose weight.

威克菲尔德先生：所有这些酒已经让我体重增加了，如果我削减饮酒量会更加健康并且减轻体重。

Nurse：Are evenings the only time that you have a drink?

护士：您只是在晚上饮酒吗？

Mr. W：Yes，when I'm on my own.

威克菲尔德先生：是的，当只有我自己的时候.

Nurse：What can you do to change the pattern?

护士：您怎样才会改变这种方式？

Mr. W：I used to enjoy a walk round the farm of an evening and my grandsons keep badgering me to take them out.

威克菲尔德先生：过去我常常喜欢晚上在农场上转转，孙子们总是缠着我带他们出去。

Nurse：Do you think that's possible?

护士：您觉得现在有可能吗？

Mr. W：Yes，and I think it would help.

威克菲尔德先生：是的，并且我认为那样是有好处的。

Nurse：I would like to see how you get on. Perhaps we can make another appointment and while you're here we can make you an appointment with Doctor Welch. She can arrange for support from a counsellor，and she might think that you would benefit from some medication.

护士：我想看看您如何取得进展。或许我们可以约好，当您再来这里我们帮您预约韦尔契医生。她能给您安排顾问的帮助，她可能会认为服用些药物应该有效。

Mr. W：Yes，I know I need some proper help and it's such a relief to have told someone about my drinking. I could never tell Tom. It would cause too much bother.

威克菲尔德先生：是的，我知道我需要一些帮助。与您谈了我喝酒的事情后感觉很轻松。我不会告诉汤姆，因为这会给他带来很多的麻烦。

# 36. Uracratia

# 尿失禁

Nurse: What sort of problem with your waterworks?

护士：您排尿有什么问题？

Mrs. C: I can't hold on and I leak urine. It's so embarrassing.

卡特太太：我憋不住而且漏尿，真是令人难为情。

Nurse: It sounds like you have two separate problems.

护士：听起来您是有两个问题。

Mrs. C: I hadn't thought of it as two problems, but it does happen at different times. The main problem is the need to pass water so often and when I need the toilet it is all of a rush. Sometimes I don't make it in time and wet myself. The leaking happens when I cough or laugh.

卡特太太：我还没有把它们当做两个问题，但它的确在不同的时候发生。主要的问题是我如此频繁地想小便，这时我就匆忙地需要上盥洗室。有时我还没有来得及找到厕所，就会弄湿了自己。漏尿通常发生在我咳嗽或大笑时。

Nurse: How often do you pass water?

护士：您多长时间小便一次？

Mrs. C: Every couple of hours or so during the day.

卡特太太：白天大约每两小时一次。

Nurse: What about at night, do you have to get up in the night?

护士：晚上呢？晚上要起床小便吗？

Mrs. C: Oh yes, I have to keep getting up. Always twice a night and sometimes more often.

卡特太太：哦，是的。我总是不得不起床。常常每晚两次，有时更多。

Nurse: When did you start having problems?

护士：您什么时候出现这问题的？

Mrs. C: Just after I retired. I'm 68 now, so it must be about four years ago.

卡特太太：就在我退休之后。现在我68岁了，这样大概是在4年前。

Nurse: Have you told your GP or the practice nurse?

护士：您已经告诉您的医生或开业护士了吗？

Mrs. C: I felt too embarrassed and it's something that happens when you get older isn't it? It really limits my social life and it worries me that I might smell.

卡特太太：我觉得太不好意思了，并且人变老了就是要发生一些这样的事情的，不是吗？

这的确限制了我的社交活动，并且我担心我的身上可能有什么气味。

Nurse： It is more common in older people，but there are different causes and many can be successfully treated. How do you normally cope with the problem?

护士： 这种情况在老年人当中是更加普遍，但有不同的病因，许多是可以成功地治疗的。通常您怎样解决这个问题呢？

Mrs. C： I try to be near a toilet，but that's not always easy if I'm out. There are not many public toilets and some of them are not very clean. I wear a sanitary towel in my knickers to cope with the leaks，but I still have plenty of washing to do.

卡特太太： 我尽可能离盥洗室近一些，但如果在外面就没那么容易了。没有那么多的公厕，并且有些不很干净。我又在短衬裤里用了卫生巾来对付漏尿，但是仍然要做很多清洗工作。

Nurse： I will add all this to your care plan and make sure that everyone knows to bring the commode as soon as you ask. Would you like a supply of towels and disposal bags to keep in the locker?

护士： 我会把这个写到护理计划当中，以保证大家都知道只要您一要求就送便盆过去。您愿意在抽屉里放些纸巾和污物袋吗？

Mrs. C： Yes please.

卡特太太： 好的。

Nurse： When your angina has settled down and you are feeling better I will arrange for the continence nurse specialist to come to see you. She is the expert and will be able to do a full assessment and suggest ways of improving the situation.

护士： 当您心绞痛病情稳定下来、感觉好转的时候，我会安排失禁护理专家来看望您。她是专家，能做出完整的评估并提出改善这种情况的建议措施。

Mrs. C： I wish I'd told someone earlier，but I thought that you had to grin and bear it. I had no idea that anything could be done.

卡特太太： 我倒是希望早一点告诉别人了，但我原来认为对这种毛病你只能忍耐它。我不知道该怎么办。

Nurse： While we're waiting I'd like to have a specimen of your water to test，and if that shows that you might have an infection we can collect a midstream specimen of urine for the laboratory.

护士： 我们在这儿等着的时候，我要为您取尿样去检查，如果表明您有可能感染，我们可以再收集中段尿送实验室化验。

Mrs. C： Is that the test where you have to pee into a pot?

卡特太太： 是那种必须尿在一个小瓶子里的检查吗？

Nurse： Yes，that's the one，but we only need the middle bit of the flow，not the urine that comes out first. Have you noticed any blood in your urine or an unusual smell?

护士： 是的，就是那种。但我们只需要尿液的中段，不是最先排出的尿液。您注意到尿液中有血或者其他的气味吗？

Mrs. C： No，nothing like that.

卡特太太： 没有，没有那样。

Nurse： What about pain when you pass urine? Does it burn or sting?

护士： 您小便时疼吗？是烧灼痛还是刺痛？

Mrs. C： No，I had cystitis when I was younger and I know how painful it is when you go.

卡特太太： 不疼，我年轻时得过膀胱炎，知道如果是膀胱炎的话小便时有多痛。

Nurse： We also need to know how often you are passing urine and how much fluid you are having，but as we are already recording fluid balance for you we will have that information.

护士： 我们还需要知道您现在的小便次数、摄入液体量，因为我们要记录您的液体平衡，我们需要了解这些信息。

Mrs. C： You will tell the nurses about how urgent it is when I ask for the commode?

卡特太太： 你会告诉其他护士当我要用便盆时有多急吗？

Nurse： Don't worry I'm putting it on the care plan now，and I will tell the nurse who takes over from me tonight. Do you think you could give me that sample now?

护士： 不必担心，我正把它写到护理计划中。我会告诉今晚接我班的护士。您现在可以给我尿样吗？

Mrs. C： Yes.

卡特太太： 是的。

Nurse： Have you any questions before I go and get the commode?

护士： 在我离开去拿便盆之前您还有什么问题吗？

Mrs. C： No，I'm looking forward to feeling better and seeing the specialist nurse about the waterworks.

卡特太太： 没了。我期望着病情好转，然后就这个问题看一下护理专家。

# 37. Dyschesia

# 大便困难

Mr. N: I feel terrible, really out of sorts.

诺顿先生：我觉得很糟，真的不正常。

Nurse: What's the trouble?

护士：哪里不舒服？

Mr. N: I haven't been properly for days.

诺顿先生：我已经好几天没大便了。

Nurse: When did you last have your bowels open?

护士：您最后一次大便是在什么时候？

Mr. N: Saturday was OK, so that's four days ago.I wish I'd said earlier, but it seemed stupid to be worried about not going when I'm laid-up with a leg that's broke.

诺顿先生：周六大便了，也就是 4 天前。我本想早些说，可是又觉得一条腿受伤卧床时还去担心没有大便，看起来很愚蠢。

Nurse: How often do you usually go?

护士：平时您多长时间大便一次？

Mr. N: Every day without fail.

诺顿先生：正常的话每天一次。

Nurse: It's probably happened because you're not as active as usual and having to use a bedpan doesn't help.

护士：可能是因为您现在的活动量不如平常的活动量大，而且只能用便盆引起的。

Mr. N: Well I can't do much with the traction and stuff.

诺顿先生：由于牵引治疗我没有办法。

Nurse: How is it making you feel?

护士：您感觉如何？

Mr. N: I'm all blown up and full of wind. Look at my stomach, it's huge. I couldn't eat nothing and my mum had brought in a Chinese as a treat.

诺顿先生：我肚子里都是气，你看看我的胃，很大。我不能不吃东西，我妈妈带来中国饭菜给我作为改善。

Nurse: Yes. your abdomen is a bit distended. Have you any pain?

护士：是的，您的腹部饱满，疼吗？

Mr. N: A bit. It feels like colic.

诺顿先生： 有一点，像绞疼。

Nurse： What's your motion like on Saturday?

护士： 周六您的大便是什么样的？

Mr. N： Just a few hard bits and I had to strain to get that out.

诺顿先生： 只是一些硬块，我不得不用力才能排出来。

nurse： What it's like normally?

护士： 平时是什么样的？

Mr. N： Normal-soft and not having to strain. Except when I've got the runs after too much beer and a curry.

诺顿先生： 平时是软的，不用费力，除了我喝太多啤酒、吃咖喱食品时泻肚外。

Nurse： Was there any pain passing the hard motion，or blood when you cleaned yourself.

护士： 用力排便时疼吗？您擦拭时有血吗？

Mr. N： No pain and I didn't see any blood. If I had l would have said straight away.

诺顿先生： 不疼，也没有看到血。如果有我马上就说了。

Nurse： Did you feel that you hadn't passed a complete motion?

护士： 有排便不完全的感觉吗？

Mr. N： Yeah，my back passage felt full just as if there was more to come.

诺顿先生： 是的，感觉下段肠子是满的，就好像还有大便。

Nurse： I'll get Dr Cox to write you up for some medicine to make you go and we can ask the physio to suggest some exercises to help.

护士： 我会通知考克斯大夫，给您药帮助排便。我们还会找理疗师为您提供一些有帮助的运动疗法。

Mr. N： My gran swears by her bottle of bowel medicine.

诺顿先生： 我奶奶信赖她的瓶装通便药物。

Nurse： You might need some suppositories or a micro enema to get things started and then a few doses of an oral laxative. Hopefully you won't need a whole bottle. It will also help if you drink more water and choose food high in fibre from the menu.

护士： 可能您需要一些栓剂或一次灌肠启动排便，之后再来一些口服通便药。希望您不需要一整瓶药。如果您多喝水，多吃富含纤维的食物也会有帮助的。

Mr. N： Yeah alright，but I don't want salad every meal.

诺顿先生： 好吧，可是我不喜欢每顿都吃沙拉。

# 38. Personal Care

# 个人护理

Nurse: Hello Mrs. McBride. I'm Nurse Ramos. I think you are expecting me. I've come in to see how you are managing at home.

护士: 麦布莱德夫人，您好！我是罗穆丝护士，我想您是在等我。我来看看您在家里的情况。

Mrs. M: Hello，dear，come in. Yes，I knew you were coming. Sue mentioned it earlier when she was in with my lunch. She's a good girl to me.

麦布莱德夫人: 你好，亲爱的！进来吧。是的，我知道你要来。苏刚才吃午饭的时候跟我说过了。她是个好女孩。

Nurse: I've got a checklist to complete，but it's usually better if you tell me in your own words how you think you are managing. What about if we start with any difficulties you might be having with washing and dressing?

护士: 这里有个检查单要完成。如果您自己告诉我您怎么样会更好。我们从您对洗漱及穿衣时遇到的困难开始怎么样？

Mrs. M: Yes，that's fine. I've always been as fit as a fiddle，but since the winter it's got more and more difficult. Well I am 83. It's all down to old age I suppose.

麦布莱德夫人: 可以。我一直身体极好，但自从冬天以来，我感到越来越困难。我已经 83 岁了，我想这是衰老引起的。

Nurse: What's more difficult?

护士: 什么更困难些呢？

Mrs. M: I struggle a bit with a strip wash at the sink，but I get by. My feet and back don't get done，and it's hard to stand up to wash down below. I need to hold on to the sink and then I can't soap the flannel.

麦布莱德夫人: 用浴盆洗澡时需要费些劲，不过还可以应付。我的脚和背都不灵活，站起来洗下身比较困难，我得扶住浴盆但这样就不能给毛巾打上肥皂了。

Nurse: Are you able to have a bath or shower?

护士: 您能淋浴吗？

Mrs. M: No，I'm not strong enough to get in and out of the bath. I'm frightened of slipping，or getting in and not getting out again.

麦布莱德夫人: 不能，我身体较弱不能进出浴室，我怕滑，怕走进去却出不来了。

Nurse: How often did you have a bath when you were able to manage?

护士： 您能洗澡时多久沐浴一次？

Mrs. M： Two or three times a week. Heating the water with the immersion heater costs too much to have a bath every day.

麦布莱德夫人： 一周2～3次，用浸没式加热器烧水花费太大，不能每天洗。

Nurse： How do you heat the water for your strip wash?

护士： 您用盆洗时怎么烧水？

Mrs. M： Boil a kettle. I've got one in the bedroom for a cuppa in the morning. Would you like a cup of tea now?

麦布莱德夫人： 用壶烧。卧室有一个用来早晨烧茶。现在来杯茶吗？

Nurse： No，thanks. I had one just before I came out to see you. Would you like to have a bath if it was possible?

护士： 不，谢谢。我来看您之前喝过一杯了。如果可能您想进浴室洗个澡吗？

Mrs. M： Oh yes，there's nothing like a soak in the bath for getting clean and relaxing you.

麦布莱德夫人： 当然。没有什么比得上泡澡既能清洁又放松的了。

Nurse： I quite agree. Is there anyone who could help you?

护士： 是这样。有谁可以帮助您吗？

Mrs. M： I can't ask Sue. She has three children to get off to school，and I can't want to sit in my dressing gown until she can get here.

麦布莱德夫人： 我不能麻烦苏，她要送三个孩子上学。我不想穿着睡衣等着她来。

Nurse： Would you consider having a bath seat that lowers you into the bath and then goes up when you're ready to get out?

护士： 您想过用洗澡椅吗？可以放低进入浴池，等您准备出来时再升高。

Mrs. M： I'm hopeless with machines. How easy are they to use?

麦布莱德夫人： 我对机器不熟悉。使用起来简单吗？

Nurse： Very easy.You have a button to push that lowers and raises the seat. If you like we can arrange for someone from Social Services to come out and do an assessment.What about washing your hair?

护士： 很简单。有一个按钮控制椅子的起落。如果您需要我们可以安排社会服务机构的人来做评估。您洗头发怎么样啊？

Mrs. M： That's no problem. I can do it at the sink. My neighbour used to be a hairdresser and she comes in every few weeks and gives it a cut and set.

麦布莱德夫人： 那没问题。我能用水池洗。我的邻居过去是理发师，她每隔几周就来给我打理一下。

Nurse： That's handy.

护士： 那很便利。

Mrs. M： It certainly is. I can't get down the town these day's unless Sue takes me. I haven't been shopping on my own for ages.

麦布莱德夫人： 当然，这些日子，如果没有苏陪着我不能进城。有很长时间我没有自己买东西了。

Nurse: Do you have any problems getting dressed and undressed?

护士：穿脱衣服有困难吗？

Mrs. M: Some things take for ever, like putting on tights or trousers.

麦布莱德夫人：有些事情要费些时间，像穿紧身衣或裤子。

Nurse: What about doing things up—buttons and zips, etc.?

护士：完成像扣扣子或拉拉链这些事情怎么样呢？

Mrs. M: I make sure that clothes do up at the front—no good struggling with a zip at the back of a dress.

麦布莱德夫人：我都要衣服前面开口——拉背后的拉链很费劲。

Nurse: The occupational therapist can suggest some simple gadgets to help with dressing and show you about easier ways of doing things. Would you like me to arrange for her to come?

护士：职业治疗师可以提供些简单工具帮助你穿衣，并给你指出做事的简单方法。您希望我帮你安排她来看你吗？

Mrs. M: Yes please. Another neighbour, Mrs Smith at number 80, had a visit from one of them and she got on very well.

麦布莱德夫人：好的。我的另一个邻居，80 号的史密斯太太接受过她们的访视，她过得很好。

# 39. Eczema

# 湿疹

Mr. D： I'm worried about my eczema when I come into hospital. It's important to follow my usual routine or it will flare up again.

戴尼斯先生： 我对住院后我的湿疹很担心，按我的日常习惯作息很重要，否则它会突然恶化。

Nurse： How long have you had eczema?

护士： 您患湿疹多久了？

Mr. D： For years，it's chronic now but some things make it worse.

戴尼斯先生： 有几年了。是慢性的，不过一些东西可以使它恶化。

Nurse： What sort of things?

护士： 什么方面的东西呢？

Mr. D： In my case it's things like getting too hot，such as from the sun shining through a window.

戴尼斯先生： 我觉得是一些加温的东西，比如透过窗户的阳光。

Nurse： We can arrange for you to have a bed well away from any windows. Is there anything else?

护士： 我们会安排您的病床远离所有的窗户，还有其他东西吗？

Mr. D： Alcohol starts up the itching，but l never touch it nowadays.

戴尼斯先生： 酒可以引起发痒，不过我现在不碰它了。

Nurse： What's your skin like now?

护士： 现在您的皮肤是什么样的？

Mr. D： Not very good. It's very red and the itching and scratching is much worse. I put it down to the stress of having to have the operation.

戴尼斯先生： 不太好，很红，瘙痒和搔抓会更糟。我认为是由于要做手术的压力所致。

Nurse： Which areas are worse affected?

护士： 哪些地方最厉害？

Mr. D： Mainly my face，as you can see，and my back is very itchy.

戴尼斯先生： 主要是我的脸，你看，我的背也很痒。

Nurse： Have you any sore areas or weeping areas?

护士： 您有脱屑或者渗出的地方吗？

Mr. D： No，my skin is just dry and very itchy. Any vesicles and broken areas would mean I was open to infection. Is that why you're asking?

戴尼斯先生：没有，我的皮肤只是干燥发痒。任何的囊泡或是破损都意味着我容易感染，这是你之所以问我的原因吧？

Nurse：Yes, exactly. But to be on the safe side I'll get the doctor to have a look now. What measures are you taking to reduce the flare up?

护士：确实是。但为了安全，我现在要请大夫来看看。如果突然复发，您有什么方法缓解吗？

Mr. D：I never use soap because it takes out my natural skin oils，so I use soap substitute，and at the moment I'm using an oily moisturizer nearly every hour，but it won't be so bad by the time I come into the ward.

戴尼斯先生：我从来不用肥皂，因为它会带走皮肤的油脂，所以我用肥皂替代品，并且我几乎每小时都用润肤油。希望我住进病房时不会很差。

Nurse：Are you using anything other than the emollient on your skin?

护士：除了润肤剂您还在皮肤上用其他什么东西吗？

Mr. D：No.

戴尼斯先生：不用。

Nurse：Have you used steroid ointments lately?

护士：您最近用过类固醇类的软膏吗？

Mr. D：No，not for months. I only have them as a last resort.

戴尼斯先生：几个月没用了，我只把它们当做最后的方案。

Nurse：What about other medicines?

护士：其他药物呢？

Mr. D：I'm taking an antihistamine so the scratching is reduced and I can get some sleep.

戴尼斯先生：我正在用抗组胺药，可以减少搔抓以利于睡眠。

Nurse：I'll make sure that your skin management is written in the care plan. Have you any questions?

护士：我会确保您的皮肤处理方法列入护理计划中，您还有什么问题吗？

Mr. D：What if my eczema gets really bad before I'm due to come in?

戴尼斯先生：如果我入院前，湿疹恶化了怎么办？

Nurse：If it gets any worse please let us know. I'll be giving you some printed information with the unit telephone number in any case.

护士：如果恶化了请让我们知道，无论如何，我会给您一些印有单位电话号码的资料。

Mr. D：OK，thanks.

戴尼斯先生：好的，谢谢。

# 40. Sleep

# 睡眠

Nurse：Good morning Mrs. Bell，how are you settling in?

护士：贝尔夫人，早上好！入住后感觉如何？

Mrs. B：Not too bad I suppose，but it feels a bit strange still.

贝尔夫人：我觉得还可以。可还是感觉有点不习惯。

Nurse：I thought it would be helpful for us to have a chat now that you have been here for a few days.You said that it feels strange.

护士：既然您已经来这里一些日子了，我认为聊聊会对我们有帮助。您刚说您感觉不习惯。

Mrs. B：I'm not complaining and everyone is so kind，but I miss the ladies from the sheltered housing.

贝尔夫人：我不是抱怨，每个人都很好。可我想小区的朋友们。

Nurse：Have any of them visited you yet?

护士：她们来看过您吗？

Mrs. B：The warden came yesterday and it was nice to hear all the gossip. My special friends are away on their hols until next week，so I expect they will be round then.

贝尔夫人：昨天管理员来了，听到些闲谈真好。我的密友度假去了，要到下周回来，所以我期待那时她们会来。

Nurse：That's good.What about your sons?

护士：那很好，您儿子呢？

Mrs. B：John brought me in，and he came yesterday on his way home from work. Nigel works away during the week，but he will be in on Saturday.

贝尔夫人：是约翰送我来的，昨天他下班回家的路上来了，尼格尔这周外出了，不过他周六会来。

Nurse：Have you got to know the other residents yet?

护士：您认识其他人了吗？

Mrs. B：I had tea with Mrs. Forbes and she was very friendly.

贝尔夫人：我和法博斯夫人一起喝茶，她非常友好。

Nurse：How are you sleeping?

护士：您睡眠如何？

Mrs. B：Not very well，I'm awake half the night.

贝尔夫人：不很好，半夜会醒。

Nurse：Is that usual for you?

护士：您经常这样吗？

Mrs. B：Nor really. I used to have the odd night when I would wake up，but most nights I would sleep right through until about half past six.

贝尔夫人：不，过去曾偶尔有过半夜醒来的不正常的夜晚，不过大多数夜晚我会一直睡到早晨 6：30。

Nurse：Do you have trouble falling asleep or do you wake up in the night?

护士：您入睡有困难还是夜里醒来？

Mrs. B：I'm really tired，but as soon as I put the light out I'm wide awake again.

贝尔夫人：我很累，可是一旦我熄灯，我又完全醒了。

Nurse：Do you get to sleep eventually?

护士：您最后能睡着吗？

Mrs. B：Yes，but then I wake up feeling whacked and groggy，I don't feel rested.

贝尔夫人：是的。可是那样我醒来感觉疲惫不堪、头晕眼花，觉得没有解乏。

Nurse：Do you wake up earlier than usual?

护士：您比平时醒得早吗？

Mrs. B：I did this morning，There was a lot of coming and going because the lady in the next room was poorly.

贝尔夫人：今天早晨是这样，因为隔壁的女士不太好，进进出出的次数很多。

Nurse：Yes，she had to go into hospital.

护士：是的，她已经去医院了。

Mrs. B：And I'm so tired in the day I keep dozing off in the chair.

贝尔夫人：我白天真累，以致于在椅子上不停地瞌睡。

Nurse：Did you usually have a short nap during the day before you came to us?

护士：您来之前在白天经常小睡吗？

Mrs. B：Well，if I'm honest，I did sometimes put my feet up after the lunchtime Archers and lose myself for a bit.

贝尔夫人：老实说，有时在午间 Archers 后我会放松休息一会。

Nurse：What time have you been falling asleep in the chair?

护士：您什么时候在椅子上睡觉？

Mrs. B：After supper，so when I come to it's time to start thinking about going to bed. That's a bit late for a nap I know.

贝尔夫人：晚饭后，所以当我醒来时已经是考虑上床睡觉的时候了。我知道对于小睡来说是晚了点。

Nurse：Do you have a bedtime routine—things that help you get to sleep?

护士：您晚间有规律的安排吗？可以帮助睡眠的。

Mrs. B：I used to have a bath last thing and take a milky drink to bed. Then read until I felt drowsy.

贝尔夫人：过去我总是洗个澡，喝杯奶就上床。然后看书直到感觉昏昏欲睡。

Nurse: What sort of time would you usually have the bath?

护士：您平时洗澡大约是几点？

Mrs. B: After the news at ten and be in bed by eleven. I'm not sure if it's all right to have a bath that late here. I expect the girls are too busy to help with baths.

贝尔夫人：晚上 10 点新闻之后，11 点之前上床。我不清楚这么晚洗澡是否可以。我想晚上的护理人员太忙不能帮我洗。

Nurse: I will have a word with the nurse in charge tonight about sure you can have a bath if you want, and get a milky drink. It is so important to get a good night's sleep.

护士：我会和晚上负责的护士讨论这件事，确保只要您需要就可以洗澡以及饮用奶制品，拥有良好的睡眠非常重要。

Mrs. B: You can say that again. I would be very grateful if they could help me with a bath.

贝尔夫人：您可以再说一遍。如果她们可以帮我洗澡我非常感激。

Nurse: Is there anything else that can be done to help you sleep properly?

护士：还有其他可以帮助您舒适睡眠的吗？

Mrs. B: It is quite warm in my room. I'm not used to having the radiator so hot in the bedroom.

贝尔夫人：屋里非常暖，我不习惯卧室的散热器开得太热。

Nurse: We can turn the thermostat down, so it just takes the chill off the room.

护士：我们可以转动温度调节钮去调低，只要暖和暖和房间就行了。

Mrs. B: They tried last night, but it was too stiff to turn.

贝尔夫人：他们昨晚试了，可是太紧了调不动。

Nurse: I'll get on to the maintenance staff right away.

护士：我会立刻与维修人员联系。

Mrs. B: It was so hot I pushed the duvetine off me.

贝尔夫人：因为太热了我把薄毯掀掉了。

Nurse: What about when you get up in the morning, will you be warm enough?

护士：您早晨起来呢，也很热吗？

Mrs. B: Oh yes, my boys treated me to some new clothes to come in here and that included a fleecy dressing gown. Look it's on the chair. Do you think it's too bright?

贝尔夫人：哦，是的。为了来这里我儿子给我买了些新衣服，有一件毛绒睡衣，看，就在椅子上，你觉不觉得它太鲜亮了？

Nurse: I like that dark pink. It's such a warm colour.

护士：我喜欢那种深粉红色，这么温暖的颜色。

Mrs. B: Yes, I like it. I did wonder about pink at my age, but then I thought 'Why not?'.

贝尔夫人：是啊，我喜欢。在我这个年纪穿粉红色我确实犹豫，可是转念就想为什么不呢？

Nurse: Is there anything else that stops you sleeping?

护士：还有什么其他事影响您睡觉吗？

Mrs. B: I still need to get used to the light coming in from the corridor.

贝尔夫人：我还需要适应从走廊射进来的灯光。

Nurse: Were you used to sleeping in complete darkness?

护士：　您习惯在全黑的环境中睡觉吗？

Mrs. B：　Yes, the sheltered housing is on the edge of the village right out in the sticks.

贝尔夫人：　是的，小区的房子在村庄边上，远离城镇。

Nurse：　We need to keep the light on in the corridor, so that everyone can move about safely.

护士：　我们需要让走廊的灯开着，这样每个人都能安全地行走。

Mrs. B：　Yes, I know. I don't suppose it will bother me for long.

贝尔夫人：　我知道。我认为不会打扰我很久的。

# 41. Recovery

# 康复

Mr. K： Nurse Brown，have you got a minute to talk?

韩先生： 布朗护士，有空聊会儿吗？

Nurse： I need to give a painkiller to another patient. I'll be back in five minutes.

护士： 我要给另一个病人服止痛药，我会在五分钟后回来。

Mr. K： OK.

韩先生： 好的。

Nurse： Right，Mr. Khan，I'm back. What would you like to talk about？

护士： 韩先生我回来了。您想谈点什么呢？

Mr. K： I'm really worried about how I'll manage to run my part of the business after the heart attack.

韩先生： 心脏病之后我真的很担心我该如何应付生意。

Nurse： Did you speak to the cardiac nurse specialist?

护士： 您和心内科护理专家说过了吗？

Mr. K： Yes，on Tuesday. She explained everything and I asked lots of questions. It all seemed quite straightforward，but now that I'm dressed and ready to go home I'm not so sure.

韩先生： 是的，在周二。我问了很多问题，她都解释了，听起来很简单。可是现在我换好衣服准备回家了，我还是不放心。

Nurse： Did she leave the printed information?

护士： 她给您印刷的材料了吗？

Mr. K： Yes.

韩先生： 是的。

Nurse： What bits are worrying you?

护士： 什么让您担心呢？

Mr. K： Well，mainly the driving and getting back to work. I drive about 20，000 miles a year on business. There is something in the leaflet about driving，but I'm worried that Swansea will take my licence away.

韩先生： 主要是开车和回去工作。忙生意我一年要开车走两万英里，材料上有关于驾驶的东西，可是我担心斯旺西会把我的驾照收回。

Nurse： Is yours an ordinary licence?

护士： 您的驾照是普通驾照吗？

Mr. K： I should think so.

韩先生： 我想应该是。

Nurse： You don't drive a bus or a lorry, do you?

护士： 您不是驾驶公交车或是卡车，是吗？

Mr. K： No, just the car and sometimes the minibus for the Community Centre.

韩先生： 不是，我只是开小汽车，有时候为社区活动中心开小巴。

Nurse： You will need to stop driving for at least four weeks and you don't have to notify DVLA.You have an appointment to see Dr Bradey next month. He will advise you about when you can start driving again.

护士： 您至少4个星期不能开车，您不需要告知车辆驾驶与车辆证照机构。下个月，您有一个预约，要去见布拉德利医生，他会就您什么时候才能开车提出建议。

Mr. K： I hope it's not much longer than four weeks, My dad and brother can visit the customers for a few weeks, but nor for ever.

韩先生： 我希望不要超过4个星期。我父亲和兄弟可以拜访客户几周，但是时间不能太长。

Nurse： So far your recovery has gone well. There's no reason to think you won't be fit to drive in a month. It might be a good idea to tell your insurance company about the heart attack.

护士： 到目前为止您恢复得不错，没有理由认为您在一个月内身体不会恢复到可以开车。把这次心脏病发作通知保险公司是个不错的提议。

Mr. K： Yes, that's sensible. I don't want to drive without insurance. That means a fine and six points on your licence.

韩先生： 是的，这是明智的，我不想在没有保险的情况下开车。那意味着罚款和扣6分。

Nurse： You mentioned getting back to work.

护士： 您提到要回去工作。

Mr. K： We run a small family business, so one person off sick puts a real strain on everyone else.

韩先生： 我们经营着一个小型家族企业，一个人病倒了，其他人的负担会加重。

Nurse： Yes, I can see that. Do you do most of the customer visiting?

护士： 是，我明白，大部分客户都是您去拜访吗？

Mr. K： Yes, my dad doesn't really like driving long distances and my brother is better at the day-to-day business.

韩先生： 是的，我父亲不喜欢跑长途，而我兄弟更擅长日常业务。

Nurse： Again Dr Bradley will advise you about going back to work, but most people gradually increase their activity and are back at work in four to six weeks. It would be longer if you had a job with a lot of physical activity.

护士： 布拉德利医生会对您是否回去工作提出建议，但大部分病人会逐渐加大他们的活动量，会在4～6周内回去工作。如果您从事需要大量体力劳动的工作，那时间也会相应延长。

Mr. K： No, if I'm in the office it's mainly computer work and telephoning customers. My job isn't very active, but I'm keen on sports.

韩先生：不，如果我在办公室，那我的主要工作是计算机操作和电话联系客户，我的工作不是非常用力，但是我热衷于运动。

Nurse: What kind of sports do you do?

护士：您做什么运动？

Mr. K: I play some cricket and coach some lads in a local football team.

韩先生：我玩板球而且在当地一家青少年足球队当教练。

Nurse: How active is the coaching?

护士：教练工作的运动量怎么样？

Mr. K: Well I work-out with the boys. I'm keen to keep on with both the cricket and the coaching.

韩先生：我同队员一起训练，我喜欢继续从事板球和足球教练。

Nurse: The staff running the formal sessions of the cardiac rehabilitation programme will be able to give you information about safe levels of exercise and playing sport. When do you start?

护士：组织心脏病康复项目正式活动的专业人员会告诉您关于练习和运动安全水平的信息。您什么时候开始？

Mr. K: The specialist nurse said that she will give me a ring next week to see how we're getting on at home and by then she will know the dates for the exercise sessions.

韩先生：护理专家说她会在下周打电话给我，看我们如何在家中进行锻炼，到那时候她就知道训练活动的日期。

Nurse: Don't forget the cardiac nurses have a telephone helpline if you have any worries once you get home, and you can also use their e-mail.

护士：回到家里您有什么担心不要忘了您有心脏病护士的求助电话，您也可以用电子邮件。

Mr. K: Yes, it's very reassuring to know that there is some back-up.

韩先生：好的，知道有这些帮助我非常放心。

Nurse: Have you any questions about your drugs and the dietary changes, or anything else?

护士：您有关于用药和饮食变化方面的问题吗？

Mr. K: No, that's all the worries for now. I just needed to get those things straight in my mind.

韩先生：没有了，现在就是这些担心了，我只是需要把那些事直接记在脑子里。

# 42. Diabetic Control

# 糖尿病控制

Nurse： Hello Mrs. Hamilton. It doesn't seem like a year since we last saw you.

护士： 您好，汉密尔顿夫人。从上次见到您到现在好像不到一年。

Mrs. H： Yes, time for the annual eye check again.

汉密尔顿夫人： 是一年，又到了每年的眼科检查时间了。

Nurse： Not everyone is so reliable about attending as you.

护士： 不是每个人都像您一样如此信赖检查。

Mrs. H： I'd be daft not to. Finding problems early is so important. My sight is already bad, I don't want to get any worse.

汉密尔顿夫人： 我不会那么愚蠢，早期发现问题很重要。我的视力已经不好了，我不想再恶化了。

Nurse： I will be putting the eye drops in to dilate your pupil, so we can examine the back of your eye. How has your sight been since last years check?

护士： 我给您滴眼药水散大瞳孔，这样我们可以检查你的眼睛后面，去年检查后您的视力怎么样？

Mrs. H： I'm finding it more difficult to read small print and I've got patchy blurring of vision. It does make life difficult.

汉密尔顿夫人： 我觉得看小字更困难了，而且视力有斑片状模糊，这确实给生活带来不便。

Nurse： How does it affect you on a day-to-day basis?

护士： 它是如何影响您的基础日常生活的？

Mrs. H： Now Jim and I have given up working we have time to do our garden. I have always had green fingers and we like walking in the countryside, but it's not much fun with my poor vision. I have to rely on Jim to read the labels on weed killer for the garden and the plant labels at the garden centre. He doesn't mind, but I mind very much. I feel so helpless and frustrated about losing my independence.

汉密尔顿夫人： 现在吉姆和我已经退休了，我们有时间去做我们喜欢的园艺而且我们喜欢在郊外散步。但是因为我的眼睛，使这些活动没有多大乐趣。我要依赖吉姆来识别花园除草剂的标签和公园中心的植物标签。虽然他不介意，但我非常介意。失去了独立性，我感觉非常无助和灰心。

Nurse： Yes, it must be frustrating.

护士： 是的，的确令人沮丧。

Mrs. H： I'm really cheesed off. It's reading books as well. I like to relax with a book after supper while Jim has a pint. But now I can only see if the print is very large and every light in the room is on. It's not very relaxing.

汉密尔顿夫人： 我非常心烦，看书也是这样，我喜欢晚饭后看书放松一下，而吉姆喜欢在附近喝一品脱。但是现在我只能在每一盏灯都亮着的房间看很大的字，这一点也不轻松。

Nurse： No，it doesn't sound very relaxing. Have you got any low vision aids.

护士： 听起来是不轻松，您没有任何辅助视力的工具吗？

Mrs. H： I've got my glasses and a magnifier and I make sure that the lighting is right for what I'm doing.

汉密尔顿夫人： 我已经配了眼镜和放大镜，而且我保证光线适合我做事。

Nurse： How is your diabetic control?

护士： 您的糖尿病控制得怎么样了？

Mrs. H： OK. I'm doing quite well with the sugar control and the insulin injections are no problem now I use a preloaded insulin pen.

汉密尔顿夫人： 我对糖控制得很好，胰岛素的注射也没问题了，现在我使用胰岛素笔。

Nurse： I'm sure you know how important this is to help stop the retinopathy from getting worse.

护士： 我确信您知道注射胰岛素对防止视网膜病恶化是多么重要。

Mrs. H： Oh yes，the diabetic nurse specialists are always harping on about the importance of managing the diabetes properly.

汉密尔顿夫人： 是的，糖尿病护士专家经常喋喋不休地说适当控制糖尿病的重要性。

Nurse： We all nag you，don't we?

护士： 我们都唠叨您，是吗？

Mrs. H： I don't mind. But just think，if I hadn't gone after the area manager post and had to have a medical it might have been ages before they found the diabetes and I started the insulin and a proper diet.

汉密尔顿夫人： 我不介意。但是只要一想，如果我没有申请地区经理的岗位，不得不做体格检查，那可能好长时间也不会发现我患有糖尿病，也就不会使用胰岛素和注意合理饮食了。

# 43. Dysmenorrhoea

# 痛经

Nurse: Hello again Mrs. Hall. I've come to answer any questions you might have about having the examination as a day case.

护士：霍尔夫人您好，又见到您了。如果您有关于检查方面的任何问题可以问我。

Mrs. H: You and the consultant explained that he would look inside the womb with a special instrument and then do a scrape to get a sample for testing, so I'm fairly clear about what will happen.

霍尔夫人：你和专家解释了会用特殊仪器探查子宫里面，而且会做刮片来取样检查。我非常清楚会发生什么。

Nurse: Have you any questions about the possible complications of the procedure?

护士：您对检查过程中可能出现的复杂情况还有问题吗？

Mrs. H: No, I'm fully aware, that there is a risk of the womb being perforated.

霍尔夫人：没有了。我清楚意识到会有子宫穿孔的危险。

Nurse: You signed your consent form and consented to a general anaesthetic.

护士：您在同意书上签字，并同意使用全身麻醉药。

Mrs. H: I didn't fancy having it done in outpatients, I'd rather be put to sleep first.

霍尔夫人：我不喜欢在门诊中做，我宁可先被麻醉。

Nurse: It will only be a short anaesthetic. You should be able to go home later that afternoon or evening. Will your partner be collecting you?

护士：只是一个小麻醉，您当天下午或晚上就应该可以回家了，您丈夫来接您吗？

Mrs. H: Yes, he'll come straight from work. His shift finishes at 3 o'clock, so it will be about 4 o'clock. Is that OK?

霍尔夫人：是的，他直接从工作单位过来。他的工作 3 点结束，过来可能要 4 点了。可以吗？

Nurse: No problem, but he should ring first just to see if you are recover enough to go home. You might still be a bit sleepy.

护士：没问题。但是他应该先打个电话看看您是否恢复得足够好并可以回家，您可能仍会有想睡觉的感觉。

Mrs. H: Mr. Bainbridge said you could give me a date for the examination.

霍尔夫人：班医生说你会告诉我检查日期。

Nurse: Yes, I'll get the dates up on the computer, but first I need to check a few things with you.

护士： 是。我会在电脑上预约日期，但是我首先要问您一些问题。

Mrs. H: OK.

霍尔夫人： 好的。

Nurse: We do the examinations on a Wednesday morning. Are there any dates that we need to avoid?

护士： 我们在星期三早上做检查，我们需要避开什么日子吗？

Mrs. H: No, we're not going away until the problems with my periods have been sorted out.

霍尔夫人： 不，我们不会外出，直到我月经的问题解决。

Nurse: We will need to avoid dates when you have your period, as it makes it difficult to get a good view of the inside of the womb. Are your periods regular?

护士： 我们需要避开您行经的日子，因为它会妨碍子宫内部视野清晰。您的月经规律吗？

Mrs. H: Fairly. It usually comes every thirty days or so. The real problem is that it lasts much longer.

霍尔夫人： 规律。它差不多 30 天左右来一次，实际问题是持续时间太长了。

Nurse: How long?

护士： 多长呢？

Mrs. H: The last three months have been dreadful, with the heavy bleeding going on for 7 or 8 days.

霍尔夫人： 前 3 个月非常糟，月经过多持续了七八天。

Nurse: Does that make things difficult for you?

护士： 给您带来什么麻烦了吗？

Mrs. H: Yes, very difficult, because I keep flooding. Sometimes the blood comes through the pad and my clothes, so I'm scared to go out. Plus I'm forever washing clothes and the bedding.

霍尔夫人： 是，非常麻烦。因为我持续出血，有时血渗透护垫和衣服，所以我害怕外出，另外我要不停地洗衣服和床上用品。

Nurse: It sounds as if your daily activities are seriously affected.

护士： 听上去您的日常活动严重受影响。

Mrs. H: Yes, they are. I can't plan to do anything for a whole week every month.

霍尔夫人： 没错，每个月有一个星期什么都做不了。

Nurse: Do you have any spotting, such as after having sexual intercourse?

护士： 您还有其他时间流血吗？比如性交后？

Mrs. H: No, only the heavy bleeding and flooding during my period. But it's affecting our sex life; either I'm bleeding or too tired.

霍尔夫人： 不，只有月经过多，但它已经影响了我的性生活，因为月经过多或是太疲劳了。

Nurse: The blood test we took will show if you are anaemic. Heavy periods often cause anaemia and that would make you tired.

护士： 我们做的血液检查会显示您是否有贫血。月经过多经常会导致贫血，所以您会感到疲劳。

Mrs. H: I really want the bleeding sorted. It's really dragging me down.

霍尔夫人：我真想马上解决这个问题，它真的拖垮我了。

Nurse: The examination will help to find a physical cause, but as you know Mr. Bainbridge thinks that you may have dysfunctional uterine bleeding and he might not find a physical cause.

护士：检查有助于找出生理上的原因。但正如您所知道的，班医生认为您可能是功能性子宫出血，而且可能找不到生理原因。

Mrs. H: I'm in agony with period pains as well. I used to have pain with my periods when I was young, but this pain is much worse.

霍尔夫人：我由于痛经而极度苦恼。我年轻的时候曾经有痛经，但是现在疼痛更严重。

Nurse: What do you take for it?

护士：您吃什么药？

Mrs. H: Just paracetamol, but they don't do much good. I know I said that I want it sorted, but I'm worried in case he says I need a hysterectomy.

霍尔夫人：就吃对乙酰氨基酚。但不是很有效。我想把问题解决，但担心万一他说要把子宫切除掉。

Nurse: There are several different treatments for heavy bleeding, such as tablets, hormones and a fairly new technique called ablation, where the lining of the womb is removed. There is lots to try before hysterectomy needs to be considered.

护士：有几种不同的治疗方案，像药物、激素和一种新的叫剥离术的技术，就是刮除子宫内膜。在考虑子宫切除之前还会有好多可尝试的办法。

Mrs. H: I do hope so. You hear about women having a hysterectomy and never really getting over it, plus all those things that happen to you.

霍尔夫人：我希望如此。听说子宫切除的妇女永远不会真正恢复，以及所有那些可能发生的事情。

Nurse: What sort of things?

护士：什么事？

Mrs. H: Well you put on weight.

霍尔夫人：体重会增加。

Nurse: There is no reason for anyone to put on weight after a hysterectomy other than the usual reasons of eating too much and not getting enough exercise.

护士：子宫切除后体重是不可能增加的，除了那些常见的原因，像吃得太多，运动太少。

Mrs. H: It wouldn't feel right somehow.

霍尔夫人：总之不会感觉很好。

Nurse: In what way?

护士：在哪些方面？

Mrs. H: You know—not feeling like a proper woman.

霍尔夫人：你知道，感觉不像正常女人。

Nurse: If Mr. Bainbridge advised a hysterectomy and you were considering it, the usual thing would be for you to see one of specialist nurses again to have a proper discussion about the operation before it went ahead. But we could talk it through now if you would like to.

护士：如果班先生建议您做子宫切除，而且您也考虑做的话，在手术前，您会再见一下护理专家，同您对手术进行适当讨论，如果您愿意，我们现在也可以仔细讨论。

Mrs. H: Yes please, if you've got time now.

霍尔夫人：好的，如果你现在有时间。

# 44. Sexual Disorder

# 性功能障碍

Mr J： I've been under the doctor for my blood pressure. She said to make an appointment for you to check me over and do the blood pressure.

约翰斯先生： 医生已经关注我的血压情况，她说已跟您预约测量我的血压。

Nurse： What has the doctor prescribed?

护士： 医生开的什么药？

Mr. J： Innovace.

约翰斯先生： 依挪威斯。

Nurse： How have you been?

护士： 您感觉怎么样？

Mr. J： Not bad.

约翰斯先生： 不是很糟。

Nurse： What，not feeling really well?

护士： 什么，真的感觉不好？

Mr J： A bit seedy，but nothing specific.

约翰斯先生： 有一点不好，但没特殊的地方。

Nurse： Is there anything worrying you?

护士： 您有什么担忧的吗？

Mr. J： I've met a nice lady，we really hit it off. She likes all the same things as me，music，food and everything.

约翰斯先生： 我遇到了一个优雅的女士，我们合得来，她喜欢的事我也喜欢，音乐、饮食、所有一切。

Nurse： Had you been on your own for long?

护士： 您独身多长时间了？

Mr. J： A long time. Jenny died of cancer ten years ago. I didn't want anyone else at first，but when the kids married and moved away I felt a bit lonely and that.

约翰斯先生： 很长时间了。珍妮 10 年前死于癌症。开始我并不想要任何人，但是当孩子们结婚并离开我，我真的感觉有点孤单了。

Nurse： Yes.

护士： 是这样。

Mr J： I met someone at work，but that soon fizzled out.

约翰逊先生：我工作时遇到过一个，但那很快就结束了。

Nurse：Some men can have difficulty with erections when taking the medicine you are on. Have you had any trouble?

护士：一些男人在服用您正在服用的这种药时，可能会有勃起障碍。您有这方面的问题吗？

Mr. J：It's difficult to talk about it，but I was impotent and couldn't do it. I told myself it was just nerves being with someone new and tiredness.

约翰斯先生：很难启齿。但是我是有勃起障碍并且不能过性生活。我告诉自己这只是因为跟一个不熟悉的人过性生活导致的紧张再加上疲劳造成的。

Nurse：Yes，it's difficult to talk about intimate things.

护士：讨论这些隐私话题是有点困难。

Mr. J：I'm worried about my new relationship. I don't want anything to go wrong like last time.

约翰斯先生：我担心我的新恋爱关系，我不想像上次一样出任何差错。

Nurse：We're lucky in this area to have a nurse who specialises in the management of erectile dysfunction，that's the medical term for problems with erections.Would you like me to arrange an assessment appointment with him?

护士：在这方面我们幸运地拥有一位治疗勃起障碍的护理专家，我们为您预约他怎么样？

Mr. J：Yes please，I need to talk to someone. When the doctor gave me the script she said one of the side-effects was trouble with erections，but how could I ask her any questions? it was so embarrassing.

约翰斯先生：好，我需要与别人谈谈。当医生给我开药时，她告诉我药的一个副作用是勃起障碍，但我没法问有关问题，太尴尬了。

# 45. Discussing Diet and Drug Therapy with a High Blood Pressure Patient

# 与高血压病人讨论饮食和用药

Nurse： Mrs. Williams，your doctor has prescribed a medication for your high blood pressure.

护士： 威廉姆斯夫人，您的医生为您的高血压开药了。

Patient： What is it?

病人： 什么药？

Nurse： It is called Hydrodiuril more often used theses days. It is a diuretic.

护士： 目前常用的一种叫噻嗪的药，是一种利尿药。

Patient： I think I have heard of those before. Is it a water pill?

病人： 我想我听说过这种药，是一种利尿药吧？

Nurse： Yes. It helps the body get rid of water and salt. It will make you urinate more so you should take it early in the morning.

护士： 对。它能帮助身体排出水和盐。它会使人排更多的尿，所以您要在上午早些时候服用。

Patient： What if take it at night?

病人： 如果我晚上服用呢？

Nurse： You will need to go to the bathroom several times during the night.

护士： 那您夜间就要去好几次卫生间。

Patient： Oh，I guess I'll take it in the morning.

病人： 哦，我想我还是早上服用吧。

Nurse： Diuril will also make your body lose potassium. Potassium is important to your body，so you will need to eat more high potassium foods.

护士： 噻嗪会使您的身体损失钾。钾对身体很重要，所以您要吃一些高钾的食物。

Patient： What kind of food contains more potassium?

病人： 什么食物含钾多？

Nurse： Fresh and dried fruits，vegetables，and fish. Bananas and oranges are good. Some people experience side effects of the drug. If you feel weak，have palpitation，or get a skin rash，call your doctor.

护士： 新鲜水果和干果、蔬菜和鱼。香蕉和橘子也不错。有些人会发生副作用。如果您感觉虚弱、心悸或皮疹，请找医生。

Patient： What would that mean?

病人： 这是什么意思？

Nurse： You could be having a reaction to the medication or you could have lost too much potassium. That is why you need to eat more foods that are high potassium. You also need to eat less salt. You should be on a low-salt diet，so you just don't add salt to your food while you are cooking or at the table.

护士： 您可能有药物反应，也可能失去了太多的钾。这就是您需要吃高钾食物的原因。您还要少吃盐，需要执行低盐饮食。这意味着您在做饭和吃饭的时候不要多放盐。

Patient： Can I add MSG?

病人： 我能加味精吗？

Nurse： No. MSG has salt in it and may have other side effects. Try to use other spices，but not MSG or salt. If you take your medication regularly and follow the diet，you should have no problems with your blood pressure. Here is some more information from the Dietary Department that you can read. If you have any questions，don't hesitate to ask.

护士： 不行，味精中含有盐并可能有其他副作用。试着用其他调料，不要用味精和盐。如果您按时吃药并注意饮食，您的血压会没事的。这是营养部给的一些资料，您可以看看。如果存任何问题，尽管问。

# 46. Cancer Care

# 癌症护理

Nurse： You look sad today Mr Bradley. I wonder if there is anything I could do to help?

护士： 您看起来挺悲痛的，布莱德利先生。我能帮您什么忙吗？

Patient： The doctor told me yesterday that I had cancer.

病人： 医生昨天告诉我患了癌症。

Nurse： How do you feel about it?

护士： 您感觉怎么样？

Patient： Well，I have known that it was serious before my surgery. My family began to stop talking about my health and didn't answer my questions. Still，when the doctor said cancer，it was awful! I felt like my lungs stopped working and my heart stopped beating. I felt cold.

病人： 唉，手术前我就知道很严重。我的家人已经不再谈论我的健康，也不再回答我的问题。而且，当医生说到癌症时，简直太可怕了。我感觉我的肺停止了呼吸，心脏也停止了跳动。我感觉冷。

Nurse： It must have been awful. What do you understand about cancer?

护士： 那一定很可怕。您了解癌症吗？

Patient： Well，the surgery probably removed it all. The tests have not shown cancer anywhere else. So they are going to start a new kind of antibody treatment along with chemotherapy.

病人： 这个，手术也许能把它完全切除，而且检查显示癌症并没有扩散。所以，他们要开始一种新的抗体治疗，跟化疗一起做。

Nurse： Yes，that is the standard treatment for some kinds of cancer.

护士： 对，这是对某些癌症的标准疗法。

Patient： I have heard that chemotherapy makes people sick.

病人： 我听说化疗会使人难受。

Nurse： Yes，unfortunately，because the chemotherapy is very toxic to cells，it affects cancer cells along with healthy cells of the body. Many patients will have nausea and vomiting. Part of the treatment includes medicine to reduce the nausea.

护士： 是的，很不幸，因为化疗对细胞有很强的毒性，它影响癌细胞，也影响身体的其他正常细胞。许多人会恶心和呕吐。治疗的一部分包括降低恶心的药物。

Patient： But I still feel nauseated.

病人： 但我仍有恶心。

Nurse： Many patients do. You can reduce the problem by do not eating very hot or cold food, by not eating spicy food or foods with lots of fiber like raw fruit vegetables. Drink fluids between. Don't eat fried foods. Things that are good to eat include eggs, white rice, and bananas. It is important to eat well. If you have good nutrition, you will get better faster.

护士： 许多病人都这样。别吃特别热的和冷的食物就能好一些。还不能吃辛辣的食物和富含纤维的食物，如生的水果和蔬菜，两餐之间要喝水，不要吃油炸的食物。鸡蛋、白米饭和香蕉可以吃。吃好非常重要。如果有好的营养，您就能更快好起来。

Patient： OK. Thank you for talking with me.

病人： 好，谢谢您跟我谈话。

Nurse： You are welcome. I'm here if you want to talk more.

护士： 别客气，如果您想说话，叫我就行。

# 47. Refusing Treatment

# 拒绝治疗

Patient：Nurse，don't give me shots again.

痛人：护士，不要再给我打针了。

Nurse：Why?

护士：为什么？

Patient：I think it is of no use.

病人：我觉得打针没用。

Nurse：Don't say that. You'll be well soon after the operation.

护士：别这么说，手术后您很快就会好起来的。

Patient：Perhaps you're right，but I'm always feeling anxious. I think I'm a heavy burden on others. Don't bother any more.

病人：也许你说得对，但我总是有些担心。我想我对别人是个负担，不想再给别人添麻烦了。

Nurse：Mrs. Jones，you know we all care about you，especially your husband and children. Do what the doctors tell you，and you will recover soon.

护士：琼斯夫人，您知道我们都在关心您，尤其是您的丈夫和孩子。按照医生要求的做，您就会很快好起来。

Patient：No，I feel that everything in the world is meaningless. I don't want to live in the world to bother others.

病人：不，我觉得世界上的一切都没有意义。我不想活在世上麻烦别人。

Nurse：Mrs. Jones，I understand your concerns，but please don't worry too much. I'm sure your condition will soon be better—if you cooperate with us.

护士：琼斯夫人，我很理解您，但是请不要太担心，如果您能与我们合作，我肯定您的病情会很快好转。

Patient：Thank you for your kindness.

病人：谢谢你的好意。

Nurse：Look at the people around you. They are all full of confidence. Mrs. Williams' condition was worse than yours before operation，but you see，she can take care of herself now.

护士：看看您周围的人，大家都满怀信心。威廉姆斯夫人手术前的病情比您差，但您看她已经能自理一切了。

Patient：I see. Nurse，give me the shot please.

病人：我明白了。护士，给我打针吧。

# 48. Health Consultation

# 健康咨询

Nurse: What's troubling you, Mr. Francis?

护士：您哪难受。弗朗西斯先生？

Patient: I have had a bed cough and my heart is beating very fast. My blood pressure is probably high.

病人：我咳嗽很厉害，心跳得很快，血压也高。

Nurse: How old are you?

护士：您多大岁数了？

Patient: I'm sixty-five years old.

病人：我 65 岁。

Nurse: Have you been taking the medications the doctor gave you? Have you given up smoking and alcohol?

护士：您吃了医生给开的药了吗？您戒烟和酒了吗？

Patient: No, I have not by now.

病人：没有，我至今还未戒掉。

Nurse: Now you may have suffered emphysema and your blood pressure and heart are abnormal. So from now on, you must stop smoking forever. There is very strong evidence that smoking is a hazard to health. Smoking irritates the throat and respiratory passages. It is sometimes linked to loss of appetite, nausea, shortness of breath, and irregularity of the heartbeat. But even more important, smoking-particularly cigarette smoking-is related to chronic and often fatal diseases of the respiratory tract. Overwhelming statistical evidence shows that smokers are more likely to develop cancer of the the lung, throat, tongue, and jaw than nonsmokers. They are also more likely to suffer from emphysema and bronchitis. In addition, apart from the tobacco tar contained in tobacco smoke, the effects of tobacco depend almost entirely upon its nicotine content. Smoking is very harmful to people young or old, especially to older people who suffered from emphysema or heart disease, and hypertension. In just three seconds a cigarette makes your heart beat faster, shoots your blood pressure up.

护士：现在您患的可能是肺气肿，此外血压和心脏也不正常，因此，从现在起您必须马上戒掉烟，以后再不能吸烟。现在已有可靠的证据表明，吸烟对健康十分有害，它刺激咽喉和呼吸道，有时还会引起食欲缺乏、恶心、呼吸急促、心律不齐。但更为重要的是呼吸道的慢性病，而且常常是致命性的疾病与抽烟尤其与卷烟有关。大多数资料统计证明，吸烟者较不吸烟者更易患肺、咽喉、舌的癌症，也更容易患肺气肿和支气管炎。此外，烟草对健康的损害，除了烟雾中所含的烟油造成的以外几乎完全是烟草中含有的尼古丁造成的。吸烟对于人，无论是年轻人还是老年人都是有害无益的。特别是对已患有肺气肿、心脏病和高血压的老龄病人来说更是危险极大。一支烟可以仅在三秒钟之内，就使您的心跳加快，血压上升。

Patient: Oh, I see. Then, how do I stay healthy as an guy?

病人：是的，我明白了，那么像我这样的人怎样才能保持健康呢？

Nurse: To a considerable extent, the individual is responsible for his own health. You must establish a definite pattern of healthy living if you are to maintain a satisfactory level of well-being.

护士：从某种程度上来说，每个人都应对自己的身体健康负责。如果您想保持良好的健康水平，就必须有一定的正常生活方式。

1. Exercise regularly such as doing Tai-Chi, going for a walk in the morning, etc.
   要经常锻炼身体，如打一打太极拳，早晨起来散散步。
2. Be on a diet that provides a proper balance of proteins, carbohydrates, fats, and a lot of vegetables and fruits which not only help to prevent constipation, but also give you the energy, vitamins and minerals that you need for daily activities.
   要吃含适量蛋白质、糖和脂肪的食物。多吃蔬菜和水果，这不仅可以防止便秘，而且提供日常生活维生素物质。
3. Obtain sufficient sleep and rest. Individuals vary in their need for sleep, with most adults averaging about eight hours a night.
   要有足够的睡眠和休息。每个人所需要的睡眠时间长短不一，大多数成年人平均每天睡眠约 8 个小时。
4. Schedule regular visits to your doctor.
   定期到医院进行体检。
5. Pay close attention to your health. Familiarize yourself with the warning signs of illness and seek medical attention promptly if you should become ill.
   随时注意您的身体状况，熟悉您要生病的种种征兆，一旦生病就马上去医院。
6. Finally, most important, maintaining a healthy mental is essential to health.
   最后，也是最为重要的一点，即保持心情舒畅，这是保证健康的最基本条件。

Patient: Well, thanks.

病人：明白了，谢谢。

# 49. Interactions

# 交流

Nurse: Hello, Mr. Adams, you're such a hard worker. You're still working even in the hospital.

护士：您好，亚当斯先生。您真是努力工作，在医院还在工作呀。

Patient: I can't help it. Since I've been sick, the company hasn't been able to function normally. As you see, there are many documents that haven't been read for the past three days.

病人：我止不住。由于我生病，公司一直不能正常运转。你看，还有这么多前三天的文件没有看呢。

Nurse: So your health is very important. Because of the myocardial infarction, you must get sufficient rest. Otherwise, your prognosis will be affected.

护士：所以，您的健康是非常重要的。由于心肌梗死，您必须得到足够的休息. 否则您的预后会受影响。

Patient: Yes, I know that. But I am so busy. I had no time to rest and had to smoke two packs of cigarettes to work through the night. I don't know what I should do now I'm suffering from this disease.

病人：是的，我知道这些。但我太忙了，我没有时间休息，晚上要抽两盒烟才能通宵工作。现在生病了，我也不知道该怎么办了。

Nurse: But this kind of lifestyle is not good for your health. Smoking can increase the rate of sudden death in coronary heart disease (CHD) by fifty percent, Fatty and high-calorie foods, which you usually eat, also increase the risk of early CHD.

护士：但这种生活方式对您的健康不好。吸烟使冠心病患者的猝死率提高 50%。肥胖和您经常的高热量饮食也会增加冠心病突发的风险。

Patient: Really? I thought smoking could only be harmful to the lung. I didn't know it was so harmful to the heart.

病人：真的？以前我只知道吸烟对肺有害，我不知道还会伤害心脏。

Nurse: In addition to affecting the heart, lung and stomach, smoking can also endanger the people around you.

护士：除了影响心脏、肺和胃之外，吸烟还危害您周围的人。

Patient: So I'm not only hurting myself but also hurting everyone else around me. I really should give up smoking.

病人： 那我不仅在伤害我自己，还在伤害我身边的人。我真应该戒烟。

Nurse: Yes. You should begin quitting right now since you seem to have made up your mind. Please give me the cigarettes you have hidden under your pillow. I am confiscating them.

护士： 对，既然您下了决心，马上就该戒烟。把您藏在枕头下的香烟交给我，我要没收他们。

Patient: Miss，you are great. You've discovered my secret. OK，here you are. What else should I pay attention to besides giving up smoking?

病人： 护士小姐，你真厉害，发现了我的秘密。好，给你。除了戒烟，我还要注意其他什么吗？

Nurse: First，you must choose a proper diet: low fat，low salt，low sugar and low calorie intake，and eat more fruits and vegetables. Second，you should exercise moderately. And finally，you have to take your medicine on time.

护士： 首先您必须科学饮食，低脂肪、低盐、低糖、低热量摄入，多吃水果和蔬菜。其次，适度锻炼。最后，要按时服药。

Patient: I see. I'll follow your advice

病人： 好，我明白了。我会按你的建议做。

# 50. Before Discharge

# 出院前

**(1)**

Nurse： Mr. Johnson，you look so fresh.

护士： 约翰逊先生，您看起来精神很好。

Patient： I really feel strong and fit。

病人： 我真觉得又健康，又强壮。

Nurse： Have you lost weight since you were ill?

护士： 您生病以来瘦了些吗？

Patient： No，I don't think so。

病人： 我想没有。

Nurse： You can go home tomorrow. Congratulations !

护士： 明天您可以出院了，祝贺您！

Patient： Thank you. All doctors and nurses here are very kind. I'll always remember you.

病人： 谢谢你们，这里的医生和护士都很好，我会记住大家的。

Nurse： It's our responsibility.

护士： 这是我们的职责。

Patient： May I ask a few question about exercises?

病人： 我可以问几个关于锻炼的问题吗？

Nurse： By all means.

护士： 当然可以。

Patient： What kinds of exercises are there?

病人： 运动能分多少种？

Nurse： There are three main groups of exercises：aerobic exercises，calisthenics and anaerobic exercises.

护士： 主要有三种运动：有氧运动、健美操和无氧运动。

Patient： What are aerobic exercises?

病人： 什么是有氧运动？

Nurse： Jogging，running，rowing，skating，badminton，rope-jumping，martial arts and other endurance exercises are all called aerobic exercises. They enhance the ability of muscles to use oxygen and improve heart and lung fitness.

护士：散步、跑步、划船、滑冰、打羽毛球，跳绳和武术等耐力性活动都是有氧运动。这些运动能提高肌肉运输氧气的能力，改善心肺功能。

Patient: Then the exercises which occur without oxygen are called anaerobic?

病人：那运动中不需要氧气的就是无氧运动了？

Nurse: That's right. Such exercises as weightlifting are anaerobic, which require brief spurts of intense effort. They improve muscles strength or build up speed.

护士：对，比如举重就是无氧运动，它需要短时间内用力屏气，这种运动能增强肌肉的力量，提高运动速度。

Patient: What is the purpose of calisthenics?

病人：做健美操的目的是什么？

Nurse: You use calisthenics to warm up before and cool down after aerobic exercises; it can improve joint flexibility and muscle tone.

护士：主要是为了在有氧运动前使身体活动开，运动后使身体平静下来。这能提高关节的柔韧性和肌肉运动的协调性。

Patient: How should I set the length for each exercises session?

病人：我要怎样安排每次运动的时间呢？

Nurse: Five minutes of warming up will prepare your body for vigorous exercises. Then fifteen to sixty minutes of aerobic exercises. You need to exercise hard until you sweat or have to breathe deeply but are not breathless. In the end, you have to take five minutes to cool down; this will prevent dizziness and fainting which may result from stopping vigorous exercises too suddenly.

护士：先做 5 分钟的预备活动，然后做 15～60 分钟的有氧运动。您必须尽力运动，直至全身出汗、呼吸加深而又不至于上气不接下气。最后您还得用 5 分钟平静下来以防因突然停止剧烈运动而导致的头晕和昏倒。

Patient: I've learned a lot from your advise, Thank you very much.

病人：与您交谈让我学到了许多，非常感谢。

### （2）

Nurse: Good morning, Mr. White. I'm Li Lin, your nurse today.

护士：早上好，怀特先生。我是李林，今天是您的护士。

Patient: Good morning, Miss Li.

病人：早上好，李小姐。

Nurse: How are you feeling today?

护士：您感觉怎么样？

Patient: I feel great!

病人：感觉非常好！

Nurse: Good. You will be discharged tomorrow.

护士：好。您明天就可以出院了。

Patient: Terrific! I'm so eager to go home.

病人：太好了！我就盼着回家呢。

Nurse： Mr. White，you need to continue being on a low-salt diet after your discharge.

护士： 怀特先生，出院后您需要坚持低盐饮食。

Patient： Why?

病人： 为什么？

Nurse： The test findings of your kidney functions have just got normal. Too much salt will hurt your kidney，so you need to be careful about having salt or sodium.

护士： 您的肾功能检查指标刚刚恢复正常。过多的盐会伤肾。因此您吃含盐或含钠的食物必须小心。

Patient： What kind of food should I eat?

病人： 我应该吃什么东西呢？

Nurse： You should have light food，a lot of vegetables and fruits. Here is a list of foods you can and should not eat. And what's more，you'd better stay away from alcohol and give up smoking.

护士： 您的饮食要清淡，多吃蔬菜水果。这里是您能吃和不适合吃的食物清单。此外，最好少碰酒并戒烟。

Patient： I'll try my best to do all of these.

病人： 我尽量做到这一切。

Nurse： Here is an explanation of the medicines prescribed by the doctor for you to take home.

护士： 这是大夫给您开的带回家服用的药的说明。

Patient： I'll read it later.

病人： 我过一会儿看。

Nurse： Besides，there is another list on this paper. If you have any of the symptoms on this list，call your doctor.

护士： 此外，这张纸上还有一个清单。如果您出现清单上的任何症状，请打电话给您的医生。

Patient： I see.

病人： 我明白。

Nurse： Don't forget to inform your wife so that she can make necessary arrangements for you to leave the hospital. If you have any question don't hesitate to ask.

护士： 别忘了打电话通知您太太，以便她为您出院做必要的安排。如果您有其他问题，请随时问。

Patient： I will. Thank you.

病人： 我会的。谢谢。

Nurse： You're welcome.

护士： 不客气。

# 51. Leaving Hospital 离院

Nurse: Good morning, Mr. White. How are you feeling now?

护士：早上好，怀特先生。现在您感觉怎么样？

Patient: I feel all my trouble has gone.

病人：我感觉病全好了。

Nurse: Congratulations. Here is the discharge form for you. Has your wife arrived yet?

护士：恭喜您。这是您的出院通知。您太太到了吗？

（The patient's wife comes in.）

（病人的妻子进来。）

Patient: Here she is.

病人：她来了。

Wife: I'm going to the Admission Office to get the account closed.

妻子：我这就去住院处结账。

Nurse: Don't forget to have Mr. White's medical assurance card with you.

护士：别忘记带怀特先生的医疗保险卡。

Wife: Thank you for reminding me. See you in a little while.

妻子：多谢提醒。待会见。

Patient: When can I go back to work?

病人：我什么时候能恢复工作？

Nurse: Just take your time. You have to wait for some days.

护士：别心急。您还得等些日子。

Patient: How long?

病人：多长时间？

Nurse: It will take you at least one month's rest to recover completely. You need to ask your doctor's advice before you decide to return to your work. You must avoid mental stress and tiring work from now on.

护士：您至少需要休息一个月才会完全康复。您决定回去工作前得先问问医生的建议。从现在起，您必须避免精神紧张和太累的工作。

Patient: Can I go out for a walk?

病人：我能出去走动吗？

Nurse: You'd better stay at home most of time during the first week. You can go out more and more to walk around. After a week you can begin to do some light exercises.

护士： 第一周您最好大部分时间待在家里，逐渐增加出去四处走动的时间。一周后您可以开始做一些轻微运动。

Patient: I see.

病人： 我懂了。

Nurse: Here are your medicines. Have you read the explanation I gave you yesterday? Do you understand it?

护士： 这是您的药。我昨天给您的说明您看了。看得懂吗？

Patient: I've read it. It's very clear.

病人： 看了，写得很清楚。

Nurse: Before you take each of them, please check the name of the medicine and instruction label I put on. Let me show you. Take one tablet of this medic-cine three times a day before meals. And that one two tablets once daily in the morning. Drink plenty of water with medicines.

护士： 服用每种药前都要检查一下药名和我贴在上面的服用方法标签。我一个个指给您看。这个药每天三次，每次一片，饭前服，那个药每天早晨服两片。服药时多喝水。

Patient: I will remember. When will these tablets be finished?

病人： 我会记住的。这些药什么时候吃完？

Nurse: In seven days, and then you have to come to the outpatient department for a consultation and get another prescription.

护士： 七天吃完，然后您得来门诊复诊再开方取药。

Patient: I've got it. Thank you.

病人： 我明白了。谢谢。

(The patient's wife comes back.)

（病人的妻子回来了。）

Wife: I've got all settled. Can we leave now?

妻子： 我都办妥了。我们现在能走吗？

Nurse: Of course. By the way, have you returned the utensils you rented and got your deposit money back?

护士： 当然。对了，你们归还你们租的用具并取回押金了吗？

Wife: Yes, we have.

妻子： 是的，取回了。

Nurse: That's fine.

护士： 那就好。

Patient: I appreciate everything you and other staff here did for me。

病人： 真的很感激您和这里的其他医生、护士为我做的一切。

Nurse: It's our pleasure. We all hope you will recover in no time.

护士： 我们乐意为您服务。我们都祝您早日康复。

# Part Four

## Model Sentences for Overseas Nursing

## 海外护理典型语句篇

# Medical and Health History
# 病史和健康史

## 1. History of the Present Illness

## 现病史

**Onset　起病**

（1） When did it begin（start）?
什么时候开始的？

（2） Did it come on suddenly?
突然出现的吗？

（3） When did you first notice it?
你第一次注意到这种情况是什么时候？

（4） When did you last feel well?
你最近一次感觉良好是什么时候？

（5） Does this happen more at night or in the morning?
这种情况在夜间要比白天发生得多些吗？

（6） Is there a particular time of day that it happens more or less?
一天当中有没有某个时候这种情况要多些或是少些？

（7） When did Mary first complain?
玛丽一开始是什么时候有症状的？

（8） Mrs. Smith，can you think of how Mike got this?
史密斯夫人，你能想起麦克是怎么得的这个病吗？

（9） How long has this been a problem?
这个问题有多长时间了？

（10） How long has each episode last?
每次发作持续多久？

（11） Does it get better the more you move around?
你来回地多走些，这种情况是否要好一些？

（12） Was it better or worse during the summer?
在夏天里它要好些还是更糟？

（13） How long does it bother Johnny each time?
它每次要烦扰约翰尼多长时间？

(14) How many times have you had this before?
你以前发作过几次？

(15) How often does it happen, once a day, week, or month?
这种情况多久发生一次，一天一次，一周一次还是一个月一次？

(16) Has this happened before?
这种情况以前发生过吗？

(17) Is there a particular time of year when it happens more often?
一年当中有没有某个时候这种情况发生得多些？

(18) Is anyone else in the family also sick?
家里边还有其他人也病了吗？

**Provoke or palliates 诱因或缓解因素**

(19) Is it getting better or worse?
这种情况变好些了还是变差些了？

(20) Have you noticed anything that makes it worse?
你注意到有什么事情让这种症状加重了吗？

(21) What do you think provokes it?
你认为是什么诱发出这种症状的？

(22) What seems to make it better?
有什么看来能让这症状好些？

(23) Is there anything you do that makes it better?
有没有什么事你做的话能让这症状好些？

(24) What sort of things have you tried to make it better?
你试过做什么来让这症状好些？

(25) What have other doctors suggested that seemed to help?
其他医生的看来有帮助的建议是什么？

(26) What medicines have you been using (taking)?
你已经用(吃)过什么药？

(27) What sort of things have you done that make Frank feel better?
你做过的什么事能让弗兰克感觉好点？

**Region 范围**

(28) Where does it hurt?
哪儿痛？

(29) Tell me exactly where it hurts.
告诉我疼痛的准确部位。

(30) Show point to where it hurts.
给我看看哪痛。

(31) Will you point to where it hurt?
你指一下哪儿痛好吗？

(32) Mrs. Smith.Where does it seem to bother James?
史密斯女士，让詹姆斯不舒服的地方在哪儿？

（33）Tell me where is the Boo-Boo.
告诉我哪儿痛。

（34）Where is the ouch（or sting）?
痛得哎哟叫（或刺痛）的地方在哪儿？

（35）Your mother tells me that you have a tummy ache.Tell me where it hurt?
你妈妈告诉我你肚子痛，告诉我痛的地方在哪儿？

（36）Does the pain move?
疼痛有转移吗？

（37）Does the pain seem to move to your shoulder or back?"
疼痛是不是转移到你的肩膀或者后背去了？

**Severity 严重度**

（38）What does your pain feel like?
你的疼痛是什么样的感觉？

（39）What sorts of pain have you been having?
你的疼痛是哪种？

（40）Have you felt anything like this before?
以前你有没有过类似的感觉？

（41）Can you describe what it feels like?
你能描述一下它感觉像什么吗？

（42）How bad is it?
有多糟？

（43）Can you sleep?
你能睡觉吗？

（44）Would you explain how bad it is?
你能解释一下它有多糟吗？

（45）Does it keep you from working?
它是否让你无法工作？

（46）Is the problem getting worse，better，or staying the same?
这个问题变得更糟了，变好些了，还是保持原样？

（47）Does it wake Johnny from sleep?
它把约翰尼弄醒了吗？

（48）What does Andy complain of?
安迪在抱怨什么？

（49）Does it keep Cindy from playing?
它让辛迪不能玩耍吗？

（50）Has he been getting worse?
他变得更糟了吗？

# 2. Patient Profile
# 个人史

**General questions　一般问题**

(1) Now, can you tell me about yourself?
现在，你能跟我谈谈你自己吗？

(2) Tell me where you were born.
告诉我你在哪儿出生。

(3) What country does your family come from?
你们一家是从哪个国家来的？

(4) Are you married?
你结婚了吗？

(5) Do you have any children? How many?
你有小孩吗？有几个？

(6) Does your child have health problems?
你的孩子有健康问题吗？

(7) What is your occupation and where do you work?
你从事什么工作？在哪儿上班？

(8) Tell me about jobs you have had in the past.
告诉我你过去都干过些什么工作。

(9) How far did you go in school?
你的最终学历是什么？

(10) Do you practice a specific religion?
你信教吗？

(11) What do you do for fun or relaxation?
你干什么来找乐或放松？

(12) What type of exercise do you do, walking, biking, swimming, or jogging?
你做哪种运动？散步、骑自行车、游泳还是慢跑？

**Family history　家族史**

(13) Now, I would like so ask some questions about your family.
现在，我想问一些有关你的家族的问题。

(14) Tell me about your family.
告诉我有关你家族的事。

(15) Has anyone in your family been seriously ill?
你的家人中有人得过重病吗？

(16) Are your parents still living?
你的父母还在吗？

(17) Is your father/mother living? How is his/her health?
你的父亲 / 母亲还在吗？他 / 她的健康如何？

(18) How old was your father when he died?
你父亲去世的时候多少岁？

(19) What was the cause of death?
怎么死的？

(20) Do you have brothers or sisters?
你有兄弟姊妹吗？

(21) Do they have any medical problems?
他们有什么健康问题吗？

(22) Are there illnesses that seem to run in your family?
你的家族里看来有什么遗传病没有？

(23) I wonder if anyone in your family has anything like the symptoms you are having?
我想知道你的家人中有没有人有跟你类似的症状？

(24) Are you a single parent?
你是一个单亲家长吗？

(25) What is you father's name?
你父亲叫什么名字？

(26) How old is your mother?
你母亲年龄多大了？

(27) Are your parents your birth mother and father?
你的父母是你的亲生父母吗？

(28) How old was your grandfather when he died?
你祖父去世时多少岁？

(29) What did your grandmother die from?
你祖母得什么病去世的？

(30) Did your father have any chronic diseases or physical abnormalities?
你父亲有慢性病或肢体异常吗？

(31) Is there any condition which seems to run in your family?
你的家族中看来有什么遗传病吗？

(32) Is there any relative with a trait or condition that you have been told is genetic?
你的亲戚中有没有人有遗传性的特征或疾病？

(33) Is there any relative who has an unusual disease or who died of any unusual condition?
你有没有什么亲戚得了一种怪病或是谁死于怪病？

(34) Were your mother/father and their parents related by blood?
你的父母及他们的父母是近亲结婚吗？

（35）Where are your family from?
你的家族是从哪儿来的？

（36）What part of the world did your parents, grandparents, or great-grandparents come from?
你的父母，祖父母或曾祖父母来自世界的哪个地区？

# 3. Past Medical History

# 既往史

（1） Have you ever had any serious illness?
你得过什么重病没有？

（2） What past illness have you had?
过去得过什么病？

（3） Tell me about all other illnesses you have had.
告诉我你还得过的其他病症。

（4） Have you ever had surgery?
你以前做过手术吗？

（5） Have you ever been hospitalized?
你以前住过院吗？

（6） What have you been hospitalized for?
你为什么住院？

（7） Have you ever had any serious accidents or injuries?
你有没有遇到过什么严重的事故或外伤？

（8） Are you allergic to any drugs?
你对什么药物过敏吗？

（9） Do you have any allergies to food or pollen?
你对食物或花粉过敏吗？

（10） Have you had any allergic reactions to drugs?
你有过药物过敏反应吗？

（11） What immunizations have you had?
你以前做过些什么预防接种？

（12） Do you take any medicine or receive any other treatments?
你吃过什么药或接受过什么其他治疗没有？

（13） Are there any medicines that you cannot take?
有什么药你不能吃吗？

（14） What medications do you take?
你在吃什么药？

（15） Do you smoke?
你吸烟吗？

(16) How much do you smoke?
你的吸烟量是多少？

(17) How many packs a day do you smoke?
你一天吸几包烟？

(18) Do you smoke cigars or cigarettes?
你抽雪茄还是抽香烟？

(19) How long have you been smoking?
你抽烟有多久了？

(20) Does anyone in your family smoke?
你家里还有人抽烟吗？

(21) Do you think you can stop smoking?
你认为你能戒烟吗？

(22) Do you drink alcohol ?
你喝酒吗？

(23) How much alcohol do you drink in a day?
你一天喝多少酒？

(24) How often do you drink?
你多久喝一次酒？

(25) Do you drink more now than you did last year?
你现在喝得比去年喝得多吗？

(26) Are you using any street drugs?
你吸毒吗？

(27) Do you use drugs for recreational purposes?
你使用毒品来找乐吗？

(28) How often do you use them?
你多久用一次毒品？

(29) What kinds of drugs do you use?
你吸哪种毒品？

# 4. General Questions

# 一般问题

（1） Overall，how would you describe your health? Excellent，fair，good or poor?
总的来说，你怎么形容你的健康状态？很棒，可以，好还是差？

（2） Tell me about your health.
告诉我你的健康状态怎么样。

（3） Is there an activity that you would like to do but can't?
有没有一种你想做却不能做的运动？

（4） How many colds or infections did you have in the last six months?
最近 6 个月你得了几次感冒或感染？

（5） Do you tire easily?
你很容易疲劳吗？

（6） Have you noticed any changes in your energy level recently?
最近你有没有注意到你的体力有变化？

（7） How much do you weigh?
你的体重是多少？

（8） How much did you weigh last year?
你去年的体重是多少？

（9） Has your weight changed recently?
最近你的体重有没有变化？

（10）How is your appetite or eating habits? Have you noticed any change recently?
你的食欲或者饮食习惯如何？最近你注意到有什么变化没有？

（11）When did you last have a general checkup?
你最近一次做全身体检是什么时候？

（12）Do you have any problems of sleeping?
你有没有什么睡眠问题？

# 5. Skin, Hair, Nails

# 皮肤、毛发、指甲

（1） Do you have any skin problems, itching, sores, rashes, or lumps?
你的皮肤有什么问题没有，如瘙痒、疮、皮疹或者肿块？

（2） Have you noticed any changes in your skin?
你注意到你的皮肤有什么异常没有？

（3） Do you have hives or skin allergies?
你有没有荨麻疹或者皮肤过敏？

（4） Have you noticed any changes in the size or color of the warts or moles?
你注意到你的皮疣或痣的大小或颜色有什么变化没有？

（5） Have you noted any changes in your nails?
你发觉你的指甲有异常没有？

（6） Have you noticed any birthmarks?
你注意到你有什么胎记没有？

（7） Have you had shingles?
你得过带状疱疹吗？

（8） Have you noticed any hair loss?
你注意到有脱发没有？

（9） Have you noticed changes in your hair?
你注意到你的头发有什么异常没有？

# 6. Head and Neck

# 头和颈

（1） Have you ever had a head injury?
你受过头部外伤没有？

（2） Have you ever been unconscious from an injury?
你有过外伤所致的意识丧失吗？

（3） Have you ever had head or neck surgery?
你以前做过头部或颈部手术吗？

（4） Do you have headaches?
你头痛吗？

（5） How often do you have headaches?
你多久头痛一次？

（6） Where do you get he headaches?
你头的哪个地方感到痛？

（7） What do you think causes them?
你觉得引起它们（头痛）的原因是什么？

（8） Do you have migraines?
你有偏头痛吗？

（9） Do you have dizzy spells?
你有一阵阵的头晕吗？

（10） Do you have pain or stiffness in your neck?
你有颈项痛或颈项强直吗？

（11） Do you have swelling or lumps on your head or neck?
你的头或颈有肿胀或肿块吗？

（12） Do you have swollen glands?
你有肿胀的腺体吗？

# 7. Nose and Sinuses

# 鼻和鼻窦

（1） Do you have any trouble with your nose or sinuses?
你的鼻子或鼻窦有什么问题没有？

（2） Does your nose get stuffy or bleed?
你的鼻子是不是不通气或者有出血？

（3） Do you have a stuffy nose?
你鼻子不通气吗？

（4） Do you have nosebleeds?
你出鼻血了吗？

（5） Has there been any drainage from your nose?
你鼻子有什么分泌物流出来没有？

（6） What color?
什么颜色？

（7） Do you have hay fever?
你得过枯草热(花粉症)吗？

（8） Do you have a history of sinus infections，nasal fracture or nasal injuries?
你以前有没有鼻窦感染、鼻骨骨折或鼻外伤的病史？

（9） Have you noticed a change in your ability to smell?
你有没有注意到你的嗅觉能力有异常？

（10）Have you been told that you snore?
有人告诉你你打鼾吗？

（11）Does your child wake up because of a stuffy nose?
你的小孩有没有因为鼻子不通气而惊醒？

（12）Does your child snore?
你的小孩打鼾吗？

# 8. Mouth

# 口

（1） Do you have any problems with your mouth?
你的口腔有什么问题没有？

（2） Do you have sores in your mouth?
你有口腔炎吗？

（3） Does it hurt when you open your mouth?
你张嘴的时候痛吗？

（4） Do you notice bleeding from your gums?
你注意到有牙龈出血没有？

（5） Do your gums bleed when you brush your teeth?
你刷牙时有没有牙龈出血？

（6） Is your tongue sore?
你的舌头痛吗？

（7） Have you had a change in taste?
你的味觉有什么异常没有？

（8） Do you have problems chewing?
你咀嚼有问题吗？

（9） Is your mouth dry?
你口干吗？

（10） Do you worry about having bad breath?
你担心有口臭吗？

（11） Do you have an ulcer in your mouth?
你有口腔溃疡吗？

（12） Are your lips dry?
你的嘴唇干燥吗？

（13） Do you feel that your tongue is rough?
你觉得你的舌头粗糙吗？

# 9. Teeth

# 牙齿

（1） How are your teeth?
你的牙齿如何？

（2） When did you last see dentist?
你上次去看牙医是什么时候？

（3） Who is your dentist?
你的牙医是谁？

（4） How often do you see the dentist?
你多长时间去看一次牙医？

（5） How often do you brush your teeth?
你多长时间刷一次牙？

（6） Do you have cavities or any other dental problems?
你有牙龈洞或其他牙齿问题吗？

（7） Do you have toothaches?
你牙痛吗？

（8） Do you have any loose teeth?
你有松动的牙齿吗？

（9） Do you wear dentures?
你戴假牙吗？

（10） Do you gums bleed when you brush?
你刷牙的时候有牙龈出血吗？

（11） Do you have wisdom teeth?
你长智齿了吗？

# 10. Throat

# 咽喉

（1） Do you have sore throats?
你咽喉痛吗？

（2） How long have you been having sore throats?
你咽喉痛有多长时间？

（3） Did you take any medicine?
你吃过什么药没有？

（4） Do you get hoarse?
你有声音嘶哑吗？

（5） Do you overuse your voice such as in cheering or singing?
在诸如喝彩或唱歌的时候你的嗓子有没有过度使用？

（6） How long have you had hoarseness?
你声音嘶哑有多长时间了？

（7） Has your voice changed recently?
你的嗓音最近有变化吗？

（8） Do you have difficulty in swallowing?
你有吞咽困难吗？

（9） Do you have a rough throat?
你有一个粗哑的嗓子吗？

（10）Do you have swollen tonsils?
你的扁桃体肿吗？

（11）Do you feel itchiness or a tickle in your throat?
你觉得嗓子痒吗？

（12）Do you choke when you eat solid food?
在你吃较硬的食物时是否会哽住？

# 11. Eyes
# 眼

（1） Have you had any trouble（problems）with your eyes?
你得过什么眼病没有？

（2） When was the last time you had an eye examination?
你上次做眼睛检查是什么时候？

（3） Do you wear glasses or contact lenses?
你戴眼镜或隐形眼镜吗？

（4） Have there been any eye infections?
有眼部感染吗？

（5） Has there been any injury to your eyes?
你受过眼部外伤吗？

（6） Do you have any pain in your eyes?
你眼睛痛吗？

（7） Do you have double vision，or blurry vision?
你有复视或者视物模糊吗？

（8） Has there been any drainage from your eyes?
你的眼睛里有什么分泌物没有？

（9） Do your eyes itch?
你的眼睛痒吗？

（10） Do you have swelling around your eyes?
你的眼睛周围肿胀吗？

（11） Does light bother your eyes?
你的眼睛厌光吗？

（12） Do you have trouble seeing at night?
夜里你的视力有问题吗？

（13） Have you ever seen a dark spot in front of your eye?
你的眼前看见过黑点吗？

（14） Do you see spots or flashes of light?
你看到光点或闪光了吗？

（15） Are you near-sighted or far-sighted?
你近视还是远视？

（16）Does your child have any vision problems?
你的小孩有什么视力问题没有？

（17）Does your daughter/son squint?
你女儿/儿子斜视吗？

（18）Does your child wear glasses?
你的小孩戴眼镜吗？

# 12. Ears

# 耳

（1） How is your hearing?
你的听力如何？

（2） Do you have any trouble with your ears?
你的耳朵有什么问题吗？

（3） Do your ears ache?
你耳朵痛吗？

（4） Do you have discharge from your ears?
你耳朵里有分泌物吗？

（5） Does noise bother you?
噪声使你很烦吗？

（6） Are there loud noises at work?
工作的地方是否有很大的噪声？

（7） Do you hear ringing or buzzing in your ears?
你的耳朵里听见有铃声或嗡嗡声吗？

（8） How do you clean your ears?
你怎么清洁你的耳朵？

（9） Does your child have any difficulty hearing?
你小孩的听力有困难吗？

（10） Has your child had any ear infections?
你的小孩有耳部感染吗？

（11） Do you have any concerns about your child's hearing?
你对你的小孩的听力有什么担心没有？

（12） Has there been any drainage from his/her ears?
他/她的耳朵里是否有什么排出物？

（13） When was the last time your son had hearing test?
你儿子最近一次做听力测试是什么时候？

（14） Has your child's hearing ever been tested?
你的小孩做过听力测试吗？

# 13. Respiratory

# 呼吸系统

（1） Do you have trouble breathing?
你的呼吸有问题吗？

（2） Do you have a cough?
你咳吗？

（3） Do you ever wheeze?
你有过喘息吗？

（4） Have you ever had asthma?
你得过哮喘吗？

（5） Have you ever coughed up blood?
你咳出过血吗？

（6） How much sputum do you produce?
你咳的痰有多少？

（7） Have you had a fever or chills?
你有过发烧或寒战吗？

（8） How many stairs can you climb before you are out of breath?
你能上多少级楼梯而不至于上气不接下气？

（9） Have you ever had chest pain?
你有过胸痛吗？

（10）Have you ever had pneumonia or bronchitis?
你得过肺炎或者支气管炎吗？

（11）Can your child keep up with the other children when playing?
你的小孩在玩耍时能跟上其他小孩吗？

（12）Does your child ever complain of chest pain?
你的小孩抱怨过胸痛吗？

# 14. Cardiovascular

# 心血管系统

（1） Have you ever had chest pain or discomfort?
你曾有过胸痛或胸部不适感吗？

（2） Have you ever noticed fluttering, or pounding of your heart?
你曾注意到你有心率过快或心悸吗？

（3） Have you ever had a murmur?
你有过心脏杂音吗？

（4） Do you get short of breath?
你有气喘吗？

（5） Do you ever feel lightheaded?
你曾感觉头昏目眩吗？

（6） Have you ever fainted?
你晕倒过吗？

（7） Can you climb stairs without becoming short of breath?
你能毫不气喘地上楼梯吗？

（8） Have you ever needed to sit up to breathe at night?
你曾有过夜里需要端坐才能呼吸的情况吗？

（9） Have you noted any swelling in your legs or joints?
你有发觉你的腿或关节肿胀吗？

（10） Do you legs or arms get numb or cold?
你的腿或手臂有麻木或发冷吗？

（11） Do your legs hurt when you walk?
你走路时腿痛吗？

（12） Do you ever notice your child squatting?
你曾注意到你的小孩蹲在地上吗？

（13） Does your child ever become pale?
你的小孩曾有脸色苍白的情况吗？

# 15. Breasts

# 乳房

（1） When and how did you notice a lump in your breast?
你在什么时候以及如何注意到你的乳房有肿块的？

（2） When was the last time you had your breasts examined?
你上一次做乳房检查是什么时候？

（3） Have you ever had a mammogram?
你曾做过乳房 X 线检查吗？

（4） Are your breasts painful or tender?
你乳房痛吗？有压痛吗？

（5） Have you ever noticed any tenderness or lump in your underarm area?
你曾注意到你的腋下有压痛或肿块吗？

（6） Have you noticed any changes in your breasts such as size，nipple or shape?
你注意到你的乳房有什么变化吗，如大小、乳头或者外形？

（7） Have you noticed discharge from your nipples?
你注意到你的乳头有分泌物吗？

（8） What was the discharge like?
分泌物是什么样的？

（9） Have you ever noticed a lump in your breast?
你曾注意到你的乳房有肿块吗？

（10） Have you ever breast-fed?
你曾哺乳过（小孩）吗？

（11） Has anyone in your family had breast cancer?
你的家族里有没有人得乳腺癌？

# 16. Gastrointestinal

# 胃肠道

（1） Have you ever had any problems with your stomach or bowels?
你曾得过什么胃肠病吗？

（2） How is your appetite?
你的胃口如何？

（3） How is your digestion?
你的胃肠消化功能如何？

（4） Do you have heartburn?
你有胃灼热吗？

（5） Do you frequently belch?
你经常嗳气吗？

（6） Do you have a problem with hiccups?
你有打嗝的毛病吗？

（7） How often do you have a bowel movement?
你多久解一次大便？

（8） Is there difficulty with the bowel movement?
解大便有困难吗？

（9） Do you use laxatives? What kind? How often?
你用轻泻剂吗？哪一种？多久用一次？

（10） Have you ever had an ulcer?
你得过溃疡吗？

（11） Do you have a problem with nausea or vomiting?
你有恶心或者呕吐的毛病吗？

（12） Do you have a problem with diarrhea or constipation?
你有腹泻或便秘的毛病吗？

（13） Do you have hemorrhoids?
你有痔疮吗？

（14） Do you have pain or itching around your anus?
你肛周有疼痛或瘙痒吗？

（15） Have you ever had blood in your stools?
你曾有大便带血吗？

（16）Do you have abdominal pain?
你有腹痛吗？

（17）Where does your belly hurt?
你肚子哪儿痛？

（18）Has your child complained of abdominal pain?
你的孩子闹过腹痛吗？

（19）How often does your child move his bowels?
你的小孩多长时间解一次大便？

（20）How often does your child poop?
你的小孩多久解一次大便？

（21）Is it soft，runny，or hard?
是软的、稀的、还是硬的？

（22）Is there any blood or mucus in the stool?
大便里有血或者黏液吗？

（23）Is there difficulty with formulas or foods?
喂配方奶或者食物有困难吗？

# 17. Urinary Tract

# 泌尿道

（1） Have you had any trouble with your bladder?
你的膀胱有什么毛病没有？

（2） Do you have pain when you urinate?
你排尿时痛吗？

（3） Do you have trouble starting your stream?
你排尿开始时有困难吗？

（4） Has your stream gotten smaller recently?
你的尿线最近变细了吗？

（5） Do you feel that your bladder doesn't seem to empty?
小便后你是否感觉膀胱不像排空了？

（6） Do you dribble urine?
你有尿滴沥吗？

（7） Have you ever had blood or pus in your urine?
你曾有小便带血或带脓吗？

（8） What is the color of your urine？Is it red or coffee-like?
你的尿是什么颜色的？红的还是咖啡样？

（9） Do you wake up often in the middle of the night to urinate?
你经常半夜起来小便吗？

（10） Have you been circumcised?
你做过包皮环切术吗？

（11） Have you ever had back pain?
你有过腰痛吗？

（12） Do you think you urinate too much（too little）?
你认为你的小便量太多了（太少了）吗？

（13） Do you have a problem controlling your urine?
你控制排尿有问题吗？

（14） Does your wee-wee hurt?
你小便时痛吗？

（15） Is your child toilet trained?
你的小孩受过上厕所的训练吗？

(16) Does your child have problems with urination?
你的小孩解小便有问题吗？

(17) Does your child wet the bed?
你的小孩尿床吗？

# 18. Muscular and Skeletal System

# 肌肉和骨骼系统

（1） Do your muscles（joints）ache?
你的肌肉（关节）痛吗？

（2） Have you ever had a fracture?
你曾经骨折过吗？

（3） Have you had dislocations of the bone or joint?
你有过骨或关节脱位吗？

（4） Do you have muscle cramps?
你有过肌肉抽筋吗？

（5） Do you have muscle twitching or weakness?
你有肌肉痉挛或肌力低下吗？

（6） Have you ever had joint swelling?
你曾经有过关节肿胀吗？

（7） Are your joints painful or stiff?
你的关节痛或关节强直吗？

（8） Do you have back pain?
你有腰痛吗？

（9） Do you have difficulty walking，bending or moving?
你行走、弯腰或者移动有困难吗？

（10） Have you noticed any weakness in your muscle?
你注意到你有肌力低下吗？

（11） Has your child had any injuries of muscles or bones?
你的小孩受过肌肉或者骨的外伤吗？

（12） Does your child have any spinal misalignments?
你的小孩有脊柱弯曲吗？

# 19. Nervous System

# 神经系统

（1） Have you ever been paralyzed?
你曾瘫痪过吗？

（2） Have you ever lost feeling in a part of your body? In your arm? Fingers? Leg? Foot?
你有没有过身体的某一部分失去感觉的情况？手臂？手指？腿？

（3） Do you ever feel lightheaded?
你曾感到头昏目眩吗？

（4） Do you have numbness or tingling sensations?
你有麻木感或麻刺感吗？

（5） How is your coordination and balance?
你的运动协调和平衡如何？

（6） Do you have any trouble walking?
你行走有问题吗？

（7） Did you feel like you are going to faint?
你觉得你快要昏过去了吗？

（8） Have you ever passed out?
你曾有过不省人事吗？

（9） Have you ever had any seizures or spells?
你曾有过癫痫发作吗？

（10） Have you ever had a problem speaking?
你曾有过言语问题吗？

（11） Have you ever had a problem with memory?
你曾有记忆问题吗？

（12） Have you noticed a change in vision? Taste? Smell?
你注意到有视觉异常？味觉异常？嗅觉异常吗？

（13） Have you noticed hand tremors?
你注意到有手震颤吗？

# 20. Endocrine System

# 内分泌系统

（1） Have you had any problems in the endocrine system such as thyroid?
你的内分泌系统有什么毛病没有？如甲状腺？

（2） When did you recognize the enlargement of your thyroid gland?
你什么时候意识到你的甲状腺增大了？

（3） How is your appetite? Has it increased，decreased，or stayed about the same?
你的胃口如何？增加了，减少了，还是保持原样？

（4） Has your weight changed recently?
最近你的体重有变化吗？

（5） Do you sweat a lot?
你出很多汗吗？

（6） Do your hands tremble or shake?
你的双手有震颤或抖动吗？

（7） Have you noticed excessive urination?
你注意到尿量过多了吗？

（8） Do you prefer hot or cold temperatures?
你更喜欢炎热的气候还是更喜欢寒冷的气候？

（9） Do you have a problem tolerating cold or heat?
你对寒冷或炎热的抵抗力有问题吗？

（10） Have you noticed a change in your hair texture or quantity?
你注意到你头发的质地或数量有变化吗？

（11） Have you noticed a change in your skin color?
你注意到你的肤色有变化吗？

（12） Has your skin become darker recently?
你的皮肤最近变黑些了吗？

（13） Have you noticed a change in your sex drive?
你注意到你的性欲有变化吗？

# 21. Female Reproductive System

# 女性生殖系统

**Menstruation　月经**

（1） Are your menstrual periods regular?
你的月经期有规律吗？

（2） What was the date of your last menstrual period?
你上一次月经是哪一天？

（3） At what age did you start having periods?
你初潮时是在什么年龄？

（4） How often do your periods come?
你多久来一次月经？

（5） How many days does your period last?
你的月经期持续几天？

（6） What is your usual flow，light，medium，or heavy?
通常你的月经量有多少？少、中等还是多？

（7） Do you have pain or cramps before or during your period?
在你经前或月经期你有疼痛或痉挛吗？

（8） Do they interfere with daily activities?
它们妨碍日常活动吗？

（9） How do you treat them?
你怎么对付它们？

（10） Do you have other symptoms with your periods such as bloating or moodiness?
在月经期你还有其他症状吗，如胃气胀或易怒？

（11） Have your periods slowed down?
你的月经周期慢下来了吗？

（12） Do you have spotting between periods?
你在月经期之间有点滴出血吗？

**Pregnancy　妊娠**

（13） Have you ever been pregnant?
你曾经怀过孕吗？

（14） How many times have you been pregnant?
你怀过几次孕？

（15）Have you had an abortion or miscarriage?
你有过人工流产或自然流产吗？

（16）How many times have you had miscarriage?
你有过几次自然流产？

（17）How many babies have you had?
你有几个小孩？

（18）Would you describe each pregnancy? How many months? Any complications?
请你描述每次怀孕的情况好吗？几个月、有并发症吗？分娩情况？

（19）Labor and delivery? Baby's sex and weight，Health of the baby?
分娩情况？孩子的性别和体重、孩子的健康情况？

**Menopause 绝经期**

（20）Do you think you are going through menopause?
你认为你正在经历绝经期吗？

（21）What are your symptoms? Hot flashes，palpitations，headaches，sweats，and/or mood swings?
你的症状是什么？热潮红、心悸、头痛、出汗和 / 或情绪易变？

（22）Do you have sleep problems or memory problems?
你有睡眠或记忆方面的问题吗？

（23）Do you have a discomfort during intercourse?
你在性交时感到不适吗？

（24）Do you take hormone replacement therapy?
你是否采取了激素替代治疗？

（25）Do you know the dose of the hormone?
你知道激素的剂量吗？

（26）How long have you been taking it?
你已经吃了多长时间了？

（27）When was the last time you had a gynecologic check-up?
你上次妇科检查是什么时候？

**Discharge 分泌物**

（28）Do you have any unusual vaginal discharge?
你有什么不正常的阴道分泌物没有？

（29）What color is it?
是什么颜色的？

（30）Does it have an odor?
有气味吗？

（31）Do you have itching?
你痒吗？

（32）Do you have pain with intercourse?
你性交时痛吗？

**Sex life 性生活**

（33）Are you in relationship involving sex?

你（和别人）有性关系吗？

（34）Are your partners men，women or both?
你的性伴侣是男性、女性还是两者都有？

（35）Are you satisfied with your sex life?
你对你的性生活满意吗？

（36）Is your partner satisfied with his/her sex life?
你的性伴侣对他 / 她的性生活满意吗？

（37）What type of contraception do you use?
你采用哪种避孕方式？

（38）Have you ever had difficulty becoming pregnant?
你有过不孕的问题吗？

（39）Have you ever had gonorrhea，herpes，chlamydia，veneral warts，or syphilis?
你曾得过淋病、疱疹、衣原体感染、性病疣或者梅毒吗？

（40）When did you have your examinations done?
你是什么时候完成检查的？

（41）How was treated?
怎么治的？

（42）Were there complications？
有并发症吗？

（43）Have you ever been tested for HIV?
你做过 HIV 检查吗？

# 22. Male Reproductive System

# 男性生殖系统

（1） Do you have any pain in your scrotum?
你的阴囊痛吗？

（2） Have you noticed any lump or swelling in your scrotum?
你注意到你的阴囊有什么肿块或肿胀没有？

（3） Have you noticed any changes in the size of your scrotum?
你注意到你的阴囊大小有改变吗？

（4） Do you have pain when you urinate?
你小便时痛吗？

（5） Do you have any trouble having an erection?
你勃起有困难吗？

（6） Are you in a relationship involving sex now?
现在，你（和别人）有性关系吗？

（7） Are your partners men，women or both?
你的性伴侣是男性、女性还是两者都有？

（8） Are you satisfied with your sex life?
你对你的性生活满意吗？

（9） Is your partner satisfied with his/her sex life?
你的性伴侣对他/她的性生活满意吗？

（10） Have you ever had gonorrhea，herpes，chlamydia，veneral warts or syphilis?
你曾得过淋病、疱疹、衣原体感染、性病疣或梅毒吗？

（11） When did you have it?
什么时候得的？

（12） How was it treated?
怎么治的？

（13） Were there complications?
有并发症吗？

# 23. Immune and Hemopoietic System

# 免疫和血液系统

（1） Do you have shortness of breath?
你有呼吸急促吗？

（2） Do you have trouble breathing?
你有呼吸困难吗？

（3） Have you ever had a bleeding problem?
你曾有过出血问题吗？

（4） Do you bruise easily?
你是否很容易碰伤？

（5） Do you bleed easily?
你是否很容易出血？

（6） Have you ever bled for a long time after having a tooth pulled?
你曾有过拔牙后长时间出血的情况吗？

（7） Have you had frequent nose bleeding?
你以前是否经常鼻出血？

（8） Do you take aspirin?
你吃阿司匹林吗？

（9） Is there anyone in your family who has a bleeding problem?
你的家族中有人有出血问题吗？

（10） Have you ever had a blood transfusion?
你曾输过血吗？

（11） Do you have a problem with hives or itching?
你有荨麻疹或瘙痒的毛病吗？

（12） Do you have a problem with chronic nasal stuffiness or drainage?
你有长期鼻不通气或流鼻涕的毛病吗？

（13） Do you become easily fatigued?
你是否变得很容易疲惫？

# 24. Cognition

# 认知

**Cognition, Orientation, Mood　认知、定向力、情绪**

（1） What is you mane?
你叫什么名字？

（2） What is your father name?
你父亲叫什么名字？

（3） Tell me who I am ?
告诉我我是谁？

（4） What is your occupation?
你的职业是什么？

（5） What season is it?
现在是什么季节？

（6） What month is it?
现在是几月？

（7） Where are you now?
你现在在哪儿？

（8） Where do you live?
你住哪儿？

（9） How do you feel today?
你今天感觉如何？

（10） How do you usually feel?
你平常感觉如何？

（11） Do you have a problem reading?
你有阅读问题吗？

（12） Do you have a problem hearing?
你有听觉问题吗？

**Memory　记忆**

（13） Where were you born?

你在哪儿出生的？

（14）Where did you go to grade school?
你在哪儿上小学？

（15）What was your first job?
你最初是干什么工作的？

（16）When were you married?
你什么时候结婚的？

（17）Do you live with anyone?
你和其他人住一块儿吗？

（18）Do you have any grandchildren?
你有孙儿吗？

（19）What are the names of your grandchildren?
你的孙儿叫什么名字？

（20）When was the last time you went to the doctor?
你上次看医生是什么时候？

# 25. Activity and Exercise

# 活动和运动

（1） Would you describe your usual daily activities including occupation，exercise，leisure activities and care giving responsibilities?
请你描述一下你的日常活动，包括职业、运动方式、休闲活动以及要尽职尽责的操心事。

（2） Do you have any difficulty in walking，dressing，grooming，oral hygiene，bathing yourself, or toileting?
你在行走、穿衣打扮、口腔卫生、洗澡、上厕所这些方面有困难吗？

（3） Are you able to walk without a cane?
没有手杖你能行走吗？

（4） Are you able to climb stairs?
你能上楼梯吗？

（5） What sort of exercise do you do?
你做哪种运动？

（6） Do you have difficulty breathing?
你有呼吸困难吗？

（7） Do you have a problem with feeling very wear or tired?
你有没有感觉非常虚弱或疲惫等问题？

（8） Does pain interfere with your movement?
疼痛妨碍你运动了吗？

（9） Do you use a walker，wheelchair or cane?
你用助步器、轮椅或手杖吗？

（10） Is there an activity that you wish you could do?
有没有一种活动是你希望你能做的？

# 26. Self-care

# 自理

（1） Do you have difficulty（problems）with swallowing?
你吞咽有困难（问题）吗？

（2） Do you have difficulty with chewing?
你咀嚼有困难吗？

（3） Do you have difficulty with using utensils and cutting food?
你使用器具及切食物有困难吗？

（4） Do you have difficulty with drinking from a cup?
你从杯子里喝水有困难吗？

（5） Do you have difficulty with selecting food?
你选择食物有困难吗？

（6） Do you have difficulty with seeing the food ?
你看食物有困难吗？

（7） Do you have difficulty with opening cans，cartons or boxes?
你开罐头，开盒子或开箱子有困难吗？

（8） Are you able to prepare food?
你能准备食物吗？

（9） Are you able to go to to market to buy food?
你能去超市买食物吗？

※ ※ ※

（10）Do you have difficulty（problems）with undressing to bathe?
你脱衣服洗澡有困难吗？

（11）Do you have difficulty with adjusting the water temperature?
你调水温有困难吗？

（12）Do you have difficulty with using soap or towels?
你用肥皂或毛巾有困难吗？

（13）Do you have difficulty with washing body parts?
你擦洗身体有困难吗？

（14）Are you able to dress and groom without help?
你能在没有帮助的情况下穿衣打扮吗？

（15）Do you have difficulty with putting on or taking off clothing?

你穿衣服或脱衣服有困难吗？

(16) Do you have difficulty with washing and styling hair?
你洗头发和做发型有困难吗？

(17) Do you have difficulty with shaving?
你刮脸有困难吗？

(18) Do you have difficulty with using deodorant?
你使用除臭剂有困难吗？

(19) Do you have difficulty with trimming nails?
你修指甲有困难吗？

(20) Do you have difficulty with brushing your teeth?
你刷牙有困难吗？

(21) Do you have difficulty with plugging in an electric cord?
你插插头有困难吗？

(22) Do you have difficulty with fastening clothing?
你扣衣服有困难吗？

※ ※ ※

(23) Do you have difficulty (problems) with getting to the toilet and undressing?
你到卫生间并脱衣服有困难（问题）吗？

(24) Do you have difficult with sitting on the toilet?
你坐上马桶有困难吗？

(25) Do you have difficulty with rising form the toilet?
你从马桶上起来有困难吗？

(26) Do you have difficult with cleaning yourself?
你（在大小便后）把自己擦干净有困难吗？

(27) Do you have difficulty with flushing the toilet?
你冲马桶有困难吗？

(28) Do you have difficulty with redressing?
你重新穿起衣服有困难吗？

(29) Do you have difficulty with performing hygiene (washing hand)?
你保持卫生（洗手）有困难吗？

(30) Do you have difficulty with using a tampon and/or sanitary napkin?
你使用月经棉条和/或做卫生棉有困难吗？

※ ※ ※

(31) Do you have difficulty with dialing?
你拨号有困难吗？

(32) Do you have problems answering the telephone?
你接电话有问题吗？

(33) Do you have difficulty with talking or hearing?
你说或者听有困难吗？

※ ※ ※

（34）Are you able to drive?
你能开车吗？

（35）Can you use public transportation without difficulty?
你乘坐公共交通工具没问题吧？

※ ※ ※

（36）Do you have problems with availability of a washer?
你用洗衣机有困难吗？

（37）Do you have difficulty with washing and/or ironing?
你洗衣服和 / 或熨衣服有困难吗？

（38）Do you have difficulty with putting laundry away?
你把洗好的衣服放好有困难吗？

※ ※ ※

（39）Can you do food shopping?
你能买食物吗？

（40）Do you have problems selecting foods?
你选食物有困难吗？

（41）Can you cook for yourself?
你能给自己做吃的吗？

（42）Do you have problems cleaning up?
你(吃完以后)清扫干净有问题吗？

※ ※ ※

（43）Do you remember to take your medicine?
你记得吃药吗？

（44）Can you open the bottle and take it?
你能打开药瓶并把药吃了吗？

※ ※ ※

（45）Is it difficult to write checks for paying bills?
开支票付账是否有困难？

（46）Do you have problems handling cash transactions?
你处理现金交易是否有问题？

# 27. Sleep and Rest

# 睡眠和休息

（1） Tell me about your sleeping habits.
告诉我你的睡眠习惯？

（2） What time do you usually go to bed?
你一般什么时候睡觉？

（3） Do you have problems getting to sleep?
你入睡有问题吗？

（4） How long does it take to fall asleep?
睡着要花多长时间？

（5） How often do you wake up in the night?
你夜里醒几次？

（6） What do you do when you wake up in the night?
夜里醒了以后你怎么办？

（7） Do you take sleeping pills?
你吃安眠药吗？

（8） What time do you usually wake up?
你一般什么时候醒？

（9） When you wake up do you feel rested?
早晨睡醒后你觉得休息好了吗？

（10） What interferes with your sleep: noise，the need to urinate，stress or fear?
妨碍你睡觉的是什么？噪音、尿意、紧张还是恐惧？

（11） Does something help you go to sleep: pills，food，drink，or special position?
有什么能帮助你入睡吗？药、食物、饮料还是特定的体位？

（12） Do you take a nap during the day?
白天你打盹吗？

（13） When do you take a nap?
你什么时候打盹？

（14） How long do you nap?
你打盹有多长时间？

# 28. Nutrition

# 营养

（1） How is your appetite?
你的食欲如何？

（2） Has there been a change in your appetite?
你的食欲有变化吗？

（3） Describe what you usually eat and drink for breakfast（lunch，dinner，snacks）.
说说你平常的早餐（午餐、晚餐、零食）饮食？

（4） Has your weight changed in the last year?
过去一年你的体重有变化吗？”

（5） Do you think you eat a well-balanced diet?
你认为你的饮食均衡吗？

（6） What foods don't you like to eat?
什么食物你不爱吃？

（7） How often do you eat fast foods each week?
每周你吃几次快餐？

（8） Are there foods that don't agree with you?
有没有不适合你的食物？

（9） Which foods are they?
是哪些食物？

（10） Do you have problems with nausea（vomiting，indigestion）?
您有恶心（呕吐、消化不良）的问题吗？

（11） Do you have trouble chewing?
你咀嚼有困难吗？

（12） Do you have trouble swallowing?
你吞咽有困难吗？

# 29. Elimination

# 排泄

（1） Do you have any trouble with urinating?
你排尿有什么困难没有？

（2） Do you have pain or burning when you urinate?
你在排尿时有疼痛或烧灼感吗？

（3） Do you have trouble urinating?
你有排尿困难吗？

（4） Do you have trouble controlling your urine?
你对排尿的控制有困难吗？

（5） Do you sometimes have trouble reaching the bathroom in time?
有时你是否在及时到卫生间方面有困难？

（6） Do you notice any delay in starting to pass urine?
你注意到在排尿开始时有延迟吗？

（7） How many times do you get up to urinate at night?
夜里你要起来排几次尿？

（8） Has your fluid intake changed recently?
最近你的液体摄入量有变化吗？

（9） Have you noticed any decrease in the size of your stream?
你注意到你的尿线变细了吗？

（10）Do you have any dribbling at the end of urination?
你排完尿时有尿滴沥吗？

（11）Do you know when you have to urinate?
你知道什么时候该排尿吗？

※ ※ ※

（12）How often do you have a bowel movement?
你多久解一次大便？

（13）Have you noticed any changes in your bowel habits?
你注意到你的排便习惯有改变吗？

（14）Has there been a change in your bowels?
你的大便有异常吗？

（15）Do you have difficulty with passage of stools?

你解大便有困难吗？

（16）Do you have a problem with constipation?
你有便秘的毛病吗？

（17）Do you use laxatives?
你用泻药吗？

（18）What kind of laxatives do you use?
你用哪种泻药？

（19）How often do you use laxatives?
你多久用一次泻药？

（20）Do you use enemas?
你用灌肠剂吗？

（21）What kind of enema do you use?
你用哪种灌肠剂？

（22）How often do you use enemas?
你多久用一次灌肠剂？

（23）Do you have a problems with diarrhea?
你有腹泻的毛病吗？

（24）Do you have any problems with controlling your bowels?
你控制排便有问题吗？

（25）Do you feel that there is stool remaining in the rectum?
你感觉到你的直肠里还残留有大便吗？

# 30. Sexuality
# 性功能

（1） Are you presently in a relationship involving sex?
你现在有性关系吗？

（2） Has your health problem affected your ability to function sexually?
你的健康问题影响你的性功能了吗？

（3） Please describe what has changed.
请说明一下有什么改变。

（4） Do you have erection problems?
你有勃起问题吗？

（5） Do you have ejaculation problems?
你有射精方面的问题吗？

（6） Do you have painful intercourse?
你有性交痛吗？

（7） Do you have difficulty attaining an orgasm?
你是否在达到高潮方面有困难？

（8） Do you have an inability to have an orgasm?
你不能达到高潮吗？

（9） Are you satisfied with the present situation?
你对目前的状况满意吗？

（10）Is your partner satisfied with the present situation?
你的性伴侣对目前的状况满意吗？

（11）Do you have sex with men，women or both?
你和男人、女人或两者有性行为吗？

（12）Do you have any discomfort during sexual activity?
在性事中你有什么不适吗？

（13）What type of contraception do you use?
你采取哪种避孕方式？

（14）Have you had any sexual contact with someone who has AIDS，chlamydia，venereal warts，syphilis，gonorrhea，or herpes?
你和艾滋病、衣原体感染、性病疣、梅毒、淋病、疱疹患者有性接触吗？

（15）When was it?
什么时候？

（16）How were you treated?
你是怎么治的？

# 31. Relationships

# 人际关系

(1) Do you live alone?
你一个人住吗？

(2) Whom do you live with?
你和谁住在一起？

(3) What is the health status of each person in your home?
你的家庭成员的健康状况如何？

(4) Do you take care of someone who does not live with you?
你是否要照顾一个不和你住在一起的人？

(5) To whom do you turn for help in time of need?
有必要的时候你会寻求谁的帮助？

(6) In the last year have you been hit, kicked or otherwise physically hurt by someone?
过去一年你有没有被人打过(踢过或受过其他的身体伤害)？

(7) Are you afraid of someone you know?
你害怕某个你认识的人吗？

(8) Is your family having any problems?
你的家庭有问题吗？

(9) Do you have children under eighteen years old?
你有 18 岁以下的小孩吗？

(10) What grade is your child in at school?
你的孩子在学校上几级年级了？

(11) How is he/she doing in at school?
他 / 她在学校怎么样？

(12) When your children misbehaves, how do you discipline them?
当你的孩子做错事的时候你怎么惩罚他们？

# 32. Coping

# 应对

（1） Has there been a change in your life in the past year：school，marital status，deaths，job，or health?
去年你的生活有改变吗？学习、婚姻状况、(亲属的)死亡、工作或者健康？

（2） How do you feel now?
你现在感觉怎么样？

（3） What do you do when you have too much stress?
当你压力太大的时候你怎么办？

（4） When did you have your last drink?
你上次喝酒是什么时候？

（5） How much did you drink on that day?
那天你喝了多少酒？

（6） On how many days out of the last thirty day did you consume alcohol?
过去 30 天里有多少天你喝了酒？

（7） What is your average daily intake of alcohol?
你平均一天喝多少酒？

（8） What is the most you have ever drank?
你最多喝过多少酒？

（9） Have you ever thought you should cut down your drinking?
你有没有想过你应该少喝酒？

（10） Have you ever been annoyed by criticism of your drinking?
你曾经因为别人批评你喝酒而苦恼吗？

（11） Have you ever felt guilty about your drinking?
你曾经因为喝酒而感到内疚吗？

（12） Do you drink in the morning(i.e. eye-opener)?
你早晨喝酒吗(也就是一睁眼就喝酒的人)？

（13） What kind of street drugs do you take?
你用哪种毒品？

（14） Do you use marijuana?
你抽大麻吗？

（15） Have you ever thought life is not worth living?

你有没有觉得生活不值得活下去？

（16）Have you ever thought about harming yourself？

你有没有想过伤害自己？

（17）How would you harm yourself？

你怎么伤害你自己？

# 33. Health Maintenance

# 健康维持

（1） How would you describe your health? Excellent，fair，good or poor?
你怎么形容你的健康状况？很棒、可以、好还是差？

（2） How would you describe your health at this time?
你怎么形容你现时的健康状况？

（3） What do you do to keep healthy?
你怎么保持健康？

（4） When was your most recent（or last）dental examination?
你最近一次做口腔检查是什么时候？

（5） When was your most recent（or last）eye exam?
你最近一次做眼科检查是什么时候？

（6） When was your most recent（or last）gynecologic exam?（female）
你最近一次做妇科检查是什么时候？（对女性）

（7） When was your most recent（or last）mammography done?（female）
你最近一次做乳房 X 射线造影检查是什么时候？（对女性）

（8） When was your most recent（or last）prostate screening?（male）
你最近一次做前列腺检查是什么时候？（对男性）

（9） When was your last fecal occult blood test done?
你最近一次做大便隐血试验是什么时候？

（10） When was your blood cholesterol level checked most recently?
你最近一次查血胆固醇水平是什么时候？

（11） When was your last tetanus（influenza）vaccination done?
你最近一次打破伤风（流感）疫苗是什么时候？

（12） Have you had a Hepatitis B（Hepatitis A）vaccine?
你打过乙肝（甲肝）疫苗吗？

（13） What diseases run in your family? Diabetes，cancer，hypertension，or heart disease?
你家族中都有哪些病在传播？糖尿病、癌、高血压、还是心脏病？

（14） What can you do to prevent the diseases in yourself: exercise，nutrition，self-breast exam，weight control，self-testicular exam?
为了防止你自己得这些病，你会怎么做？锻炼、（加强）营养、乳房自我检查、控制体重、睾丸自我检查？

(15) What kind of exercise do you do? How often?
你做哪种运动？多久做一次？

(16) How frequently do you have bowel irregularity?
你多久出现一次大便不规律？

(17) How frequently do you have respiratory infections?
你多久得一次呼吸道感染？

(18) How frequently do you have influenza?
你多久得一次流感？

(19) How frequently do you have skin rashes?
你多久发一次皮疹？

(20) What immunizations has your child had?
你的小孩做过哪些预防接种？

# 34. Pain

# 疼痛

**Type of pain　疼痛的类型**

(1) Now, tell me about your pain.
现在，告诉我疼痛的情况。

(2) What kind of pain do you have?
你是哪种痛？

(3) How would you describe the pain?
你怎么形容你的疼痛？

(4) Could you describe the pain?
你能描述一下疼痛的情况吗？

(5) Is the pain burning, sticking, or cramping in nature?
这个疼痛从类型上来说是灼痛，刺痛还是痉挛性痛？

(6) Where is your pain?
你哪儿痛？

(7) Point to where your pain is.
指一下你哪儿痛。

(8) Where is the boo-boo (ouch)? (to a young child)
哪儿痛啊？(对小孩)

**Pain: onset, duration and frequency　疼痛：起病、持续时间和频度**

(9) When did it begin?
什么时候开始(痛)的？

(10) When does it become painful?
什么时候变痛的？

(11) How long does it last?
它(经常)持续多久？

(12) How long did it last?
它持续了多久？

(13) How often does it come?

多久发作一次？

（14）Does it come regularly?
它（疼痛）定期发作吗？

（15）Does the pain come once a day，once an hour，or once every ten minutes?
疼痛是每天发作一次，每小时一次还是每十分钟一次？

（16）When did you first notice this problem?
你第一次注意到这个问题是什么时候？

（17）How long have you had this pain?
你有这种疼痛多长时间了？

（18）Do you feel ouch all the time?（to a young child）
你一直觉得痛吗？（对小孩）

**Pain: severity　疼痛：严重程度**

（19）How bad is you pain?
你的疼痛有多厉害？

（20）Would you rate the intensity of pain on a scale of one to ten，with ten being the most severe pain?
如果把疼痛强度分为1到10级，10级是最严重的痛，你怎么评估你的疼痛？

（21）How have you tried to relieve this pain?
你如何来缓解这个疼痛？

（22）Have you taken anything for the pain?
你为了治这个疼痛吃过什么药没有？

（23）Does deep breath affect the pain?
深呼吸会影响疼痛吗？

（24）What do you do to relieve the pain?
为了缓解疼痛你怎么做？

（25）Does the pain tingle?
这个疼痛让你有麻刺感吗？

（26）What seems to aggravate your pain?
有什么看来会加剧你的疼痛？

# 35. Specific Location of Pain

# 特殊部位的疼痛

**Chest pain　胸痛**

（1）Tell me about your chest pain. What type of pain did（do）you have?
告诉我你胸痛的情况。你是哪种痛？

（2）How long did the chest pain last?
胸痛持续了多长时间？

（3）When did you first notice it?
你第一次注意到它是什么时候？

（4）Has anyone in your family had a heart attack?
你的家族里有人曾有过心脏病发作吗？

（5）Have you ever had heart disease?
你得过心脏病吗？

（6）Have you noticed fluttering or pounding of your heart?
你注意到你有心跳过快或心悸吗？

（7）Have you had shortness of breath?
你有过呼吸急促的情况吗？

（8）Did the pain radiate to your rum，abdomen，shoulder，or jaw?
疼痛是放射到你的手臂、腹部、肩还是下颌？

（9）Do Wu have discomfort or an unpleasant feeling in your chest?
你的胸部有不适感或不快感吗？

（10）Did you have palpitations or sweating?
你有心悸或发汗吗？

（11）What makes the pain worse：eating，deep breathing，moving，exercise，coughing?
什么使疼痛恶化了？进食、深呼吸、运动、锻炼还是咳嗽？

**Headache　头痛**

（12）Tell me when these headaches started.
告诉我这些头痛是什么时候开始的。

（13）How often do you get these headaches?
这些头痛多久发作一次？

（14）Where does it hurt?
哪儿痛？

（15）What does the headache feel like?
头痛的感觉像什么？

（16）Do you have a fever，difficulty walking or difficulty seeing when you have a headache?
当你头痛的时候你有发热、行走障碍或视力障碍吗？

（17）Do you have nausea when you have these headaches?
当你头痛的时候会恶心吗？

（18）Do these headaches wake you up at night?
这些头痛夜里会把你弄醒吗？

（19）Can you think of anything that might trigger these headaches?
你能想想有什么事可能会引发这些头痛吗？

（20）Are you ever dizzy?
你曾头晕过吗？

（21）Do you have blackout?
你有过一时性黑蒙吗？

（22）Where are your headaches? Forehead，temples，or all over?
你的头痛是在哪个部位？前额、颞部还是所有地方？

（23）Is it one-sided or bilateral?
它是一侧痛还是双侧痛？

（24）Does the pain occur at the same time every day?
疼痛是否每天都在同一时间发作？

（25）Does coughing，sneezing or changing position affect the headache?
咳嗽、喷嚏或改变体位会影响头痛吗？

（26）Do certain foods cause a headache? Chocolate? Cheese? Red wine?
有没有某种食物会引起头痛？巧克力？乳酪？红葡萄酒？

**Arm or leg pain　手臂或腿痛**

（27）Do you have any problems with your hands，arms，legs，feet or joints?
你的手、手臂、腿、脚或者关节有什么问题没有？

（28）Have you had broken bones in your hands，arms，legs，or feet?
你的手、手臂、腿或脚骨折过吗？

（29）Do you have leg cramps that wake you up during the night?
你有没有夜里因为大腿痛性痉挛而惊醒？

（30）Do you have varicose veins in your legs?
你的双腿有没有静脉曲张？

（31）Do your fingers get numb，painful or change color when exposed to cold?
你的手指遇到寒冷的时候有没有变得麻木、疼痛或者变色？

（32）Does the pain interfere with your daily life?
疼痛妨碍你的日常生活了吗？

（33）Do you have problems with coordination?
你的运动协调有问题吗？

（34）Do you have pain in your buttocks?

你的臀部有疼痛吗？

（35）Do your legs or hands swell?
你的腿或手肿吗？

（36）Does he walk with a limp?
他走起路来一瘸一拐吗？

（37）Does she have deformity in her arms or legs?
她的手臂或腿有畸形吗？

**Gastric pain 胃痛**

（38）Mr. Smith，now I want to get back to your abdominal pain.
史密斯先生，现在我想回到你腹痛这个问题。

（39）Tell me what your pain is like.
告诉我你的疼痛像什么。

（40）Did the pain begin suddenly or gradually?
疼痛是突然发生的还是逐渐发生的？

（41）Point to where it hurts.
指一下哪儿痛。

（42）Does the pain move around?
疼痛有转移吗？

（43）Do you have nausea with the pain?
你疼痛时有恶心吗？

（44）Did you throw up（vomit）?
你吐了吗？

（45）Are you constipated?
你便秘吗？

（46）Do you have diarrhea?
你有腹泻吗？

（47）Do you have gas?
你有胃肠胀气吗？

（48）Do you burp often?
你经常打饱嗝吗？

（49）Do you have pain before or after you eat?
你饭前或饭后有疼痛吗？

（50）What kind of foods aggravate your pain?
哪种食物加剧了你的疼痛？

（51）Have you ever had blood in your bowel movements?
你曾有过大便带血吗？

（52）Does the pain go through to your back?（Does the pain radiate toward your back？）
疼痛转移到你背部了吗？（疼痛放射到你的背部了吗？）

（53）What do you do to relieve the pain?
你做什么来缓解疼痛？

（54）Do you take any medicine?”
你吃了什么药没有？

（55）Is the pain relieved by lying down，sitting or bending over?
疼痛是在平躺、坐立还是俯身时才有缓解？

（56）What color are you stools?
你的大便是什么颜色？

（57）Has your child complained of abdominal pain?
你的孩子抱怨过肚子痛吗？

（58）Where does your tummy hurt?（to a small child）
你的肚子哪儿痛啊？（对小孩）

**Abdominal pain　腹痛**

（59）Tell me about your abdominal pain.
告诉我你腹痛的情况。

（60）Point to where it hurts.
指一指哪儿痛。

（61）Does the pain move to another area?
疼痛转移到其他区域了吗？

（62）Did the pain begin suddenly or gradually?
疼痛是突然发作的还是逐渐发作的？

（63）How long have you had this pain?
你有这个疼痛症状多长时间了？

（64）How often?
多久痛一次？

（65）Do you have nausea or vomiting?
你有恶心或呕吐吗？

（66）Is the pain related to your periods?
这个疼痛和你的月经周期有关吗？

（67）Is the pain related to body position?
这个疼痛和体位有关吗？

（68）Do you have burning when you urinate?
当你小便时有烧灼感吗？

（69）Are you pregnant?
你怀孕了吗？

（70）Could you be pregnant?
你有怀孕能力吗？

（71）When was your last bowel movement?
你上一次大便是什么时候？

（72）What color were the stools?
大便是什么颜色？

**Dysuria: pain and irritation of the bladder and urethra　排尿困难：膀胱和尿道的疼痛和激惹**

(73) Ms.Smith，now I want to get back to your urinary problem.
史密斯女士，现在我想回过来说说你的排尿问题。

(74) When do you have the pain?
你什么时候开始痛的？

(75) Do you have trouble starting your stream?
你排尿开始的时候有麻烦吗？

(76) Has your stream gotten smaller recently?
你的尿线最近变细了没有？

(77) Do you have burning pain?
你有灼痛感吗？

(78) Do you have blood in your urine?
你的小便里有血吗？

(79) Do you dribble urine?
你有尿滴沥吗？

(80) Do you have vaginal discharge?
你有阴道分泌物吗？

(81) Do you have a discharge from your penis?
你的阴茎有分泌物吗？

(82) Does pain happen after intercourse?
性交后会出现疼痛吗？

(83) Does your back ache?
你腰痛吗？

(84) Have you had a new sexual partner?
你有一个新的性伴侣吗？

(85) Did you pee?(To a young child)
你撒尿了吗？(对小孩)

(86) Does it hurt when you pee?
当你撒尿的时候痛吗？

(87) Does it hurt when you tinkle?
当你撒尿的时候痛吗？

(88) Any blood in his?
他的小便里有血吗？

# 36. Dyspnea: Shortness of Breath

# 呼吸困难:呼吸急促

(1) Tell me about your trouble breathing.
告诉我你呼吸困难的情况。

(2) Would you describe your shortness of breath?
你能描述一下你呼吸急促的情况吗?

(3) When did it happen?
什么时候开始的?

(4) When did you first notice it?
你第一次注意到它是什么时候?

(5) In what situations do you have shortness of breath?
什么情况下你会有呼吸急促?

(6) Do you get short of breath when you exercise?
锻炼的时候你会气喘吗?

(7) How many steps can you climb without stopping to breath?
你一口气能上多少级楼梯?

(8) Is the difficulty relieved by rest or by standing upright?
是休息还是站直了能缓解呼吸困难?

(9) What helps alleviate the difficulty breathing?
有助于缓解呼吸困难的是什么?

(10) Do you wheeze when you have shortness of breath?
当你呼吸急促的时候你有喘鸣吗?

(11) Do you ever wake up short of breath at night?
你曾在夜里醒来并且气喘吁吁吗?

(12) Is your shortness of breath getting better or worse?
你呼吸急促的情况有好转了还是更差了?

(13) Have you had a chest X-ray recently?
你最近做胸部X线检查了吗?

# 37. Dizziness: Sensation of Whirling or Turning in Space

# 头晕：旋转感或空间旋转感

（1） Tell me more about your dizziness.
告诉我更多有关你头晕的情况。

（2） Did it come suddenly or gradually?
是突然发作的还是逐渐发作的？

（3） Do you feel the room spinning around you?
你是否觉得这个房间在围着你转？

（4） Do you feel like you are spinning?
你是否觉得好像你自己在旋转？

（5） Is the dizziness aggravated when you move your head?
当你摇头的时候头晕是否加重了？

（6） Does the dizziness get worse or go away when you move your body?
当你活动身体的时候头晕是更严重了还是消失了？

（7） How long have you been having vertigo?
你有眩晕症状多长时间了？

（8） Does the dizziness come and go，or does it continue?
头晕是反复发作的还是一直存在的？

（9） Do you feel like you are falling?
你是否觉得你正在往下坠落？

（10） Do you have nausea or vomiting?
你有恶心或呕吐吗？

（11） Is your hearing affected when you are dizzy?
当你头晕的时候听力是否受影响？

（12） Do you feel like you are going to faint?
你是否觉得你就要昏倒了？

（13） Are you unsteady when you walk?
你走路不稳吗？

# 38. Vomiting

# 呕吐

（1） Have you ever had a problem with vomiting?
你曾有过呕吐的问题吗？

（2） Do you feel like vomiting?
你觉得要呕吐吗？

（3） Did you throw up everything?
你是不是全吐了？

（4） How often do you throw up?
你多久呕吐一次？

（5） What does the vomit look like? Fresh blood，coffee grounds，undigested food?
呕吐物看来像什么？鲜血、咖啡渣还是未消化的食物？

（6） Was there blood in the throw-up?
呕吐物里有血吗？

（7） Did you feel better after you threw up?
你吐完以后是否感觉好一些？

（8） Do you feel sick to your stomach?
你是不是感到胃不舒服？

（9） Do you vomit after eating?
你吃完以后就吐了吗？

（10） When you vomit，do you have a headache?
当你吐的时候头痛吗？

（11） When was your last menstrual period? Was it a normal period?
你的末次月经是什么时候？月经正常吗？

（12） Did she have dry-heaves?
她有干呕吗？

（13） Did he toss what he ate?
他把他吃的都吐了吗？

# 39. Cough: Type of Cough

# 咳嗽：咳嗽的类型

（1） Tell me about your cough.
告诉我你咳嗽的情况。

（2） When did the cough start?
什么时候开始咳嗽的？

（3） Was the onset gradual or sudden?
起病急还是缓？

（4） Do you cough at a certain time of day?
你是在一天中的某个确定时间段咳的吗？

（5） What color is the sputum?
痰是什么颜色的？

（6） Does anything make the cough worse or better?
有没有什么事使得咳嗽症状加重或改善的？

（7） Does the cough start in your throat or deep in the chest?
咳嗽是从你咽喉开始的还是从胸部深处开始的？

（8） Do you have chest pain when you cough?
当你咳的时候胸痛吗？

（9） Did you cough up any sputum or blood?
你咳出痰或者血了吗？

（10） Have you had blood in the sputum?
你有过痰中带血吗？

（11） Do you wheeze or notice a whistling sound when you breathe?
当你呼吸的时候有喘鸣或是注意到口哨音了吗？

（12） Have you had frequent colds recently?
你最近经常感冒吗？

（13） Is the cough relieved if you sit up?
如果你坐直了咳嗽是否会有缓解？

（14） How long has your son/daughter been coughing?
你的儿子 / 女儿咳了多久了？

（15） Does he wake up by coughing?
他咳醒过吗？

# 40. Pruritus

# 瘙痒

(1) Do you itch?
你痒吗？

(2) Where do you itch?
你哪儿痒？

(3) How bad is your itching?
有多痒？

(4) I notice that you are scratching your neck. Do you itch?
我注意到你在抓你的脖子。你痒吗？

(5) Is the itching constant or occasional?
是经常痒还是偶尔痒？

(6) Do you have a rash?
你有皮疹吗？

(7) Do you think you have poison ivy?
你觉得你有毒葛吗？

(8) Are you allergic to anything?
你是不是对什么东西过敏？

(9) Are you using a new cosmetic，soap or detergent?
你正在用一种新的化妆品、肥皂或是洗涤剂吗？

(10) Have you had contact with any chemicals?
你有接触什么化学物质吗？

(11) Have you traveled in the last 12 months?
最近一年你旅行过吗？

(12) Have you had an insect bite?
你被虫咬了吗？

# 41. Vaginal Bleeding

# 阴道出血

（1） Now tell me about your periods.
现在告诉我有关你月经的情况。

（2） How often do you have a period?
你多久来一次月经？

（3） How many days does it last?
月经要持续几天？

（4） Is your bleeding usually light，medium，or heavy?
你月经血量一般是少、中等还是多？

（5） How many pads do you use a day?
你一天要用多少卫生巾？

（6） Have you had unprotected sex?
你有无防护性行为吗？

（7） Could you be pregnant?
你有怀孕能力吗？

（8） Do you have clots?
你（的月经里）有血块吗？

（9） Do you have a vaginal discharge?
你有阴道分泌物吗？

（10）Do you use birth control pills?
你用口服避孕药吗？

（11）When did your periods stop?
你的月经什么时候完？

# 42. Dysphagia and Odynophagia

# 咽下困难和吞咽痛

（1） Now tell me about your problem with swallowing.
现在告诉我有关你吞咽的问题。

（2） When did you first notice this?
你第一次注意到这种情况是什么时候？

（3） What do you mean by difficulty in swallowing?
你说的吞咽困难是什么意思？

（4） Do you feel fullness or heaviness in your stomach?
你觉得你的胃已经胀满了或者很沉重吗？

（5） What foods do you have difficulty in swallowing?
你吃什么食物有吞咽困难？

（6） What liquids?
什么饮料？

（7） Do you have difficulty swallowing liquids，solids or both?
你对什么东西有吞咽困难，液体、固体还是两者都有？

（8） Point to where you feel the difficulty.
指一下你感到哪儿有困难。

（9） Do you always have the difficulty when you swallow something?
当你吞东西的时候总是有困难吗？

（10） Is it getting worse?
更糟了吗？

（11） Do you have pain when you swallow?
当你吞咽的时候是否疼痛？

（12） Are you nauseated when you swallow?
当你吞咽的时候是否恶心？

（13） Do you feel like the food is sticking in your throat?
你是否觉得食物粘在你的喉咙里？

# 43. Hemoptysis (Blood Sputum)

# 咯血(血痰)

（1） Do you bring up phlegm（sputum）?
你吐出痰了吗？

（2） What color is the sputum?
痰是什么颜色？

（3） When did you notice the bloody sputum?
你什么时候注意到有血痰的？

（4） Did you have a nosebleed?
你出过鼻血吗？

（5） Did you have a sore throat?
你咽喉痛吗？

（6） Have you coughed up blood recently?
你最近咳出过血没有？

（7） How much sputum did you cough up?
你咳了多少痰出来？

（8） Do you have night sweats?
你盗汗了吗？

（9） Have you had contact with anyone with tuberculosis?
你接触过结核病患者没有？

（10） Have you had a TB test?
你做过结核菌素试验吗？

（11） Was your tuberculin test negative or positive?
你的结核菌素试验是阴性还是阳性？

# 44. Fatigue：Overwhelming，Sustained Sense of Exhaustion

## 疲劳：压倒性的，持续性的衰竭感

（1） Do you get tired easily?
你很容易疲倦吗？

（2） Do you become fatigued easily?
你是不是很容易疲劳？

（3） What is your energy level like?
你的精力如何？

（4） When did you start feeling fatigue?
你什么时候开始感到疲劳的？

（5） How long have you been having fatigue?
你疲劳有多长时间了？

（6） Is it getting worse or better?
是更糟了还是好转了？

（7） When are you tired? In the morning，evening or all the time?
你什么时候会疲倦？是早晨、傍晚还是一直（都疲倦）？

（8） Does the tiredness come and go?
疲倦是反复发作的吗？

（9） What do you think is the cause of your fatigue?
你觉得你疲劳的原因是什么？

（10） How do you sleep?
你睡得如何？

（11） Do you notice any changes in appetite，sleeping pattern，or life style?
你注意到你的食欲、睡眠模式或者生活习惯有什么改变吗？

（12） Did you ever have or do you have any illness such as diabetes，infectious mononucleosis，or liver or kidney disease?
你曾得过，或者你现在患有诸如糖尿病、传染性单核细胞增多症、肝脏病或者肾脏病这类的疾病？

# 45. Fever: Type of Fever

# 发热：热型

（1） Have you had any chills?
你打过寒战吗？

（2） When did the fever start?
什么时候开始发热的？

（3） Did you have any fever or chills?
你有发热或寒战吗？

（4） Did you take your temperature?
你量过体温吗？

（5） How high was it?
有多高？

（6） Did you shiver or did your teeth chatter?
你颤抖吗或你牙齿打战吗？

（7） Do you get night sweats?
你有盗汗吗？

（8） How many days has your child had fever?
你的孩子发热几天了？

（9） Did you give him/her any medicine such as aspirin or tylenol?
你给他/她吃过什么药没有，例如阿司匹林或扑热息痛？

（10） How are his mood and appetite?
他的情绪和食欲如何？

（11） Did he have seizures or cramps?
他有癫痫发作或痛性痉挛吗？

# 46. Constipation

# 便秘

(1) How often do you move your bowels?
你多久解一次大便？

(2) Have you ever been troubled with constipation?
你曾被便秘所困扰吗？

(3) Do you have any difficulties in moving your bowels?
你解大便有什么困难没有？

(4) Has there been any changes in your bowel movements?
你的排便有什么变化吗？

(5) What color are your stools?
你的大便是什么颜色？

(6) Do you take laxatives or enemas? How often?
你吃轻泻剂或者灌肠吗？多久一次？

(7) What do you do if you are constipated?
如果你便秘了你怎么办？

(8) Do you have nausea，vomiting，weight loss or abdominal pain?
你有恶心、呕吐、体重减轻或者腹痛吗？

(9) Did he poop this morning?（Talking about a child）
今天早晨他大便了吗？（谈论一个小孩）

(10) Was your poop very hard like a marble?
你的大便硬得像大理石吗？

(11) Does it hurt when you poop?
当你大便的时候痛吗？

(12) Did she poop after the enema?
她灌肠以后解大便了吗？

(13) Did you make stink yesterday?
你昨天解大便了吗？

(14) Is his stool all backed up?
他的大便解出来了吗？

# 47. Diarrhea

# 腹泻

（1） How many times have you had diarrhea?
你有过几次腹泻？

（2） Do you have frequent loose stools?
你经常解稀便吗？

（3） Are the stools formed?
大便成形吗？

（4） Did you have cramping or gas with your BM（Bowel Movement）?
你解大便的时候有痉挛或放屁吗？

（5） Do you have a fever or abdominal pain?
你发热或者腹痛吗？

（6） Do you have a rash?
你有皮疹吗？

（7） Was there mucus or blood in the stool?
大便有黏液或血吗？

（8） Can you think of anything you ate that causes diarrhea?
你能想起什么你吃了就会引起腹泻的东西吗？

（9） Have you traveled recently?
你最近旅行过吗？

（10） Have you traveled out of the US or Canada in the last twelve months?
过去一年你去美国或加拿大以外的地方旅行过吗？

（11） How much caffeine do you drink or eat?（coffee，chocolate，soft drinks）
你喝了或吃了多少咖啡因？（咖啡、巧克力、软饮料）

（12） Do you also have a problem with constipation?
你还有便秘的问题吗？

（13） How many days did he have the runs?
他腹泻已有多少天了？

（14） Do you think he got the runs from something he ate?
你认为他是吃了什么东西才腹泻的？

（15） Did he start to get loose stools today?

他今天开始解稀大便了吗？

（16）How loose was his stool? Was it out of his diapers down to his legs?
他的大便有多稀？是不是从他的尿片流到他腿上了？

# 48. Urticaria (Hives)

# 荨麻疹

（1） Do you have any allergies?
你有过敏吗？

（2） Are you allergic to any medicine such penicillin or sulfa drugs?
你对什么药物过敏吗，如青霉素或磺胺类药物？

（3） Are you allergic to any foods?
你对什么食物过敏吗？

（4） Do you have hives?
你有荨麻疹吗？

（5） What kinds of reaction did you have when you had the allergy?
当你过敏时都有哪些反应？

（6） Did you have a rash，hives or swelling?
你有皮疹、荨麻疹或肿胀吗？

（7） Do you work around special chemicals or cleaning products?
你的工作环境有特殊化学物质或洗涤剂吗？

（8） Have you been sick recently?
你最近生病了吗？

（9） Do you have hives in cold weather，hot weather，or both?
你在什么天气会有荨麻疹，冷天、热天还是两者都会有？

（10） Have you ever experienced hoarseness，shortness of breath，wheezing，nausea，vomiting or abdominal pain?
你曾经历过声嘶、呼吸急促、喘鸣、恶心、呕吐或腹痛吗？

（11） Have you traveled in the last twelve months?
最近一年旅行过吗？

# 49. Purpura and Petechiae

# 紫癜和点状出血

（1） Do you bleed easily?
你很容易出血吗？

（2） Do you have bleeding problems?
你有出血问题吗？

（3） Is there anyone in your family who is a hemophiliac or bleeder?
你的家族中有人是血友病患者或者容易出血的人吗？

（4） Do you sometimes get black or blue spots for no reason?
你是不是有时候身上会不明原因地出现黑色或青色的斑点？

（5） When did you first notice these spots?
你什么时候第一次注意到这些斑点？

（6） Did you injure yourself?
你伤着自己了吗？

（7） Do you have nosebleeds?
你有鼻出血吗？

（8） What over-the-counter medications do you take?
你吃了些什么非处方药？

（9） Have you recently been ill?
你最近生过病吗？

# 50. Jaundice (Icterus)

# 黄疸

（1） How long have you noticed the change in your skin?
你注意到你皮肤的变化有多长时间了？

（2） What color is your urine?
你的小便是什么颜色的？

（3） What color is your stool?
你的大便是什么颜色的？

（4） Have you ever had hepatitis?
你得过肝炎吗？

（5） Do you have a history of gallstones?
你有胆石病史吗？

（6） Does anyone in your family have jaundice?
你的家族中有人得过黄疸吗？

（7） Have you ever-had liver disease?
你得过肝脏病吗？

# 51. Hematuria

# 血尿

（1） Have you noticed a change in the color of your urine?
你注意到你的小便颜色有变化没有？

（2） What color is your urine?
你的小便是什么颜色？

（3） Is the urine bloody all the time?
小便一直都带血吗？

（4） Do you have back pain?
你有腰痛吗？

（5） Does it hurt when you urinate?
你解小便的时候痛吗？

（6） Did you pass clots?
你小便里有血块吗？

（7） What medications do you take?
你吃的是什么药？

（8） Have you eaten beets or rhubarb recently?
你最近吃过甜菜或大黄没有？

（9） Do you take laxatives?
你吃了轻泻剂吗？

（10） Have you had an injury to your back or abdomen?
你的背部或腹部受过伤吗？

（11） Do you play contact sports?
你参与要与人身体接触的运动吗？

# 52. Weight Change

# 体重变化

(1) How much do you weigh?
你的体重是多少？

(2) Do you eat regularly?
你的饮食有规律吗？

(3) The nurse will measure your weight and height.
护士将会给你称体重并量身高。

(4) How much did you weigh last year?
你去年的体重是多少？

(5) How often do you check your body weight?
你多久量一次体重？

(6) Has your weight changed recently?
你的体重最近有变化吗？

(7) Why do you think that your weight has changed?
为什么你认为你的体重已经改变了？

(8) What would you like to weigh?
你希望的体重是怎样的？

(9) When did you start gaining weight?
你什么时候开始体重增加的？

(10) Describe your work activity.
描述一下你的工作情况。

(11) Describe your activities outside of work.
描述一下你工作以外的活动。

# 53. Procedures

# 操作

**Blood pressure 血压**

(1) I am going to take your blood pressure now.
现在我将给你量血压。

(2) I am going to take your blood pressure in your other arm.
我要在你的另一侧手臂上量血压。

**Pulse 脉搏**

(3) I am going to feel your pulse on your wrist.
我要在你的手腕上摸一下脉搏。

(4) I am going to feel your pulse in your neck.
我要在你的颈项上摸一下脉搏。

(5) I am going to feel your pulse behind your knee.
我要在你膝关节后面摸一下脉搏。

(6) I am going to feel your pulse in your groin.
我要在你的腹股沟处摸一下脉搏。

(7) I am going to feel your pulse at your ankle.
我要在你的踝关节处摸一下脉搏。

(8) I am going to feel your pulse on the other side.
我要在你的另一边摸一下脉搏。

**Temperature 体温**

(9) I am going to take your temperature.
我要测一下你的体温。

(10) Please open your mouth and I will place this thermometer under your tongue for a minutes.
请张开嘴，我将把这个体温计在你的舌下放一分钟。

(11) I will take your temperature by putting this instrument in your ear for less than a minutes.
我将把这个器具在你的耳朵里放上不到一分钟来量你的体温。

(12) I am going to take a rectal temperature on you. Please roll on your side.
我要给你测直肠温度。请侧着身子睡。

**Requests 请求**

（13）Please sit up.
请坐。

（14）Please lie down.
请躺下。

（15）Please roll on your left (right) side.
请向左侧(右侧)侧卧。

（16）Please bend your knees and bring them up to your chest.
请屈膝并使之挨着你的胸部。

（17）Please stand.
请站立。

（18）Please lean over this table.
请弯下身子俯在这张桌子上。

（19）Please take a deep breath and breathe out through your mouth.
请深吸一口气并从你的嘴里呼出来。

（20）Please hold your breath.
请屏住呼吸。

（21）Breathe now.
现在呼出来。

（22）Please swallow.
请吞一下。

（23）Please, cough.
请咳一下。

（24）Please do what I do.
请跟着我做。

（25）Please walk the door and back towards me.
走到门口再朝我走回来。

# 54. Diagnostic Tests 诊断性检查

**Blood test　血液检查**

（1） I am going to take your blood sample.
我要给你采血了。

（2） I would like to draw your blood.
我将给你抽血。

（3） Let me draw your blood.
让我来给你抽血。

（4） We must check your blood.
我们必须检查你的血液。

（5） Would you go to the phlebotomy room on the third floor for a blood test.
请你到三楼采血室做一个血液检查好吗？

（6） Please be seated until you are called.
在叫到你前请坐着（等）。

（7） Please sit down and stretch your arm.
请坐，把手臂伸出来。

（8） Please sit down and put your arm out.
请坐并把手臂伸出来。

（9） Give me your arm.
给我你的手臂。

（10） Please take off your jacket.
请脱去你的夹克。

（11） Please roll up your sleeve.
请把你的袖子卷起来。

（12） I will prick your ear lobe.
我要刺一下你的耳垂。

（13） I will prick your thumb.
我要刺一下你的拇指。

（14） Okay. It's done. Did it hurt?
好了。完了。痛吗？

（15） Please hold the gauze for a few minutes.

请按几分钟纱布。

（16）Please take this paper to your doctor.
请把这张纸拿给你的医生。

**Examination of the urine　尿液检查**

（17）I am going to check your urine.
我将要检查你的尿液。

（18）I would like to test your urine.
我想检查你的尿液。

（19）We will test your urine。
我们将检查你的尿液。

（20）We would like to do a urine test while you are waiting.
我们想在你等候期间给你做个尿液检查。

（21）We would like to give you urine test before you see the doctor.
我们想在你看医生之前给你做个尿液检查。

（22）We need to examine your urine.
我们需要检查你的尿液。

（23）Please bring your urine in this cup.
请把你的尿液盛在这个杯子里。

（24）Please collect your urine sample in this cup.
请把你的尿样收集到这个杯子里。

（25）Please take your urine in this cup to half way.
请把你的小便盛满这个杯子的一半。

（26）Please collect your urine in the middle part of urination.
请收集你的中段尿。

（27）As we will culture you urine，clean your penis with this wet gauze before you collect urine.
由于我们将给你做尿培养，在你收集尿液之前先用这个湿纱布清洁你的阴茎。

（28）Please collect midstream urine in this sterilized container first thing in the morning.
请将你第一次晨尿的中段尿收集到这个无菌容器里。

（29）After you collect a urine sample，please take it to the lab at Room 123.
在你取好尿样以后，请把它带到 123 室的实验室去。

**Examination of Stools　大便检查**

（30）We need to examine your stools.
我们需要检查你的大便。

（31）We would like to test your stools.
我们想检查你的大便。

（32）Would you bring your BM in this box at your next visit?
请你下次来的时候把你的大便放在这个盒子里好吗？

（33）Take your stool sample to the lab at the corer.
带着你的大便标本到转角处的实验室去。

（34）Please lie on your back and bend your knees.

请仰面躺下并屈膝。

（35）Please have your thighs and knees flexed.
请屈起你的大腿和膝盖。

（36）I will examine your bottom.
我要检查你的肛门。

（37）Please relax.
请放松。

（38）It will finish in seconds.
马上就完了。

（39）That's all.
完了。

（40）We must examine the stools of your son.
我们必须检查你儿子的大便。

（41）Please bring his poo-poo tomorrow.
明天请把他的粪便带来。

**Electrocardiogram（ECG） 心电图**

（42）I would like to take your electrocardiogram（ECG）.
我将给你做心电图。

（43）Please take off your shirt and socks，and lie down on your back.
请脱掉衬衣和袜子，然后仰面躺下。

（44）I will put these electrodes on your chests，arms and a leg.
我将把这些电极置于你的胸部，双臂和一条腿上。

（45）Please relax and don't move.
请放松，不要动。

（46）It will be finished in three minutes.
检查将在3分钟内完成。

（47）Now l would like to take another ECG after you exercise.
现在我想在你做运动以后再做一次心电图。

（48）Would you step up and down these steps twenty times？
请你在这些楼梯上下20次好吗？

（49）Would you walk on this treadmill?
请你在这架踏车上行走好吗？

（50）Tell me if you have chest pain.
如果你胸痛就告诉我.

（51）It's finished. You can get dressed.
做完了，你可以穿衣服了。

**Ultrasound examination 超声波检查**

（52）We will do ultrasound test.
我们将要做超声检查。

（53）Please get undressed and wear this paper wear.

请脱掉衣服然后穿上这件纸衣服。

(54) Don't worry. It doesn't hurt you.
别担心，不会弄痛你的。

(55) Please lie on your back.
请仰面躺下。

(56) We will put jelly on your skin.
我们将把胶冻涂在你的皮肤上。

(57) Now, hold your breath.
现在，屏住呼吸。

(58) Please lie on your left facing the wall.
请朝左侧躺，面对墙壁。

(59) Please lie on your stomach.
请俯卧。

(60) It's done. Here is tissue. You can wipe off the jelly.
做完了，这是棉纸，你可以把胶冻擦掉。

**Chest X-ray　胸部X线检查**

(61) I will take your chest X-ray.
我将给你做胸部X线检查。

(62) I would like to take your chest X-ray.
我想给你做胸部X线检查。

(63) Please take off your shirt and put it in this basket.
请脱掉你的衬衣并把它放到这个篮子里。

(64) Please undress from the waist up.
请把上衣脱了。

(65) Please put on this hospital wear.
请穿上这件病员服。

(66) Please take your watch and jewelry off.
请把手表和珠宝首饰取下来。

(67) Please stand here facing the board.
请站在这里，面对这块板。

(68) Lean your chest against the board.
把你的胸部靠在这块板上。

(69) Please put your chin on top of the board.
请把你的下颌放在这块板的顶上。

(70) Take a deep breath and hold it.
做一个深呼吸然后屏住气。

(71) You may breathe now.
现在你可以呼气了。

(72) Now I would like to take another one from a different angle.
现在我想换个角度，再照一张。

(73) Please turn to the right side and lift your arms.
请转向右侧并上举双臂。

(74) Okay. That's all.
好的，完了。

# 55. Communicating Difficult Information

# 与重病患者家属交流

（1） Please come with me.（Take person to a private place.）
请跟我来。（把他带到一个安静的地方。）

（2） Please sit down.（Sit down yourself.）
请坐。（你自己也坐下。）

（3） I am sorry but your child（son，daughter，husband，wife，mother）is very sick.
我很抱歉，但你的孩子（儿子、女儿、丈夫、妻子、母亲）病得很重。

（4） I am sorry but your son is critically ill.
我很抱歉，但你儿子病情危重。

（5） Does your wife have a living will?
你妻子签有生前遗嘱吗？

（6） Has your husband made his decision regarding the type of treatments he would want in this situation known to you?
你丈夫已经把他在这种情况下想接受的治疗决定告诉你了吗？

（7） I am sorry but your grandfather has died.（Can lightly touch shoulder.）
我很抱歉但你祖父已经过世了。（可轻触肩膀。）

（8） Is there someone we can call for you?（If the relative or person is alone.）
我们能为你叫什么人来吗？（如果家属是独自一人。）

（9） Is there someone who we can call to be with you?
我们能叫谁来陪你吗？

（10） Would you like to see your sister?（Stay with person in room with deceased person.）
你想见你姐姐吗？（陪家属待在死者的房间里。）

（11） Are you aware of your father's desires regarding organ donation?
你知道你父亲捐赠器官的意愿吗？

（12） How do you feel about organ donation?
你对器官捐赠怎么想？

# Appendix Ⅰ Nursing Staff

# 护理人员

registered nurse（RN） 注册护士

registered general nurse（RGN） 全科注册护士

licensed vocational nurse（LVN） 有照职业护士

licensed practical nurse（LPN） 有照职业护士

advanced practice nurse（APN） 高级职业护士

clinical nurse specialist（CNS） 临床专科护士

registered mental health Nurse（RMN） 精神科护士

certified nursing assistant（CAN）（=Nurse Aide） 护士助理

nurse practitioner 独立执业护士

nurse anesthetist 麻醉护士

nurse midwife 助产士

community nurse 社区护士

nursing director 护理部主任

head nurse 护士长

specialist nurse 特别护士

nurse in charge 主班护士

student nurse 实习护士

service care associate 护工

# Appendix Ⅱ Commonly Used Nursing Terms

# 常用护理术语

**Nursing processes 护理过程**

assessment 估计

nursing diagnosis 护理诊断

planning 计划

intervention(implementation, management) 措施(实施、管理)

evaluation 评价

**Daily care of the patient 对病人的日常护理**

morning(evening)care, AM(HS)care 晨(晚)间护理

bed making 整理床铺

oral hygiene(mouth care) 口腔卫生

brushing the teeth 刷牙

flossing the teeth 清牙垢

denture care 清洗假牙

bathing 洗澡

cleanliness and skin care 清洁与皮肤护理

perineal care 洗会阴

hair care 梳头

shaving 刮脸

care of nails and feet 指甲修剪和洗脚

changing hospital gowns 更换住院服装

massage 按摩

bedsore care 褥疮护理

**Measurement of vital signs 测量生命体征**

taking oral(rectal, axillary)temperature 量口腔(直肠、腋下)体温

taking a radial pulse 测量桡动脉脉搏

counting respirations 计呼吸次数

measuring(taking)blood pressure 量血压

**Catheterization 导管插入术**

cardiac catheterization 心导管插入术

laryngeal catheterization, intubation 喉插管术

retro-urethral catheterization 逆行导尿管插入术

urethral catheterization 尿道导管插入术

**Clean techniques, medical asepsis 消毒灭菌**

asepsis 无菌(法)

integral asepsis 完全无菌

disinfection 消毒

concomitant(concurrent)disinfection 随时消毒，即时消毒

steam disinfection 蒸汽消毒

terminal disinfection 终末消毒

disinfection by ultraviolet light 紫外线消毒

**Sterilization 灭菌，消毒**

chemical sterilization 化学灭菌法

fractional sterilization 间歇灭菌法

intermittent sterilization 间歇灭菌法

mechanical sterilization 器械灭菌法

**Decompression 减压(术)**

cardiac decompression 心减压术

cerebral decompression 脑减压术

orbital decompression 眼眶减压术

decompression of pericardium 心包减压术

gastro-intestinal decompression 胃肠减压术

decompression of rectum 直肠减压术

decompression of spinal cord 脊髓减压术

**Dialysis 透析**

peritoneal dialysis 腹膜透析
hemodialysis 血液透析

**Drainage 引流、导液**

aspiration (suction) drainage 吸引导液(引流)
closed drainage 关闭引流法
negative pressure drainage 负压吸引法
open drainage 开放引流法
postural drainage 体位引流法
vaginal drainage 阴道引流法
vesicocelomic drainage 膀胱腹腔引流

**Enema 灌肠**

barium enema 钡灌肠
blind enema 肛管排气(法)
contrast enema 对比灌肠
glycerin enema 甘油灌肠
high (low) enema 高(低)位灌肠
magnesium sulfate enema 硫酸镁灌肠
retention (non-retention) enema 保留(无保留)灌肠
soapsuds enema 肥皂水灌肠
turpentine enema 松节油灌肠

**Feeding 饲、喂养**

Forced (forcible) feeding 强制喂养
intubation (tube) feeding 管饲法
nasal feeding 鼻饲法
rectal feeding 直肠营养法

**Heat and clod applications 冷、热敷**

applying hot compresses 热敷
applying hot soaks 湿热敷
assisting the patient to take a sitz-bath 帮病人坐浴
applying hot water bottles 用热水瓶
applying an ice bag (collar) 用冰袋
applying cold compresses 冷敷
giving a cold (an alcohol) sponge bath 冷水(酒精)擦浴

**Infusion 输入、注入**

glucose infusion 葡萄糖液输注
glucose-saline infusion 葡萄糖 盐水输注
saline infusion 盐水输注

**Injection 注射**

endermic intracutaneous injection 皮内注射
hypertonic saline injection 高渗盐水注射
hypodermic injection 皮下注射
intramuscular injection 肌内注射
intraocular injection 眼球注射
intrapleural injection 胸膜腔注射
intrauterine injection 子宫内注射
intravesical injection 膀胱注射
nasal injection 鼻内注射
peritoneal injection 腹膜腔注射
rectal injection 直肠注射
subconjunctival injection 结膜下注射
urethral injection 尿道注射
vaginal injection 阴道注射

**Irrigation 冲洗**

vaginal irrigation 阴道冲洗
bladder irrigation 膀胱冲洗
continuous irrigation 连续冲洗法
mediate irrigation 间接冲洗法

**Isolation 隔离、分离**

strict isolation 严密隔离
contact isolation 接触隔离
respiratory isolation 呼吸隔离
drainage (secretion) precautions 引流预防措施
enteric precautions 肠道预防措施
blood (body fluid) precautions 血液(体液)预防措施
protective isolation 保护性隔离

**Lavage 灌洗、洗出去**

blood (systemic) lavage 血液毒素清洗法
ether lavage (腹腔内) 乙醚洗法
gastric lavage 洗胃
intestinal lavage 洗肠
peritoneal lavage 腹膜腔灌洗
pleural lavage 胸膜腔灌洗

**Medication 药疗、投药、给药**

Endermic medication 皮内透药法
Epidermic medication 皮上投药法
Hypodermatic medication 皮下投药法
Intramuscular medication 肌肉投药法
ionic medication 离子透药疗法
nasal medication 鼻内投药法
oral medication 口服法
rectal medication 直肠投药法
sublingual medication 舌下投药法
transduodenal medication 十二指肠内投药法
vaginal medication 阴道投药法

**Suctioning 吸气引液**

upper airway suctioning 上呼吸道抽吸
nasogastric suctioning 鼻胃抽吸
wound suctioning 伤口吸引

**Transfusion 输血、输液**

arterial transfusion 动脉输血
blood transfusion 输血
direct (immediate) transfusion 直接输血
drip transfusion 滴注输（血）液
indirect transfusion 间接输血
plasma transfusion 输血浆
serum transfusion 输血清
venous transfusion 静脉输血，静脉输液

**Diet nursing 饮食护理**

absolute diet (fasting) 禁食
balanced diet 均衡饮食
convalescent diet 恢复期饮食
diabetic diet 糖尿病饮食
fat-free diet 无脂饮食
salt-free diet 无盐饮食
fever diet 热病饮食
full diet 全食，普通饮食
half diet 半食
high caloric diet 高热量饮食
high-carbohydrate diet 高糖类饮食
high-protein (protein rich) diet 高蛋白饮食
invalid diet 病弱者饮食
light diet 易消化饮食
liquid diet 流质饮食
high fat diet 高脂饮食
low fat diet 低脂饮食
low caloric diet 低热量饮食
low-protein diet 低蛋白饮食
low-residue diet 低渣饮食
nourishing diet 滋补饮食
obesity diet 肥胖病饮食
prenatal diet 孕期饮食
regimen diet 规定食谱
smooth (soft) diet 细软饮食

**Preparing the patient for the surgery 为病人手术前做准备**

shaving the patient's skin (skin prep) 备皮
anesthesia 麻醉

**Postoperative care 手术后护理**

coughing and deep-breathing exercises 咳嗽呼吸练习
applying elastic stockings 穿弹性袜
applying elastic bandages 用弹性绷带

**Emergency care( first aid )急救护理**

cardiopulmonary resuscitation 心肺循环复苏术
mouth-to-mouth (mouth-to-nose, mouth-to-stoma) resuscitation 口对口（口对鼻，口对颈部小口）循环复苏术
emergency care for fainting (shock, stroke) victims 晕厥（休克、中风）患者急救
emergency care used to control hemorrhage 止血急救
emergency care given to help a patient who is vomiting 呕吐患者急救
emergency care for a patient during a seizure 癫痫发作急救
hospice care 临终护理
postmortem care 死后护理

# Appendix Ⅲ Common Clinical Nursing Abbreviation

# 常用英语临床护理缩写

## A

| | | |
|---|---|---|
| A&E | accident and emergency | 事故急救部(急诊科) |
| A/N | assistant nurse | 助理护士 |
| AB | apex beat | 心尖搏动 |
| Abd | abdomen | 腹部 |
| a.c. | before meals | 餐前 |
| adm | admission | 入院 |
| ADL | activity of daily living | 日常生活活动 |
| ad lib | as desired | 适宜 |
| ADON | assistant director of nursing | 护士长助理 |
| AFS | activity flowsheet | 操作流程 |
| a.m. | in the morning | 上午 |
| Anaesth | anaesthetist | 麻醉师 |
| ant | anterior | 前面的 |
| ante | antenatal | 胎儿期的 |
| AOR | at own risk | 自负风险 |
| AP | anterior-posterior | 前后的 |
| appt | appointment | 预约 |
| ARM | artificial rupture of membranes | 人工破膜 |
| ARP | arterial blood pressure | 动脉血压 |
| asp | aspiration | 吸气 |
| Ab | antibody | 抗体 |
| AFB | acid fast bacilli | 抗酸杆菌 |
| AFP | alpha feto protein | 甲胎蛋白 |
| Ag | antigen | 抗原 |
| ANA | anti-nuclear antibody test | 抗细胞核抗体 |
| ASOT | anti-streptolysin titre | 链球菌溶血素滴度 |
| ATⅢ | anti thrombin iii | 第三抗凝血素 |
| AXR | abdominal X-ray | 腹部X线 |

## B

| | | |
|---|---|---|
| b/f | brought forward | 承前 |
| BBA | birth before arrival | 到达时已出生 |
| BF | breast feeding | 母乳喂养 |
| bld | blood | 血 |
| BNO | bowels not opened | 便秘 |
| BO | bowels open | 排便 |
| BP | blood pressure | 血压 |
| BRP | bathroom privileges | 浴室优先权 |
| BWO | bladder washout | 膀胱冲洗 |
| Bx | biopsy | 活组织检查 |
| Bil | bilirubin | 胆红素 |
| BT | bleeding time | 出血时间 |
| BUN | blood urea nitrogen | 血浆尿素氮 |
| Bd/bid | twice a day | 一天两次 |
| BMX | barium meal X-ray | 钡餐X线 |
| BEX | barium enema | 钡剂灌肠 |

## C

| | | |
|---|---|---|
| C | centigrade | 摄氏温度计 |
| C.A.T | computerised axia tomography（scan） | X线电脑断层扫描 |
| cap | capsule | 胶囊 |
| C.O. | cardiac output | 心排出量 |
| C.S.U. | catheter specimen of urine | 导尿标本 |
| c/f | carried forward | 转下 |
| c/o | complain of | 抱怨，主诉 |
| c/s | culture and sensitivity | 文化和敏感性 |
| $C_1$ | cervical vertebra（used with number） | 颈椎1 |
| cal | calorie | 卡 |
| cath | catheter/catheterization | 导管、导管检查 |
| CBI | continuous bladder irrigation | 持续膀胱冲洗 |
| CCT | controlled cord traction | 脊椎牵引 |
| CCU | coronary care unit | 心脏病监护病房 |
| CEA | carcino embryonic antigen | 癌胚抗原 |
| ceph | cephalic | 头的，头侧的 |
| CEU | continuing education unit | 继续教育部 |
| CLD | clear liquor drained | 引流通畅 |
| CMV | controlled mandatory ventilation | 控制强制性通气 |
| CNS | central nervous system | 中枢神经系统 |

| | | |
|---|---|---|
| $CO_2$ | carbon dioxide | 二氧化碳 |
| con，d | continued | 继续 |
| CPAP | continuous positive airway pressure | 持续气道正压通气 |
| CPM | continuous passive movement | 连续被动活动 |
| CPR | cardiopulmonary resuscitation | 心肺复苏法 |
| CRIB | complete rest in bed | 绝对卧床休息 |
| CRN | cord round neck | 脐绕颈 |
| CRP | c-reactive protein | C 反应蛋白 |
| CSF | cerebral spinal fluid | 脑脊液 |
| CSSD | central sterile supply department | 中心消毒供应室 |
| CTG | cardiotocography | 胎心宫缩监护 |
| CT | computerised tomography/clotting time | 计算机体层摄影 / 凝血时间时间 |
| CXR | chest X-ray | 胸部 X 线 |
| cm | centimeter | 厘米 |
| CVL | central venous line | 中心静脉导管 |
| CVP | central venous pressure | 中心静脉压 |
| Cx | cervix | 颈部，子宫颈 |

## D

| | | |
|---|---|---|
| D&C | dilation and curettage | 扩宫刮宫术 |
| D/C | discontinue | 终止 |
| DC | differential count | 分类计数 |
| DCT | direct coombs test | 直接抗球蛋白试验 |
| D/D | diabetic diet | 糖尿病饮食 |
| D/L | double light（applicable to phototherapy） | 双光源（用于光照疗法） |
| D/S | dextrose saline | 葡萄糖盐水 |
| D/S（M） | dextrose saline（maintenance） | 葡萄糖盐水（保养） |
| D/S（R） | dextrose saline（replacement） | 葡萄糖盐水（替换） |
| D5% | dextrose 5% | 5% 葡萄糖 |
| DD | date of delivery | 分娩日期 |
| DDON | deputy director of nursing | 护理部副主任 |
| Defib | defibrillation | 除颤 |
| Del | delivery/delivered | 分娩 |
| Del. Suite | delivery suite | 产房 |
| Dept | department | 部门 / 区 |
| DIL | dangerously ill list | 危重患者名单 |
| Disch | discharge | 出院 |
| DIVC/DIC | disseminated intra-Vascular coagulation | 弥散性血管内凝血 |
| DM | diabetes mellitus | 糖尿病 |

| | | |
|---|---|---|
| DNA | deoxyribonucleic acid | 脱氧核糖核酸 |
| DOA | dead on arrival | 到达时已死亡 |
| DOB | date of birth | 出生日期 |
| DOC | diet of choice | 饮食选择 |
| dpm | drops per minute | 每分钟滴数 |
| DPT vaccin | diptheria，pertussis，tetanus vaccine | 百白破疫苗 |
| Dr | doctor | 医生 |
| DTA | deep transverse arrest | 深位横阻 |
| DVT | deep vein thrombosis | 深部静脉血栓形成 |
| DW | dayward | 日间病房 |
| Dx | diagnosis | 诊断 |
| DXT | deep X-ray therapy | 深部X线治疗 |

## E

| | | |
|---|---|---|
| E. coli | escherichia coli | 大肠埃希菌，大肠杆菌 |
| ECG/EKG | electrocardiogram | 心电图 |
| ECT | electro-convulsive therapy | 电惊厥治疗 |
| EDD | expected date of delivery | 预产期 |
| EEG | electroencephalogram | 脑电图 |
| EHL | electro-hydro lithotripsy | 水下电击碎石术 |
| EI | elective | 选修的 |
| elix | elixir | 酏剂 |
| Em | emergency | 急诊 |
| EMG | electromyogram | 肌电图 |
| EMS | emergency medical services | 急诊医疗服务 |
| EMV | expired minute volume | 分钟通气量 |
| EN | enrolled nurse | 注册护士 |
| Endo | endoscopy | 内镜检查 |
| ENT | ear，norse and throat | 五官科 |
| eod | every other day | 每隔一天 |
| EP | eusol paraffin | 优苏石蜡 |
| Epi | episiotomy | 外阴切开术，侧切 |
| ER | emergency room | 急诊室 |
| ESR | erythrocyte sedimentation rate | 红细胞沉降速度 |
| ERCP | endoscopic retrograde cholangiopancreatography | 内镜逆行胰胆管造影 |
| ESRF/D | end stage renal failure/disease | 终末期肾脏疾病 |
| ESWL | electro shock wave lithotripsy | 体外震波碎石术 |
| et | and | 和 |
| ET $CO_2$ | expired tidal carbon dioxide | 呼气末二氧化碳 |
| ETT | endotracheal tube | 气管导管 |

| | | |
|---|---|---|
| ETV | expired tidal volume | 潮气量 |
| EUA | examination under anaesthesia | 麻醉下检查 |
| Exam | examination | 检查 |

## F

| | | |
|---|---|---|
| F | fahrenheit | 华氏 |
| F/st | full strength | 充足的力量 |
| FB | foreign body | 异物 |
| FBC | full blood count | 全血细胞计数 |
| FD | forceps delivery | 产钳分娩 |
| FDP | fibrinogen degradation products or fibrin | 纤维蛋白原降解产物 |
| Fe | iron | 铁 |
| FESS | functional endoscopic sinus surgery | 功能性鼻窦内镜手术 |
| FFP | fresh frozen plasma | 新鲜冰冻血浆 |
| FH | fetal heart | 胎心 |
| FHHR | fetal heart heard®ular | 听诊胎心规律 |
| FHR | fractional inspired oxygen | 吸入氧分数（百比分） |
| FHR | fetal heart rate | 胎心率 |
| Fld | fluid | 液体 |
| FS | frozen section | 冷冻切片 |
| Ft | feet | 英尺 |
| FT | fallot's tetralogy | 法洛四联症 |
| FWB | full weight bearing | 全重量支撑 |

## G

| | | |
|---|---|---|
| G | gravida | 孕妇 |
| GA | general anaesthesia | 全身麻醉 |
| Ga | gadolinium | 钆 |
| Gal | gallon | 加仑 |
| GB | gall bladder | 胆囊 |
| G/C | general condition | 一般情况 |
| GE | gastro-enteritis | 胃肠炎 |
| Gest | gestation | 妊娠 |
| GM | general manager | 总经理 |
| Gm | gram | 克 |
| GMS | glycerine magnesium sulphate | 甘油硫酸镁 |
| GIT | gastro-intestine tract | 胃肠道 |
| GP | general practice/ general practitioner | 全科医学、全科医生 |
| G6PD | glucose-6-phosphate dehydrogenase | 葡萄糖 -6- 磷酸脱氢酶 |

| | | |
|---|---|---|
| gutt（gtt） | drops | 滴剂 |
| G/W | glucose water | 葡萄糖溶液 |
| GXM | group and cross match | 分组匹配 |
| GYN | gynaecology | 妇科学 |

## H

| | | |
|---|---|---|
| /hr | per hour | 每小时 |
| H/O | history of | 史 |
| $H_2O$ | water | 水 |
| $H_2O_2$ | hydrogen peroxide | 过氧化氢 |
| HA | hospital assistant | 医院助理 |
| Hb | haemoglobin | 血红蛋白 |
| HBs | heavily blood stained | 大出血污染的 |
| HC | head circumference | 头围 |
| HCA | health care assistant | 保健员 |
| Hct | hematocrit | 红细胞压积 |
| Hep | hepatitis | 肝炎 |
| Hg | mercury | 汞 |
| HGT | haemo glucose test | 血糖检测 |
| Histo | histology | 组织学 |
| HIV | human immunodeficiency virus | 人类免疫缺陷病毒（艾滋病病毒） |
| HKA | housekeeping assistant | 家政助理 |
| HMD | hyaline membrane disease | 肺透明膜疾病 |
| HN | head nurse | 护士长 |
| hosp | hospital/hospitalized/hospitalization | 医院 |
| HPM | has passed meconium | 已排胎便 |
| HPU | has passed urine | 已排尿 |
| HR | heart rate | 心率 |
| Hr | hour | 小时 |
| Ht | height | 体重 |
| HVS | high vaginal swab | 高位阴道拭子 |
| Hypt | hyperectension | 膝关节脱位 |
| Hyst | hysterectomy | 子宫切开术 |

## I

| | | |
|---|---|---|
| I & D | incision and drainage | 切开引流术 |
| i.e. | that is | 即 |
| I/N | intra-nasal | 鼻腔 |
| InTT | insulin tolerance test | 胰岛素耐量试验 |

| | | |
|---|---|---|
| I/O | intake and output | 出入量 |
| IA | intra-arterial | 动脉内 |
| IABP | intra-aortic balloon pump | 主动脉内球囊反搏 |
| ICP | intra-cranial pressure | 脑压增高 |
| ICU | intensive care unit | 重症监护病房 |
| ID | identification | 鉴定 |
| IDC | indwelling catheter | 留置导管 |
| IDM | infant of diabete mother | 患糖尿病母亲的婴儿 |
| IHD | ischemic heart discase | 缺血性心脏病 |
| IM | intra-muscular | 肌内 |
| INA | intra-nasal antrostomy | 鼻内上颌窦开窗术 |
| Inj | injection | 注射 |
| Invx/invest | investigation | 调查 |
| IOP | Intra-ocular pressure | 眼(球)内压 |
| IPPR | intermittent positive pressure respiration | 间歇性正压呼吸 |
| IPPV | intermittent positive pressure ventilation | 间歇性正压换气 |
| Irreg | irregular | 无规律 |
| ISG | immune serum globulin | 免疫血清球蛋白 |
| IT | intra-thecal/inferior turbinectomy | 鞘内/下鼻甲切除术 |
| ITP | idiopathic thrombocytopenic purpura | 特发性血小板减少性紫癜 |
| IUCD | intra-uterine contraceptive device | 子宫内避孕装置 |
| IUD | intra-uterine death | 子宫内死亡 |
| IUGR | intra-uterine growth retardation | 宫内生长迟缓 |
| IV | intravenous | 静脉内 |
| IVI | intravenous infusion | 静脉注射 |
| IVP | intravenous pyelogram | 静脉注射肾盂造影图 |
| IVT | intravenous therapy | 静脉注射疗法 |
| IVU | intravenous urogram | 静脉尿路造影 |

## J

| | | |
|---|---|---|
| JVP | jugular venous pulse | 颈静脉搏动 |

## K

| | | |
|---|---|---|
| KCI | potassium chloride | 氯化钾 |
| kg | kilogram | 千克 |
| K wire | Kirschner wire | 基尔希纳丝(骨骼牵引时用) |
| KIV | keep in view | 记在心上 |
| KUB | kidneys, ureters, bladder | 肾、输尿管及膀胱 |
| KVO | keep vein open | 保持静脉通畅 |

## L

| | | |
|---|---|---|
| l | litre | 升 |
| L | length | 长度 |
| L & D | labour and delivery | 分娩（经阴道生产） |
| L/S | lumbosacral | 腰骶的 |
| L1 | lumbar vertebra（used with number） | 腰椎 1 |
| LA | local anaesthesia/left arm | 局部麻醉 / 左上肢 |
| Lab | laboratory | 实验室 |
| LAD | left anterior descending | （冠状动脉）左前降支 |
| Lap | laparotomy | 剖腹术 |
| LAP | left atrial pressure | 左心房压 |
| Lat | lateral | 侧面的 |
| LB | left buttock | 左臀 |
| lb | pound | 磅 |
| LFT | liver function test | 肝功能检查 |
| LGA | large for gestational age | 过期妊娠 |
| LIMA | left internal mammary artery | 左乳内动脉 |
| lin | liniment | 搽剂 |
| linct | linctus | 舐膏剂 |
| liq | liquid | 液体 |
| LMP | last menstrual period | 末次月经 |
| LOA | left occipital anterior | 左枕前位 |
| LOC | loss of consciousness | 意识丧失 |
| LOL | left occipital lateral | 左枕侧 |
| LOP | left occipital posterior | 左枕后 |
| LOT | left occipital transverse | 左枕横位 |
| LOW | lotion | 洗剂 |
| lot | loss of weight | 体重减轻 |
| LP | lumbar puncture | 腰椎穿刺 |
| LSCS | lower segment cesarean section | （子宫）下段剖宫产术 |
| Lt | left | 左侧 |
| LT | left thigh | 左股，左大腿 |

## M

| | | |
|---|---|---|
| M | male | 女性 |
| MAP | mean airway pressure | 平均气道压 |
| MAS | meconium aspiration syndrom | 胎粪吸入综合症 |
| Mat | maternity | 产妇的 |
| max | maximum | 最大 |

| | | |
|---|---|---|
| MBS | moderately blood stained | 中度染血 |
| MCH | mean cell haemoglobin | 红细胞平均血红蛋白量 |
| MCHC | mean cell haemoglobin concentration | 红细胞平均血红蛋白浓度 |
| MCU | micturating cysto-urethrogram | 排尿膀胱造影 |
| MCV | mean cell volume | 平均细胞容积 |
| mcgm | microgram | 微克 |
| MDP | manic depression psychosis | 躁狂抑郁症 |
| Mec | meconium | 胎粪 |
| Med/Surg | medical/surgical | 内 / 外科 |
| mEq/L | milliequivalent per litre | 每升毫（克）当量 |
| mEq | milliequivalent | 毫（克）当量 |
| mg | milligram | 毫克 |
| Mgt | management | （疾病等的）处理（法） |
| M.I. | membrane intact | 膜完整 |
| ml | milliliter | 毫升 |
| mm | millimeter | 毫米 |
| min | minute | 分钟 |
| mixt | mixture | 混合物 |
| MMS | moderate meconium stained | 中度羊水粪染 |
| MMT | mixture magnesium trisilicate | 三硅酸镁合剂 |
| mod | moderate | 适量 |
| M&R | manipulation and reduction | 推拿复位 |
| MR | membrane ruptured | 破裂的膜 |
| MRI | magnetic resonance imaging | 磁共振成像 |
| MRSA | methicillin resistant staph aureus | 耐甲氧西林金葡菌 |
| MSU | mid-stream urin | 中段尿 |
| Multip | multiparity | 经产，多胎产 |
| MV | minute volume | 分钟通气量 |
| MVP | mitral valve prolapse | 二尖瓣脱垂 |
| MVR | mitral valve replacement | 二尖瓣置换术 |
| MW | midwife | 助产士 |

## N

| | | |
|---|---|---|
| NaCl | sodium chloride | 氯化钠 |
| $NaHCO_3$ | sodium bicarbonate | 碳酸氢钠 |
| N.B. | note bene（footnote） | 脚注 |
| N/G | naso-gastric | 鼻胃 |
| N/S | normal saline | 生理盐水 |
| NA | not applicable | 不适用 |
| NAD | no abnormality detected | 没有查到不正常情况 / 未见异常 |

| | | |
|---|---|---|
| NB | newborn | 婴儿 |
| NBFD | Neville Barnes forceps delivery | 巴恩斯·内维尔钳分娩 |
| NBM/NPO | nil by mouth/nil per orally | 禁食 / 未口服 |
| NCP | nursing care plan | 护理计划 |
| ND | night duty | 夜班 |
| N/D | normal delivery | 正常分娩 |
| Neb | nebulizer | 雾化器 |
| Neg | negative | 否定的，反面的 |
| Neuro | neurology，neurologically | 神经病学的 |
| NIBP | non-invasive blood pressure | 无创血压 |
| NWB | non weight bearing | 非承重 |
| NNJ | neonatal jaundice | 新生儿黄疸 |
| noct | at night | 晚上 |
| NP Mec | not passed meconium | 未排胎粪 |
| NPC | naso-pharyngeal carcinoma | 鼻咽癌 |
| NPU | not passed urine | 未排尿液 |

## O

| | | |
|---|---|---|
| O.T. | occupational therapy | 职业治疗 |
| O/A | on admission | 入院时 |
| O/E | on examination | 进行检查 |
| $O_2$ | oxygen | 氧气 |
| OA | occipito-anterior | 枕前(胎位) |
| Obs/Gyn | obstetrics and gynaecology | 妇产科学 |
| OCG | oral cholecystogram | 口服造影剂胆囊照片 |
| OD | overdose | 过量 |
| Om | every morning | 每天早上 |
| On | every night | 每天晚上 |
| OP | occipito-posterior | 枕后(胎位) |
| Op | operation | 手术 |
| OPD | out-patient department | 门诊部 |
| OR | operating room | 手术室 |
| ORIF | open reduction internal fixation | 切开复位内固定 |
| Ortho | orthopaedic | 整形外科的 |
| OT | operating theatre | 手术室 |
| Outpt | outpatient | 门诊患者 |
| oz | ounce | 盎司 |

## P

| | | |
|---|---|---|
| P | pulse | 脉搏 |

| | | |
|---|---|---|
| P&M | placenta and membrane | 胎膜 |
| PA | posterior-anterior | 前后 |
| PAC | premature atrial contraction | 房性过早收缩 |
| Paeds | paediatrics | 儿科学 |
| PAP | pulmonary artery pressure | 肺动脉压 |
| PAP Smear | papanicolaou smear | 巴氏涂片 / 帕帕尼古拉乌涂片 |
| Para | parity（used with number of deliveries） | 产次（指分娩次数） |
| PAT | paroxysmal atrial tachycardia | 阵发性房性心动过速 |
| Path | pathology | 病理学 |
| PAWP | pulmonary artery wedge pressure | 肺动脉楔压 |
| PCV | packed cell volume | 血细胞压积 |
| Pc | after meals | 餐后 |
| PDA | patent ductus arteriosus | 动脉导管未闭 |
| pm | afternoon | 下午 |
| Per | through | 通过 |
| PET | pelvic floor repair | 盆底修复 |
| PEG | percutaneous endoscopic gastrostomy | 经皮内镜下胃造瘘术 |
| pH | measure of acid base balance | 测量酸碱平衡 |
| Physio | physiotherapy | 物理疗法 |
| PI | prothrombin index | 凝血酶原指数 |
| PID | pelvic inflammatory disease | 盆腔炎 |
| PIE | pulmonary interstitial emphysema | 间质性肺气肿 |
| PIH | pregnancy induced hypertension | 妊娠性高血压 |
| PIVD | prolapsed inter-vertebral disc | 椎间盘脱出 |
| PKU | phenylketonuria | 苯丙酮尿症 |
| PNL | percutaneous nephro-lithotripsy | 经皮肾镜激光碎石术 |
| po | per orally or by mouth | 口服 |
| $PO_4$ | phosphate | 磷酸盐 |
| POP | plaster of paris | 熟石膏 |
| pos | positive | 积极的，正面的 |
| post | posterior | 前面的 |
| postop | after operation | 术后 |
| POT | post-operative treatment | 术后康复治疗 |
| PPH | postpartum haemorrhage | 产后出血 |
| PPL | postpartum ligation | 产后结扎 |
| PP wash | potassium permanganate wash | 高锰酸钾冲洗 |
| PR | per rectum | 经直肠 |
| Pre | before | 以前 |
| Pre-op | before operation | 术前 |
| Prem | premature | 早产儿 |

| | | |
|---|---|---|
| Primip | primigravida | 初孕妇 |
| Prn | pro nata/as necessary | 必要时 |
| PROM | premature rupture of membranes | 胎膜早破 |
| Pt | patient | 病人 |
| PT | prothrombin time | 凝血酶原时间 |
| PTB | pulmonary tuberculosis | 肺结核 |
| PTC | percutaneous transluminal cholangiography | 经皮胆管造影 |
| PTCA | percutaneous transluminal coronary angioplasty | 经皮冠状动脉成形术 |
| pte | private | 私人的 |
| PTT | partial thromboplastin time | 部分凝血激酶时间 |
| PU | passed urine | 排尿 |
| PUO | pyrexia of unknown origin | 不明原因的发热 |
| PV | per vagina | 经阴道 |
| PVC | premature ventricular contraction | 心室早发性收缩 |
| PVD | peripheral vascular disease | 周围性血管疾病 |
| PWB | partial weight bearing | 部分承重 |

## Q

| | | |
|---|---|---|
| qds/qid | four times a day | 一天四次 |

## R

| | | |
|---|---|---|
| RA | right arm | 右上肢 |
| RA Factor | rheumatoid arthritis factor | 风湿性关节炎因子 |
| R/B | right buttock | 右臀 |
| RCC | red cell count | 红细胞计数 |
| R/O | removal off | 切除 |
| RDS | respiratory distress syndrome | 呼吸窘迫综合征 |
| reg | regular | 规律 |
| resp | respiration | 呼吸音 |
| Rh | rhesus factor | 猕因子，Rh 因子 |
| RHC | right hypochondriac | 右季肋部 |
| RIB | rest in bed | 卧床休息 |
| RIB&BP | rest in bed with bathroom privileges | 卧床休息与浴室优先权 |
| RIF | right iliac fossa | 右髂窝 |
| RLF | retrolental fibroplasia | 晶状体后纤维组织增生 |
| RLL | right lower lobe | 右下叶 |
| RLQ | right lower quadrant | 右下象限 |
| Rm | room | 房间 |
| RML | right mediolateral | 右中外侧的 |

| | | |
|---|---|---|
| RMO | resident medical officer | 驻地医疗主任 |
| RN | registered nurse | 注册护士 |
| ROA | right occiput anterior | 右枕前 |
| ROP | right occiput posterior | 右枕后 |
| ROT | right occiput transverse | 右枕横位 |
| RR | respiration rate | 呼吸频率 |
| Rt | right | 右 |
| RT | right thigh | 右大腿 |
| RTA | road traffic accident | 交通事故 |
| RTW | return to ward | 返回病房 |
| RUL | right upper lobe | 右上叶 |
| RUQ | right upper quadrant | 右上象限 |
| RWO | rectal washout | 直肠灌洗 |
| Rx | treatment/recipe | 治疗 / 处方 |

## S

| | | |
|---|---|---|
| Sl | sacral vertebra（by number） | 骶椎Ⅰ |
| S.I. | soluble insulin | 可溶解胰岛素 |
| S/B | seen by | 被看到 |
| SB | serum bilirubin | 血清胆红素 |
| S/L | single light（for use with phototherapy）/sublingual | 单光（光照疗法）/ 舌下 |
| $Sao_2$ | oxygen saturation | 氧饱和度 |
| SBS | slight blood stained | 中等血污的 |
| SC | subcutaneous | 皮下的 |
| SD | soft diet | 软食 |
| Sec. | Second | 第二 |
| SEN | senior enrolled nurse | 高级注册护士 |
| SFD | small for date | 小于胎龄儿 |
| SG | specific gravity | 比重 |
| SGA | small for gestational age | 小于胎龄 |
| SGOT | Serum glutamic oxaloacetic transaminase | 血清谷草转氨酶 |
| SGPT | serum glutamic pyruvic transaminase | 血清谷丙转氨酶 |
| SI | surgical induction（applies to labour & delivery） | 手术诱导（用于分娩） |
| SIMV | synchronize intermittent mandatory ventilation | 同步间歇指令通气 |
| SLE | systemic lupus erythematosus | 系统性红斑狼疮 |
| SMD | save measure drainage/sub-mucous diathermy | 保留引流 / 下透气热疗法 |
| SOB | short of breath | 呼吸短促 |
| soln | solution | 解决方案 |
| SSG | split skin grafting | 分层皮片移植 |
| ST | sofra tulle/sinus tachycardia | 凡士林纱布 / 窦性心动过速 |

| | | |
|---|---|---|
| stat | immediately/at once | 立刻，马上 |
| spec | specimen | 标本 |
| S.R. | sinus rhythm | 窦性节律 |
| SR | ward sister | 护士 |
| SRM | spontaneous rupture of membranes | 自发性胞膜破裂 |
| SSN | senior staff nurse | 资深护士 |
| Staph | staphylococcus | 葡萄球菌属 |
| std | standard | 标准，单位 |
| STO | stitches to be out | 拆线 |
| strep | streptococcus | 链球菌 |
| supp | suppository | 栓剂 |
| $SVO_2$ | Surface venous oxygen | 表面静脉血氧含量 |
| SVT | supra ventricular tachycardia | 室上性心动过速 |
| SWD | short wave diathermy | 短波透热疗法 |
| SWO | stomach washout | 洗胃 |
| SXR | skull X-ray | 头颅平片 |
| Syr | syrup | 糖浆 |

## T

| | | |
|---|---|---|
| Tab | tablet | 片剂 |
| TB | tuberculosis | 结核 |
| TBC | thyroid binding capacity | 甲状腺结合力 |
| TBG | thyroid binding globulin | 甲状腺素结合球蛋白 |
| tbsp | tablespoon | 大汤匙 |
| TCM | transcutaneous monitoring | 经皮检测 |
| TCU | to come up（follow up appointment） | 拿出（后续任命） |
| TCT | thrombin clotting time | 凝血酶凝血时间 |
| T & S | toilet and suture | 清创缝合 |
| T.V. | tidal volume | 潮气量 |
| T/V | time/volume | 时间 / 容量 |
| T1 | thoracic vertebra（by number） | 胸椎 1 |
| tds/tid | three times a day | 一天三次 |
| Temp | temperature | 体温 |
| TG | tulle gras | 敷伤巾 |
| TH | total hysterectomy | 全子宫切除术 |
| THBSO | total hysterectomy with bilateral salphingo-oopherectomy | 全子宫切除术及两侧输卵管及卵巢切除术 |
| TIA | transient ischemic attack | 短暂性脑缺血发作 |
| tinct | tincture | 酊（剂） |
| TMS | thick meconium stained | 重度胎粪吸入 |

| | | |
|---|---|---|
| TOL | trial of labour | 分娩途径 |
| TOP | termination of pregnancy | 终止妊娠 |
| TPN | total parental nutrition | 全胃肠外营养 |
| TPR | temperature，pulse，respiration | 体温，脉搏，呼吸 |
| TPHA | treponema pallidum hemagglutination assay | 梅毒螺旋体血凝试验 |
| TSSU | theater sterile supplies unit | 手术消毒供应中心 |
| tsp | teaspoon | 茶匙 |
| Ts&As | tonsillectomy and adenoidectomy | 扁桃体切除术和增殖腺切除术 |
| TT | thrombo test | 凝血酶时间 |
| TTNB | transient tachypnoea of newborn | 新生儿短暂性呼吸过速 |
| TTO | to take out | 取出 |
| TUR | transurethral resection | 经尿道切除术 |
| TURBT | transurethral resection of bladder tumour | 经尿道膀胱肿瘤切除术 |
| TURP | transurethral resection of prostate | 经尿道前列腺切除术 |
| TURT | transurethral resection of tumor | 经尿道肿瘤切除术 |
| TW/DC | total white/differential count | 白细胞总数 / 分类计数 |

## U

| | | |
|---|---|---|
| U | unit | 单位 |
| U/E | urea/electrolytes | 尿素和电解质 |
| U/R | urine routine | 尿液常规检查 |
| URTI | upper respiratory tract infection | 上呼吸道感染 |
| u/s | ultrasound | 超声 |
| UTI | urinary tract infection | 泌尿道感染 |
| UAC | umbilical arterial catheterization | 脐动脉插管(法) |
| ung | ointment | 软膏 |
| UV | ultraviolet | 紫外的，紫外线的 |
| UVC | umbilical vein catheterization | 脐静脉插管(法) |

## V

| | | |
|---|---|---|
| Vac Ext | vacuum extraction | 真空吸出 |
| VD | venereal disease | 性病 |
| VE | vaginal examination | 阴道检查 |
| VP shunt | ventricular-peritoneal shunt | 脑室腹腔分流术 |
| VSD | ventricular septal defect | 室间隔缺损 |
| VS | vital signs | 生命体征 |
| VT | ventricular tachycardia | 室性心动过速 |
| Vtx | vertex | 顶(先露) |
| v/o | verbal order | 口头命令 |

## W

| | | |
|---|---|---|
| WBC | white blood cell | 白血细胞 |
| WCC | white cell count | 白细胞计数 |
| Wt | weight | 体重 |
| Wd | ward | 病区，病房 |

## Y

| | | |
|---|---|---|
| Y | year | 年 |

# Appendix Ⅳ Vocabulary Commonly Used in Hospital

# 医院常用词汇

## A

admission 入院
air conditioner 空调
allergist 过敏反应科医生
assistant 助手
associate chief physician 副主任医师
attending physician 主治医师

## B

backing 靠背
back of a chair 椅背
basement 地下室
blood bank 血库
body rest 靠背
bone density 骨密度
book shelf 书架

## C

cabinet 柜子
canteen 食堂
CDFI 彩色多普勒血流成像
ceiling 天花板
ceiling fan 吊扇
cellar 地下室
chairman 主席
changing room 更衣室
charge 收费
chief superintendent nurse 主任护师
chief physician 主任医师
clean room 洁净室
colonoscope 结肠镜
combustible 易燃物
conchoscope 鼻镜
contaminated zone 污染区
corridor 走廊
CR 计算机X线摄影术
cranial reflex 脑反射
critical region 危险区域
crutch 拐杖
CT 计算机断层扫描仪
cystoscope 膀胱镜

## D

dentist 牙科医生
dermatologist 皮肤医生
department of gynecology 妇科
department of pediatrics 儿科
department of dermatology 皮肤科
department of neurology 神经科
department of obstetrics 产科
department of urology 泌尿科
department of radiology 放射科
department of ultrasonography 超声科
department of orthopaedics 骨科
department of physiotherapy 理疗科
department of acupuncture 针灸科
department of TCM 中医科
director 主任
discharge 出院
disinfection room 消毒室
dispensary of TCM 中药房

door 门
dormitory 宿舍
DR 数字 X 线摄影术
drawer 抽屉
dustbin 垃圾桶

## E

ECG 心电图
ECG room 心电图室
EEG 脑电图
electric fan 电扇
elevator 电梯
EMG 肌电图
emergency room（ER） 急诊室
emergency ward 急诊病房
endocrinologist 内分泌医生
endoscope 内镜
enteroscope 肠镜
E.N.T specialist 耳鼻喉医生
entrance 入口
exit 出口
explosive 易爆的
extern 医科实习学生

## F

floor 地板
frozen section 冷冻切片
funduscope 眼底镜

## G

garbage can 垃圾桶
garden 花园
gastroscope 胃镜
ground 广场
gynecologic examination 妇检
gynecologist 妇科医生

## H

head nurse 护士长
health bureau 卫生局
health department 卫生厅
hospital room 病房
human resources 人力资源部

## I

image center 影像中心
inflammable 易燃的
information desk 问询处
injection room 注射室
inpatient 住院病人
inpatient department 住院部
instructor 讲师
intensive care unit 重症室
internist 内科医师

## L

Laboratory（lab） 实验室
laryngeal endoscope 喉镜
lavatory 厕所（文雅）
lobby 休息室

## M

massage department 按摩科
measuring pot 量杯
medical department 医学部
medical examination center 体验中心
men’s room 男厕所
microwave oven 微波炉
minister 部长
Ministry of Personnel 人事部
morgue 太平间
moving bed 移动床 / 车床
moxibustion 艾灸
MRI 磁共振成像

## N

neurologist 神经科医生
nuclear medicine 核医学
nurse 护士

nurse in charge 主管护师
nurse station 护士站

## O

observation nursing unit 观察室
obstetrician 产科医生
oculist 眼科医生
office 诊室
operating room 手术室
osteopath 骨科医生
Outpatient Clinic/Department 门诊部
oven 烤箱

## P

parking lot 停车场
parlor 大厅
passageway 通道
patho-center 病理中心
patients bed 病床
patients'room 病房
pediatrician 儿科医生
pharmacy 药房 / 西药房
physical examination center 体检中心
pillow 枕头
plain abdominal radiograph 腹部平片
pool 水池
prescription 药方
president 主席（院长）
price 计价
primary nurse 护师
Prof.（professor） 教授

## R

refrigerator 冰箱
registration office 挂号处
registry 挂号处
remote control 遥控器
research worker 研究人员
resident 住院医师
resting room 休息室

## S

school of nursing 护士学校
seat cushion 坐垫
section chief 科长
sewerage 下水道
square 广场
staircase 楼梯
sterilizing room 消毒室
storage room 储藏室
stretcher 担架
subscription center 预约中心
surgeon 外科医生
surgery 外科学

## T

TCD 经颅多普勒
teaching assistant 助教
telecontrol instrument 遥控器
television 电视
toilet 厕所
top floor 顶楼
tracheoscope 气管镜
Traditional Chinese Doctor 中医师

## U

UCG 超声心动图
UCG room 超声心动图室
ultrasound machine 超声仪
urologist 泌尿科医生

## W

waiting room 候诊室
walking stick 拐杖
wall 墙
ward 病房
washing machine（washer） 洗衣机
water closet 厕所
windowsill 窗台
wheelchair 轮椅
women's room 女厕所